Emergency Surgery

Emergency Surgery

R Rajamahendran
MBBS (Government Kilpauk Medical College)
MS (General Surgery—Government Kilpauk Medical College)
MRCS (Edinburgh) MCh (Surgical Gastroenterology—Madras Medical College) FMAS
Director, Founder and Faculty
RRM Next PG/SS Medical Coaching Institute, Tamil Nadu
Senior Assistant Professor
Department of Surgical Gastroenterology
Villupuram Medical College
Director/ Consultant Surgical Gastroenterologist
RRM Gastro Super Speciality Hospital, Villupuram
Consultant GI and HBP Surgeon, Villupuram
Advanced Laparoscopic Surgeon
Surgery Faculty—Doctutorials Online Platform

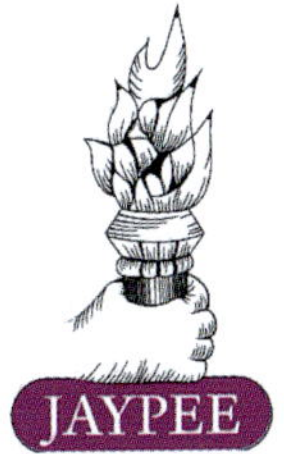

JAYPEE BROTHERS MEDICAL PUBLISHERS
The Health Sciences Publisher
New Delhi | London

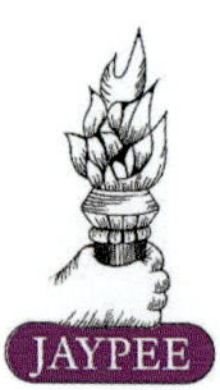

JAYPEE **Jaypee Brothers Medical Publishers (P) Ltd.**

Headquarters
EMCA House, 23/23-B
Ansari Road, Daryaganj
New Delhi 110 002, India
Landline: +91-11-23272143, +91-11-23272703
+91-11-23282021, +91-11-23245672
e-mail: jaypee@jaypeebrothers.com

Corporate Office
4838/24, Ansari Road, Daryaganj
New Delhi 110 002, India
Phone: +91-11-43574357
Fax: +91-11-43574314
e-mail: jaypee@jaypeebrothers.com

Overseas Office
JP Medical Ltd.
83, Victoria Street, London
SW1H 0HW (UK)
Phone: +44-20 3170 8910
e-mail: info@jpmedpub.com

EU GPSR Authorised Representative
Logos Europe, 9 rue Nicolas Poussin
17000, La Rochelle, France
Phone: +33 (0) 6 67 93 73 78
e-mail: contact@logoseurope.eu

Website: www.jaypeebrothers.com
Website: www.jaypeedigital.com

Emergency Surgery

First Edition: **2026**

ISBN: 978-93-7202-150-9

Printed at: Samrat Offset Pvt. Ltd.

Dedication

This book is dedicated to my close friend, *Late Dr S Karthikeyan MD (Anesthesia)*, whom I missed in a road traffic accident. This book is written with memories of my beloved friend.

Contributors

KS Saravana Krushna Raja MS MCh DrNB
Head, Cardiothoracic Surgery
Kalaignar Centenary Super Speciality Hospital
Chennai, Tamil Nadu, India

M Murali MS MCh DNB (Vascular Surgery) MRCSEd
Consultant Vascular and Endovascular Surgeon
Assistant Professor
Department of Vascular Surgery
Thanjavur Medical College Hospital
Chennai, Tamil Nadu, India

Premnath Susendran MS MCh (Neurosurgery)
Senior Resident
Institute of Neurosurgery
Madras Medical College
Chennai, Tamil Nadu, India

R Rajamahendran MS MRCS (Edinburgh) MCh (Surgical Gastroenterology) FMAS
Director, Founder and Faculty
RRM Next PG/SS Medical Coaching Institute, Tamil Nadu
Senior Assistant Professor
Department of Surgical Gastroenterology
Villupuram Medical College
Director/ Consultant Surgical Gastroenterologist
RRM Gastro Super Speciality Hospital, Villupuram
Consultant GI and HBP Surgeon, Villupuram
Advanced Laparoscopic Surgeon
Surgery Faculty—Doctutorials Online Platform

Raghul M MS DNB MCh (Pediatric Surgery) Chennai
University Gold Medalist in Pediatric Surgery
Professor Prasad Neonatology Medal
Professor TDR Minimally Invasive Surgery Medal
Professor Kesavan Pediatric Urology Medal Only for Indian
Selected for BAPS
Fellowship UK 2021

S Dorian Hanniel Terrence MBBS MS FIAGES MCh (Surg Onco)
Senior Resident
Department of Surgical Oncology
Govt. Arignar Anna Memorial Cancer Hospital and Research Institute
Centre of Excellence for Cancer Diseases
Kanchipuram, Tamil Nadu, India
Teaching Faculty at Doctutorials

U Venkatesh MBBS MS MCh (URO) DNB (URO)
Consultant and Head
Department of Urology, Renal Transplant, Vascular access and Robotic Surgery
Kauveri Multispeciality Hospital, Hosur
Professor Chinnasamy Gold Medal in Urology, 2015
Best Paper Award in TAPASU 2014
CPK Menon Best Paper Award, USICON 2018

Vijay Jaganathan MS MRCS DNB MCh (Plastic Surgery)
Fellow in Hand and Reconstructive Microsurgery
Professor and HOD
Saveetha Medical College Hospital
Chennai, Tamil Nadu, India

Preface

Bringing a title on *"Emergencies in General Surgery"* is really a big task, and when I got an opportunity to make this book from the Director of Jaypee Brothers Medical Publishers—I accepted the task knowing this is going to be a Himalayan Task. Yes, it took nearly 1 year to complete this project. Doing gastro and hepatobiliary part was easier for me as I am doing them routinely, but I must collect contents from concerned specialists in which I am not familiar like urology, cardiothoracic and vascular surgery (CTVS), neurosurgery etc.

Updating all the latest protocols from various standard journals and textbooks was really time taking amidst my practice and classes. Finally after a long struggle with the help of Jaypee Brothers Medical Publishers and my friends from various specialties, this book is coming out. This book is intended to make awareness among all the surgeons let it be a postgraduate or practicing surgeon regarding the emergency practices. This book will be a reference book for MS/DNB postgraduates for their final examinations and will be a day-to-day guide for practicing surgeons whenever they get a doubt in emergency managements.

The first edition will always have it's pros and cons—I request you to send your suggestions on improving the book for further editions to my *E-mail ID: minnalraja@gmail.com.*

R Rajamahendran

Acknowledgments

To start with I acknowledge the Group Chairman Sir, Mr Jitendar P Vij, for providing me this opportunity to make this book. I would like to thank the entire team of Jaypee Brothers Medical Publishers (P) Ltd., including Mr Akhilesh Saxena (Development Editor) for making this most needed content for the surgeons.

My love and thanks to all my students who used to motivate me in all my book projects past 15 years.

The biggest acknowledgments of this edition goes to the contributors of this book:

1. Dr U Venkatesh MCh (Urology), Kauveri Hospital, Hosur, Tamil Nadu
2. Dr Vijay Jaganathan MCh (Plastic Surgery), Saveetha Medical College Hospital, Kuthambakkam, Tamil Nadu
3. Dr M Murali MCh (Vascular Surgery), Tanjore Medical College Hospital, Tamil Nadu
4. Dr Raghul M MCh (Pediatric Surgery), Mehta Hospitals, Chennai, Tamil Nadu
5. Dr KS Saravana Krushna Raja, MCh (Cardiothoracic Surgery), Kalaignar Centenary Hospital, Chennai
6. Dr S Dorian Hanniel Terrence MCh (Oncosurgery), Government Arignar Anna Memorial Cancer Hospital, Kanchipuram
7. Dr Premnath Susendran MCh (Neurosurgery), Madras Medical College, Chennai

My acknowledgment never ends without my team members and hospital staffs and my family. They are the pillars of my achievements.

Contents

SECTION 1: General and Trauma

SECTION 2: Gastrointestinal Tract Emergencies

SECTION 3: Hepatobiliary Pancreatic Emergencies

SECTION

1

General and Trauma

Metabolic Responses to Injury

R Rajamahendran

INTRODUCTION

The metabolic response to injury is directly proportional to the grade of the injury in terms of rise in temperature, heart rate, respiratory rate, energy expenditure, and white blood cell (WBC) count. These changes result in systemic inflammatory response syndrome (SIRS), hypermetabolism, catabolism, shock, and finally, multiple organ dysfunction syndrome (MODS).

MEDIATORS OF METABOLIC RESPONSE TO INJURY

- Damage-associated molecular patterns (DAMPs), also known as *alarmins,* are the molecular fragments released during tissue damage.
- These DAMPs are sensed by toll-like receptors and nucleotide-binding leucine-rich repeat receptors that includes—macrophages, neutrophils, and dendritic cells.
- The above cells are called as inflammasomes, which activate key inflammatory cytokines—interleukin-1 (IL-1), IL-6, tumor necrosis factor alpha (TNF-α), interferons, chemokines and other mediators.
- This results in SIRS, cell death and tissue damage, and immune suppression.
- DAMPs also result in leaky capillaries and coagulopathy and results in acute kidney injury, acute lung injury, and MODS.

NEUROENDOCRINE RESPONSE TO INJURY

- The neurons terminate in hypothalamus in response to stress and stimulate corticotropin releasing factor (CRF).
- CRF stimulates adrenocorticotropic hormone (ACTH) from anterior pituitary, which stimulates adrenal gland to release steroids.
- Sympathetic nervous system stimulates adrenaline and glucagon.
- Metabolic response to these stress hormones is to liberate glucose from stores and break down fat and protein.
- *Other effects seen are:* Insulin release and sensitivity altered, hypersecretion of growth hormone and prolactin, inactivation of thyroid hormones and gonadal hormones, and low circulatory levels of insulin-like growth factor-1 **(Fig. 1)**.

Ultimately, the metabolic response is manifested as:

- Hypermetabolism and catabolism
- Muscle breakdown
- Immunosuppression
- Organ dysfunction and failure
- Increased susceptibility to secondary infections (nosocomial infections)
- Increased insulin resistance with increased glucose level.

The phases of insult are divided into Ebb and Flow Phase as shown **Table 1**.

METABOLIC CHANGES AFTER TRAUMA AND SURGERY

- Catabolic phase begins at the time of injury and lasts for 24–48 hours.
- Predominant hormones in catabolic phase are—catecholamines, cortisol, and aldosterone.
- The main role of catabolic phase is to conserve both circulating volume and energy stores for later recovery and repair.
- During catabolic phase, increase production of counter regulatory hormones (catecholamines, cortisol, and glucagon) and inflammatory mediators such as IL-1,6, and TNF-alpha; there is significant fat and protein

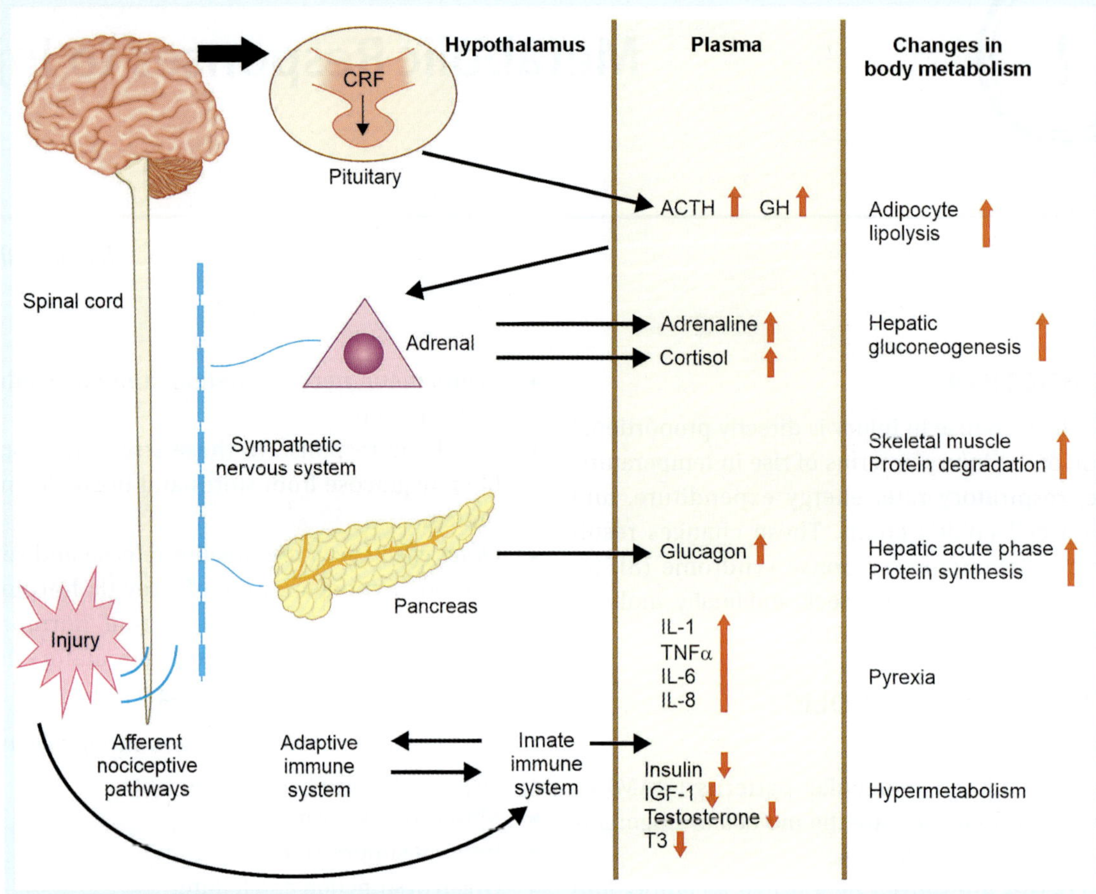

Fig. 1: Neuroendocrine stress response. (ACTH: adrenocorticotropic hormone; CRF: corticotropin releasing factor; GH: growth hormone; IGF-1: insulin-like growth factor-1; IL: interleukin; TNF: tumor necrosis factor)

TABLE 1: Comparison of Ebb and flow phases.

	Ebb phase	*Flow phase*
Duration	<24 hours	Catabolic phase—2–10 days Anabolic phase—weeks to months
Characteristic features	• Low basal metabolic rate • Hypovolemia • Hypothermia • Decreased cardiac output • Lactic acidosis	• Increased basal metabolic rate (BMR) • Hypervolemia • Hyperthermia • Increased cardiac output – Leukocytosis – Increased oxygen consumption – Increased gluconeogenesis
Hormones	Stress hormones (catecholamines, cortisol, and aldosterone)	• Stress hormones • Glucagon • Insulin+/-
Role	Conserves circulatory volume and energy stores for recovery and repair	Mobilization of body energy stores for recovery and repair

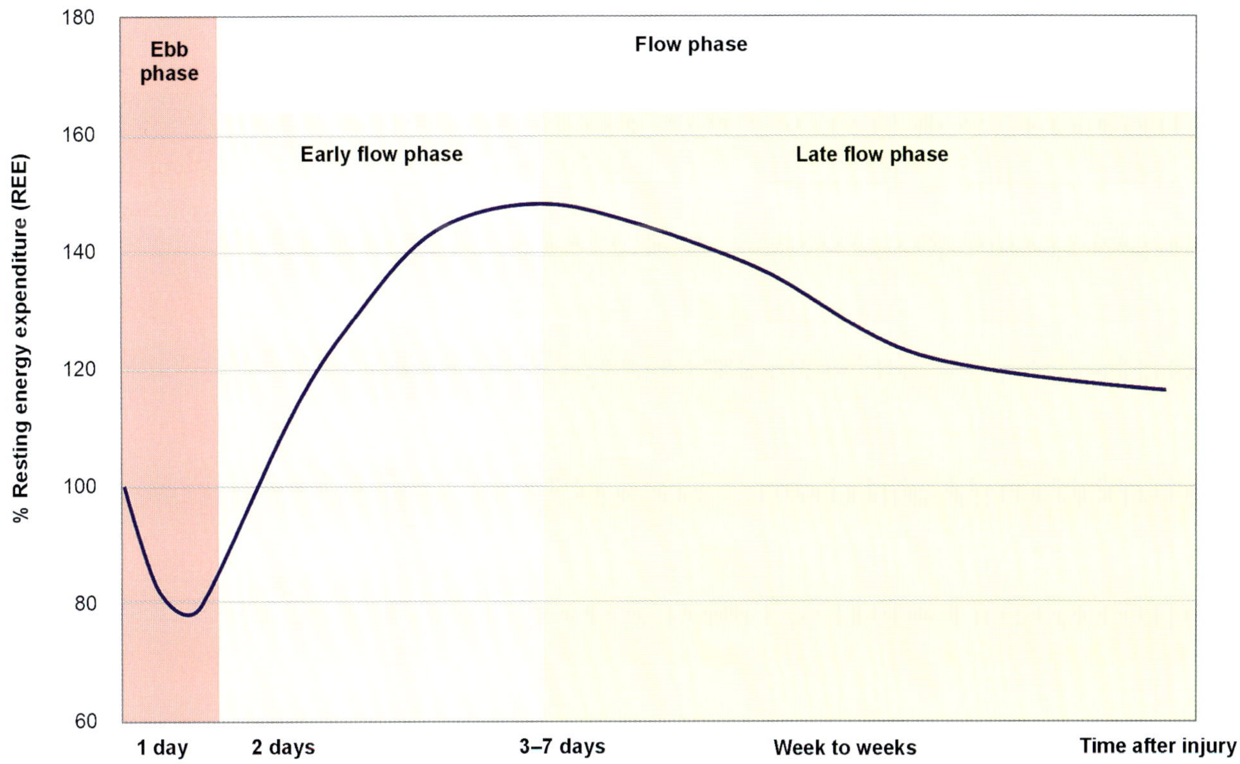

Metabolic response to injury proposed by Cuthbertson et al. A short ebb phase characterized by hypometabolism occurs immediately after the injury and is characterized by a decrease in metabolic rate, oxygen consumption, body temperature, and enzymatic activity. The ebb phase is followed by a longer hypemetabolic flow phase marked by an increased catabolism, with a high oxygen consumption and an elevated (REE) rate.

Fig. 2: Post-traumatic and postsurgical metabolic alterations.

mobilization resulting in heavy weight loss and urinary nitrogen excretion **(Fig. 2)**.

- During shock, insulin levels never rise to the expected level to lower the hyperglycemic status, in fact, insulin levels may fall low.
- During the catabolic phase, not all tissues are catabolic. Catabolism is happening in peripheral tissues (fat, muscle, and skin) with shift of amino acids toward liver, immune system, and wound.

ALTERATIONS IN SKELETAL MUSCLE PROTEIN METABOLISM

- During catabolic phase, muscle wasting is more common, especially in skeletal muscles in periphery. It can also occur in respiratory muscle further complicating the process of ventilation. Only cardiac muscle is spared.
- Urinary nitrogen loss is around 20 gm/day due to muscle catabolism.
- Hyperalimentation (excess feeding) concept is now changed to modest nutritional support.

ALTERATIONS IN HEPATIC PROTEIN—ACUTE PHASE PROTEIN RESPONSE

- The liver has higher protein turn over than muscles of around 10–20% per day.
- Albumin is the major export protein from liver.
- There is reprioritization of body proteins toward liver.
- Increased reactants like CRP, fibrinogen in serum
- Decreased reactants like albumin in serum

CHANGES IN BODY COMPOSITION FOLLOWING MAJOR SURGERY/CRITICAL ILLNESS

- Catabolism leads to a decrease in skeletal muscle and fat mass.
- Body weight may increase paradoxically because of expansion of fluid within the extracellular fluid space.

FACTORS THAT MUST BE AVOIDED TO PREVENT COMPOUNDING OF METABOLIC RESPONSE TO INJURY

- *Blood or fluid loss:* Results in aldosterone production and sodium water retention and edema.
- *Hypothermia:* Characterized by arrythmias.
- *Tissue edema:* Diminishes the oxygen delivery causing cellular hypoxia.
- Tissue under perfusion.
- *Starvation:* Now, carbohydrate rich fluid is advised 2 hours before surgery.
- *Immobility:* It has been a potent stimulus for inducing muscle wasting.

CHAPTER 2

Shock, Fluid Management, Blood Transfusion

R Rajamahendran

INTRODUCTION

- *Shock is the most common cause of death among surgical patients.*
- Shock is a systemic state of low-tissue perfusion, which is inadequate for normal cellular respiration.

FEATURES OF SHOCK

- Anaerobic metabolism results in *metabolic acidosis due to excess lactic acid.*
- Endothelial leak is high resulting in *edema.*
- Preload and afterload decrease and there is compensatory baroreceptor response resulting in increased sympathetic over activity—*tachycardia and vasoconstriction.*
- *Increased respiratory rate* and minute ventilation to excrete excess carbon dioxide
- Decreased perfusion results in *decreased urine output.*
- Activation of renin angiotensin system activates, vasopressin (antidiuretic hormone) is released leading to vasoconstriction and reabsorption of water.
- Cortisol is also released resulting in "*sodium and water reabsorption.*

CLASSIFICATION OF SHOCK

Classification of shock is given in **Figure 1.**

- *Hypovolemic:* Hemorrhagic/nonhemorrhagic (most common type of shock)
- *Cardiogenic:* Due to heart diseases
- *Obstructive:* Due to decreased preload such as tamponade, tension pneumothorax, etc.
- Distributive
- *Endocrine:* Hypo/hyperthyroidism and adrenal insufficiency.

Hemodynamic profiles of different types of shock are given in **Table 1**.

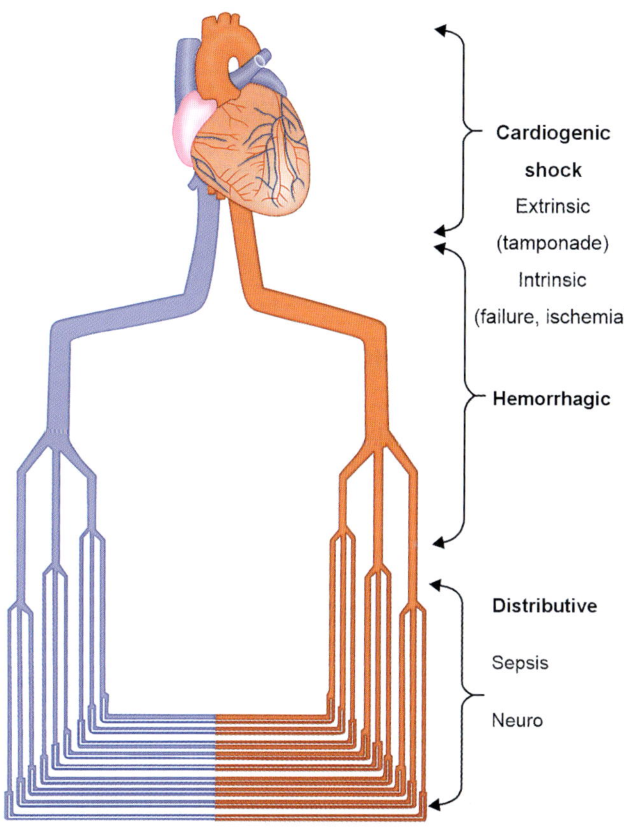

Fig. 1: Types of shock.

Extra Edge

Distributive shock:

- Includes anaphylactic shock, septic shock, and spinal cord injury (neurogenic shock)
- Inadequate organ perfusion is associated with vascular dilatation and hypotension, low systemic vascular resistance, inadequate afterload, and a resulting abnormally high cardiac output
- In anaphylaxis *vasodilatation* is *due to excess histamine release*

TABLE 1: Hemodynamic profiles of different types of shock.

Variables	*Hypovolemia*	*Cardiogenic*	*Obstructive*	*Distributive*
Cardiac output	Low	Low	Low	High
Vascular resistance	High	High	High	Low
Venous pressure	Low	High	High	Low
Mixed venous saturation	Low	Low	Low	High
Base deficit	High	High	High	High

TABLE 2: Clinical progression and severity indicators in shock states.

Variables	*Compensated*	*Mild*	*Moderate*	*Severe*
Lactic acidosis	+	++	++	+++
Urine output	Normal	Normal	Reduced	Anuria
Level of consciousness	Normal	Mild anxiety	Drowsy	Comatose
Respiratory rate	Normal	Increased	Increased	Labored
Pulse rate	Mild increase	Increased	Increased	Increased
Blood pressure	Normal	Normal	Mild hypotension	Severe hypotension

SEVERITY OF SHOCK

- *Compensated:*
  - In compensated shock, there is adequate response to maintain the blood flow to kidney, lungs, and brain.
  - *Apart from tachycardia and cool peripheries, there may be no other clinical signs of hypovolemia.*
  - This state is maintained by reducing perfusion to skin, muscle, and gastrointestinal tract **(Table 2)**.

Decompensation:

- Progressive renal, respiratory, and cardiovascular decompensation results.
- In general, loss of *15% of blood volume is compensated.*
- *Blood pressure is maintained and falls after 30–40% of circulating volume has been lost.*

COMPLICATIONS OF SHOCK

- Multiple organ failure
- Failure of two or more organ systems **(Table 3)**

RESUSCITATION

Fluid therapy:

- There is no ideal fluid for resuscitation.
- Most importantly, they both have oxygen carrying capacity as zero.

TABLE 3: Organ dysfunction in severe systemic illness.

Lung	Acute respiratory distress
Kidney	Acute renal insufficiency
Liver	Acute liver insufficiency
Clotting	Coagulopathy
Cardiac	Cardiovascular failure

- *In hemorrhagic shock, the ideal fluid for replacement is blood, but for waiting time, we give crystalloids.*

Vasopressor and inotropic support:

- They are not indicated as first-line therapy for hypovolemic shock.
- Drugs such as *phenylephrine* and *noradrenaline are used in distributive type of shock* (sepsis or neurogenic shocks). In these cases, the vasodilatation is the cause, hence, the drugs are beneficial.
- If the vasodilatation is resistant, add vasopressin.

Monitoring of response:

- *Urine output (Best monitor)*
- Level of consciousness
- Electrocardiography (ECG) and oxygen saturation.

In shock, only clinical indicators of perfusion of gastrointestinal tract (GIT) and muscular beds are the measure of lactic acidosis (lactate and base deficit) and mixed venous oxygen saturation

Mixed venous oxygen saturation (MVOS):

- The percentage saturation of oxygen returning to heart from body is a measure of oxygen delivery and extraction by tissues.
- Normal MVOS = *50–70%* **(Table 4)**

Hemodynamic parameters: Diagnostic and therapeutic roles of central venous pressure (CVP) and pulmonary capillary wedge pressure (PCWP) are given in **Table 5**.

Essential table:

- Accurate method to monitor intravenous (IV) fluids, inotropic agents, and vasodilators in shock is central venous pressure (CVP)
- Urine output is the BEST CLINICAL PARAMETER for all kinds of shock
- Adequacy of resuscitation/response is best monitored by urine output
- Please note CVP is not ideal in cardiogenic shock and septic shock—in such cases, pulmonary capillary wedge pressure is most sensitive

HEMORRHAGE

The treatment for hemorrhage is arresting the bleeding and not by fluid resuscitation or blood transfusion **(Table 6)**.

- *Primary hemorrhage:* Occurring immediately as a result of an injury or surgery.
- *Reactionary hemorrhage:* It is delayed hemorrhage within 24 hours and is usually caused by dislodgement of clot by resuscitation, normalization of blood pressure, and vasodilation.
- *Secondary hemorrhage:* Sloughing of wall of a vessel. It usually occurs *7–14 days.*

After injury and is precipitated by factors such as infection, pressure necrosis, or malignancy.

Classification

- Adult human has 5 liters blood (70 mL/kg in children and adults and 80 mL/kg in neonates.
- Hemoglobin level is a poor indicator of the degree of hemorrhage as it represents a concentration and not an absolute amount.

TABLE 4: Mixed venous oxygen saturation (MVOS).

MVOS < 50%	*MVOS > 70%*
Increased oxygen consumption by cells	Less oxygen is delivered to cells and hence more of oxygenated blood returns
Cardiogenic shock and hypovolemic shock	Septic shock and distributive shock

TABLE 5: Hemodynamic parameters: Diagnostic and therapeutic roles of central venous pressure (CVP) and pulmonary capillary wedge pressure (PCWP).

CVP	*PCWP*
Helps to distinguish between cardiogenic shock and hypovolemic shock	Best indicator for both blood volume and left ventricular function than CVP
CVP is not reliable indicator of left ventricular function because of the wide disparity between left and right ventricular functions	Helps to differentiate left and right ventricular failure, pulmonary embolism, septic shock, and ruptured mitral valve
	• Accurate therapy to monitor intravenous (IV) fluids, inotropic agents, and vasodilators • Measure cardiac output by thermodilution technique
Normal value: 0–8 mm Hg	• *Normal value:* 10 mm Hg • *Pulmonary artery pressure:* 25 mm Hg

TABLE 6: Four classes of hemorrhagic shock.

Parameter	*Class I*	*Class II*	*Class III*	*Class IV*
Blood loss (%)	0–15	15–30	30–40	>40
Central nervous system	Slightly anxious	Mildly anxious	Anxious or confused	Confused or lethargic
Pulse (beats/min)	<100	>100	>120	>140
Blood pressure	Normal	Normal	Decreased	Decreased
Pulse pressure	Normal	Decreased	Decreased	Decreased
Respiratory rate	14–20 breaths/min	20–30 breaths/min	30–40 breaths/min	>35 breaths/min
Urine output (mL/h)	>30	20–30	5–15	Negligible
Fluid requirement	Crystalloid	Crystalloid	Crystalloid + blood	Crystalloid + blood

- Pulse rate increases in Class 2 hemorrhagic shock.
- Blood pressure decreases in Class 3 hemorrhagic shock.
- Pulse pressure decreases in Class 2 hemorrhagic shock.

SEPTIC SHOCK

- It is also called vasodilatory shock.

Causes of Vasodilatory Shock

- Systemic response to infection
- Noninfectious systemic inflammation—pancreatitis and burns
- Anaphylaxis
- Acute adrenal insufficiency
- *Prolonged severe hypotension:* Hemorrhagic and cardiogenic shock.
- *Metabolic:* Lactic acidosis and carbon monoxide poisoning.

Terms in Sepsis

- *Sepsis:* Evidence of infection + systemic signs of inflammation.
- *Severe sepsis:* Hypoperfusion with signs of organ dysfunction.
- *Septic shock:* Presence of above with more significant evidence of tissue hypoperfusion and systemic hypotension.

Definitions in Shock

Systemic inflammatory response syndrome (SIRS)

Diagnosis: Two or more of the following criteria:
- Temperature >38°C or <35°C
- Heart rate >90 beats/min
- Respiratory rate >20 breaths/min or $PaCO_2$ <32 mm Hg
- White blood count (WBC) count >12,000/mm^3 or <4,000/mm^3

Sepsis: SIRS + documented infection

Severe sepsis: Sepsis + organ dysfunction or hypoperfusion(e.g., lactic acidosis, oliguria, and altered mental status)

Septic shock: Sepsis + organ dysfunction + hypotension (SBP <90 mm Hg or SBP >90 mm Hg with vasopressors)

SYSTEMIC INFLAMMATORY RESPONSE SYNDROME

- Systemic inflammatory response syndrome (SIRS) is final common pathway in shock of any cause where there is failure of inflammatory localization with vasodilation, increased endothelial damage, thrombosis, leucocyte migration, and activation.
- It is a part of severely decompensated reversible shock that eventually leads to MODS, irreversible shock wherein patient is anuric, drowsy, cold, and terminally ill.
- *SIRS carries poor prognosis.*

Sequential Organ Failure Assessment Score

Sepsis-related organ failure assessment score, also known as sequential organ failure assessment score (SOFA) score, is used to track a person's status during the stay in an intensive care unit (ICU) to determine the extent of a person's organ function or rate of failure.

The SOFA score is a complex score based on:
- Respiratory system
- Cardiovascular system
- Hepatic function
- Coagulation profile
- Renal function
- Neurological function

Quick Sequential Organ Failure Assessment (Table 7)

- The quick SOFA (qSOFA) simplifies the SOFA score and can easily and quickly be repeated serially on patients. It takes into consideration only 3 points.
- *The score ranges from 0 to 3 points.* The presence of 2 or more qSOFA points near the onset of infection was associated with a greater risk of death or prolonged ICU stay.
- These are outcomes that are more common in infected patients who may be septic than those with uncomplicated infection.

Based upon these findings, the Third International Consensus Definitions for Sepsis recommends qSOFA as a simple prompt to identify infected patients outside the ICU who are likely to be septic.

TABLE 7: Quick sequential organ failure assessment (qSOFA) Score.

Assessment	*qSOFA score*
Low blood pressure (BP) (<100 systolic)	1
High respiratory rate (>22 breaths/minute)	1
Altered mentation (GCS < 15)	1

(GCS: Glasgow coma score)

TABLE 8: Sepsis management.

Three given to patients	*Three taken from patients*
1. Intravenous (IV) fluids	1. Blood cultures
2. IV antibiotics	2. Full blood count
3. Oxygen and monitor urine output	3. Lactate

Surviving sepsis campaign (sepsis bundle or Sepsis Six):

- Sepsis bundle, also known as resuscitation bundle, is a combination of evidence based objectives that must be completed in 6 hours for patients with severe sepsis/ lactate > 4 mmol/L **(Table 8)**.

Treatment

- Airway, breathing, and circulation
- Hypotension is managed with *fluids*—balanced salt solution
- Next antibiotics are given to take care of sepsis.
- Vasopressors such as dopamine, dobutamine, epinephrine form second-line therapy.

Extra Edge

- Shock index (SI) is defined as heart rate divided by systolic blood pressure (BP). It has been shown to be a *better marker for assessing severity of shock than heart rate and BP alone*. It is a hemodynamic stability indicator
- However, SI does not take into account the diastolic BP, and thus a *modified SI (MSI)* was created
- *MSI is defined as heart rate divided by mean arterial pressure*
- High MSI indicates a value of stroke volume and low systemic vascular resistance, a sign of hypodynamic circulation
- In contrast, low MSI indicates a hyperdynamic state
- *MSI has been considered a better marker than SI for mortality rate prediction*

Recent advances:

Lactate: It is an active metabolite and is capable of moving between cells. It is postulated that lactate is transferred from its site of production in the cytosol to neighboring cells and to a variety of organs (e.g., heart, liver, and kidney), where its oxidation and continued metabolism can occur.

- Pseudo hormone
- Brain protective in total brain injury
- *Base deficit*, a measure of the number of millimoles of base required to correct the pH of a liter of whole blood to 7.4, seems to correlate well with lactate level.

HYPOTHERMIA IN SHOCK

- *Lethal triad of acidosis, hypothermia*, and *coagulopathy* is common in resuscitated patients who are bleeding or in shock from various factors.
- The optimal method to break the "vicious circle of death" is to stop the bleeding and the causes of hypothermia.
- Classification of hypothermia in trauma
  - *Mild:* 36–34°
  - *Moderate:* 34–32°
  - *Severe:* <32°

Recent advances:

- *Regional hypoperfusion:* Gastric tonometry
- *Near-infrared (NIR) spectroscopy:* Occult hypoperfusion
- *Coagulation:* Thromboelastography and rotational thromboelastometry (ROTEM) have emerged as dynamic (bestmeasures of coagulation.
- Prothrombin time (PT) and international normalized ratio (INR) are static measure of coagulation

Damage control resuscitation:

- The concept of damage control resuscitation or hemostatic resuscitation involves rapid control of bleeding as the highest priority; using permissive hypotension because this would minimize the use of acellular fluids as well as potential disruption of natural clot formation; and minimizing the use of crystalloid solutions.
- *Using hypertonic saline* (HTS) to reduce the total volume of crystalloid necessary
- *Using blood products early* and considering the use of drugs, such as recombinant activated Factor VIIa *(rFVIIa)* or *factor IX*, to stop bleeding and to reduce coagulopathy

Trauma resuscitation: 1:1:1 (balanced resuscitation)

- Plasma, platelets, and packed red blood cells in a *1:1:1*
- When red blood cells are transfused, match each unit with one unit of platelets and 1 unit fresh frozen plasma (FFP) (1:1:1)
- This balanced approach will not correct coagulopathy although it can prevent coagulopathy
- Correct underlying coagulopathy

Massive resuscitation:

- Most patients do not require massive transfusion, usually defined as a transfusion of *more than 10 units of packed red blood cells (PRBCs) in 24 hours*

Recent advances in resuscitation:

- Allowing permissive hypotension
- Minimizing crystalloid resuscitation
- Using HTS
- Aggressively using blood and blood products

FLUIDS AND ELECTROLYTES

Two types of fluids crystalloids & colloids are given in **Table 9**.

Classification of intravenous fluids by tonicity is given in **Table 10**.

TABLE 9: Types of fluids.

Crystalloids	*Colloids*
• May be isotonic/hypertonic • Expands plasma volume in less time • Cheap • Can precipitate cerebral edema	• Hypertonic solution. • Expands plasma volume for 2–4 hours • Expensive • Decreased cerebral and pulmonary edema
Examples are: • Ringer lactate • Normal saline (NS) • Glucose solution • Dextrose with NS • Hypertonic saline	*Examples are:* • Dextrans • Albumin • Gelatins • Hydroxyethyl starch • Blood replacement

TABLE 10: Classification of intravenous fluids by tonicity.

Isotonic	*Hypertonic*	*Hypotonic*
• Dextrose 5% in water • 0.9% normal saline • Ringer lactate	• 5% dextrose in half normal saline • 5% dextrose in normal saline • Dextrose 10% in water	0.45% normal saline

TABLE 11: Composition of solutions.

Solution	*Na*	*K*	*Ca*	*Cl*	*Lactate*	*Colloid*
Hartman's solution	131	5	2	111	29	
Normal saline (0.9% NaCl)	154			154		
Dextrose saline (4% dextrose in 0.18% saline)	30	30				
Gelofusine	150	150				Gelatin 4%
Haemaccel	145	5.1%	<1	145		Polygelin 75 g/L
Hetastarch						Hydroxy ethyl starch 6%

Choice of Fluid

- Ringer lactate (balanced salt solution) **(Table 11)**
  - Intestinal obstruction
  - Fluid of choice for first 24 hours of burn
  - Intra operative fluid management
- Colloids
  - Renal failure
  - Liver failure (albumin)
  - Used after 24 hours of burns
- Normal saline
  - Hyponatremia
  - Brain injury
  - Diabetic ketoacidosis
  - Hypochloremic metabolic alkalosis
- Hypertonic saline
  - Cerebral and pulmonary edema.
  - Hyponatremia **(Table 12)**

Fluids and Electrolytes

Fluid losses occur by 4 routes:

1. *Lungs:* 400 mL water in expired air is lost in 24 hours.
2. *Skin:* 600–1000 mL/day via sweat
3. *Feces:* 60–150 mL/day
4. *Urine:* 1,500 mL/day

TABLE 12: Comparison of hyperkalemia and hypokalemia.

Characteristics	*Hyperkalemia*	*Hypokalemia*
Definition	• $K^+ > 5.5$ mmol/L	• $K^+ < 3.5$ mmol/L
Etiology	• Hypoaldosteronism • Trimethoprim • Pentamidine	• Drugs (insulin, alpha blocker, and beta-2 agonist) • Metabolic alkalosis • Hyperaldosteronism • Cushing syndrome • Diabetic ketoacidosis • Bartter's syndrome • Congo adrenal hyperplasia • Hypoventilation
Clinical presentation	• Muscle weakness • Flaccid paralysis • Hypoventilation if respiratory muscle involved • Cardiac toxicity causing ventricular fibrillation or asystole	• Hypotonia and paralytic ileus • Abdominal distension • Fatigue, myalgia, and episodic muscle weakness
Electrocardiography (ECG)	• *Tall peaked T wave* • Sine wave pattern • Increased PR and increased QRS duration	• *Prominent U wave* • Flattening/inversion of wave. • ST depression • Prolonged QU interval
Treatment	• Ca-gluconate • Insulin with dextrose • Bicarbonate(severe) • Peritoneal dialysis	• Oral KCL IV KCl (severe cases)
Definition	Plasma $Na^+ > 145$ mmol/L	Plasma $Na^+ < 135$ mmol/L
Etiology	• Diarrhea • Osmatic diuresis • Decreased fluid intake • Central diabetes insipidus	• CRF • Nephrotic syndrome and cirrhosis • SIADH • Diuretic
Clinical presentation	• Altered sensorium • Irritability and seizure • Thirst and polyuria • Weakness and twitching	• Hypoaldosteronism • Nausea, headache, and confusion • Stupor, seizure, and coma • Increased intracranial tension
Treatment	• Water intake • Correct etiology	• Fluid and salt restriction • Diuretics • Hypertonic saline

(CRF: Chronic Renal Failure; SIADH: Syndrome of inappropriate antidiuretic hormone secretion)

Maintenance of fluid is essential and average human needs 30–40 mL/kg/day.

Daily requirement of electrolytes:

- *Sodium:* 50–90 millimols/day
- *Potassium:* 50 mM/day
- *Calcium:* 5 mM/day
- *Magnesium:* 1 mM/day

BLOOD TRANSFUSION AND BLOOD PRODUCTS

Transfusion

- *The amount of blood withdrawn from donor:* 450 mL
- Maximum three times/year
- Each unit of blood is screened for *hepatitis B, hepatitis C, human immunodeficiency virus (HIV 1) and HIV 2, and syphilis*

Blood Products

Whole blood	*Packed red cells*
• Rich in coagulation factors than packed cells and more metabolically active than stored blood • *Available as 450 mL pack* • Contains red blood cell (RBC), white blood cell (WBC), plasma, platelet, of which WBC and platelet are nonfunctional • Used in massive bleeding, open heart surgery, etc	• The cells are spun down and concentrated • *Each unit is 330 mL* • Hematocrit = 50–70% • Packed cells are stored in saline, adenine, glucose, mannitol (SAG-M) solution to increase their shelf life to 5 weeks at 2–6°C • *Older storage regimens:* Citrate phosphate dextrose giving cells shelf life of 2–3 weeks • 1 unit increases Hb by 1 gm/dL • Hematocrit by 3%
Fresh frozen plasma: • Rich in coagulation factors • Stored at –40 to –60°C (2-year shelf life) • Rh D positive fresh frozen plasma (FFP) can be given to Rh D negative women • Available in 200–250 mL packets	*Cryoprecipitate:* • Supernatant precipitate of FFP and is rich in factor VIII and fibrinogen • Stored at –30°C with a 2-year shelf life • Available in 15 mL
Platelets: • They are available as pooled platelet concentrate containing 250 × 10^9 cells/liter • Platelets are stored on a special agitator at 20–24°C. Half-life is only 5 days • Useful in patients with thrombocytopenia	*Prothrombin complex concentrates (PCC):* • Highly purified concentrates prepared from pooled plasma • They contain factors II, IX, and X. Factor VII may be included or produced separately

Blood storage:
- Patients who receive repeated transfusions over long periods may get iron overload.
- Each transfused unit of red blood cells (RBCs) contain approximately 250 mg elemental iron
  - If citrate phosphate dextrose (CPD) is used for storage, blood can be stored for 21 days at 1–6°C
  - If adenine is added to CPD, we can increase storage time to 35 days

Autologous blood:
- Patients undergoing elective surgery, pre donate their blood up to 3 weeks before surgery for retransfusion during operation **(Table 13)**.

TABLE 13: Perioperative blood transfusion.

Hemoglobin level (gm/dL)	*Indication*
<6 gm	Benefit from transfusion
6–8 gm	Transfusion unlikely to be beneficial in the absence of bleeding or impending surgery
>8 gm	No indication for transfusion

Complications of blood transfusion:
- Incomplete hemolytic transfusion reaction
- *Febrile nonhemolytic transfusion reaction (most common)*
- Allergic reaction
- *Infection:*
  - Bacterial infection (as a result of faulty storage)
  - Hepatitis B, C, and G
  - HIV 1 and 2
  - Human T-lymphotropic virus types (HTLV) 1 and 2
  - *Malaria*
  - West Nile virus, parvovirus B-19, human herpesvirus (HHV-8), and *Cytomegalovirus* (CMV)
- Air embolism
- Thrombocytopenia
- *Transfusion related acute lung injury (TRALI)* (usually from FFP)
- Fatal hemolysis
- Graft-versus-host disease (GVHD)
- Human leukocyte antigen (HLA) and red blood cell (RBC) allosensitization
- Patients who receive repeated transfusions over long periods may get *iron overload.* Each transfused unit of RBCs contain approximately *250 mg elemental iron.*

Management of coagulopathy:
Standard guideline for blood products infusion is given below:
- FFP if prothrombin time or partial thromboplastin time is >1.5 times normal
- Cryoprecipitate if fibrinogen < 0.8 gm/L
- Platelets if platelet count < 50 × 10^9/mL (<50,000 cells/mm^3)

Effects of storage of whole blood?
- Reduction in pH
- Raise in potassium concentration
- Progressive reduction of red cell content of 2,3 diphosphoglycerate, which results in decrease in oxygen carrying capacity
- Loss of platelet function in whole blood within 48 hours of donation
- Reduction of factor VIII to 10–20% of normal in 48 hours
- Coagulation factors VII and IX are stable in storage

TABLE 14: Blood transfusion.

Blood component	*Temperature of storage*	*Shelf life*
Whole blood	1–6°C	35 days
Packed cells	–	42 days
Platelets	20–24°C	5 days
Fresh frozen plasma (FFP)	–40°C	2 years
Cryoprecipitate	–30°C	2 years

Massive Blood Transfusion

It is defined as transfusion of greater than patient's total blood volume in 24 hours or as acute administration of more than half the patients estimated blood volume over a few hours **(Table 14)**.

Complications of massive transfusion:

- Coagulopathy
- *Hypocalcemia* (due to binding of ionized calcium by citrate used as anticoagulant)
- *Hyperkalemia* (due to RBC lysis)
- *Hypomagnesemia*
- Hypothermia
- Volume overload
- Dilutional thrombocytopenia
- Decreased oxygen delivery [due to decrease in 2,3 diphosphoglycerate (DPG)]
- *Metabolic alkalosis* (even though the stored blood contains pH 6.3, because of massive transfusion, sodium citrate is metabolized in liver to sodium bicarbonate)
- *Rare:* Metabolic acidosis

Extra Edge

Platelet transfusion:

- *Volume:* 50 mL
- Stored at room temperature
- Survived only for 5 days
- 1 unit has 5,000–10,000 platelets
- ABO compatibility is not needed for platelet and FFP
- Blood pack containing platelets will not be functioning after 24 hours

High-yield Extra Edge:

- *Threshold for platelet transfusion:* 10,000 cells/μL
- For invasive procedure, minimum platelet count must be 50,000
- For surgeries, minimum platelet count must be 1 lakh

Trauma: General Aspects (Based on Advanced Trauma Life Support, 10th Edition)

R Rajamahendran

INTRODUCTION

- The most common cause of death in the first four decades of life is trauma.
- It is the third common cause of death overall.

MECHANISMS OF INJURY

- *Overt mechanism:*
  - Penetrating trauma
  - Blunt trauma
  - Thermal trauma
  - Blast injury
- *Covert mechanism:*
  - Blunt trauma
  - Penetrating trauma
  - Penetrating knife
  - Gunshot injury

The track can be identified by the anatomy, which shows the organs injured.

Extra Edge

Overt injury:
- Some injuries are so obvious that they present even before the patient details are not known
- *Example: Singed facial hair* associated with carbonaceous sputum suggest inhalational burns and anesthetic colleague should be called as soon we identify such problem before the patient goes for larynx edema

Covert injuries:
- These cases need application of common sense and identifying the hidden injuries
- *Example: Seat belt injury*—flexion and distraction will have an overt injury of dislocated knee, chance fracture of lumbar spine, *but hidden duodenal injury and popliteal artery rupture should be sought*

Advanced Trauma Life Support (ATLS)

Steps in ATLS:
- *Primary survey:* With simultaneous resuscitation, identify which is killing the patient
- *Secondary survey:* Identify other injuries
- *Definitive care*

TRIAGE

Triage a French word that means *"to sort".*

Four color codes are given **(Fig. 1) (Table 1)**

- *Red:* First priority is a critical patient
- *Yellow*: Urgent is second priority
- *Green:* Minor and third priority
- *Black:* Dead or about-to-die patients.

BLUNT TRAUMA

- The most common cause is road traffic accident.
- Use of seat belt by the front row occupants reduces their death rate by 45%.

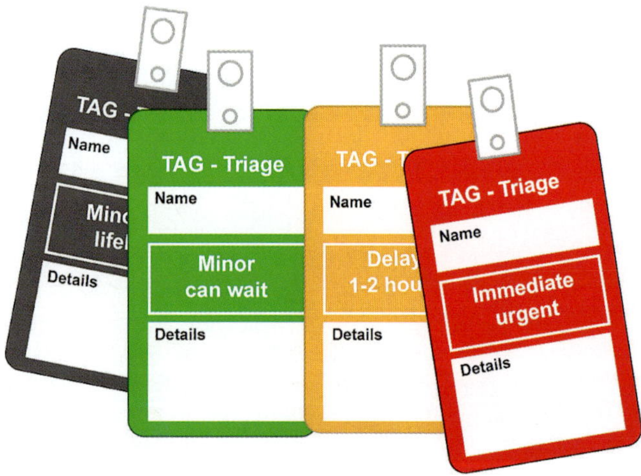

Fig. 1: Triage.

TABLE 1: Priority levels with corresponding colors.

Priority	*Color*	*Example*
I	Red	Tension pneumothorax
II	Yellow	Pelvic fracture
III	Green	Simple fracture
Last—zero priority	Black	Unsalvageable

- Remember, if the rear seat belts are worn, the death rate of front seat occupants with seat belts is reduced to 80%.
- Seat belt mark if present in thorax has *four-fold thoracic trauma* and mark in *abdomen has three fold risk* than those not having mark.

Primary Survey: cABCDE

- c—exsanguinating external hemorrhage
- A—airway
- B—breathing
- C—circulation
- D—disability and neurological status
- E—exposure

C—Exsanguinating External Hemorrhage

- Even before airway is managed, exsanguinating external hemorrhage must be controlled first by pressure or packing.
- In limbs, tourniquet must be applied for concerned time and early surgical repair must be done.

Airway with Cervical Spine Control

- For head injury with *Glasgow coma scale (GCS) score ≤8,* immediate intubation is needed.
- While maintaining the patent's airway, always maintain *cervical spine stability.*
- *Things to be done in airway:*
  - Suctioning secretions or blood from airway
  - *Airway maneuvers:* Jaw thrust, chin lift, oropharyngeal or nasopharyngeal airway insertion.

Breathing and Ventilation

- *Oxygen* must be offered to all trauma patients via reservoir mask in high flow.
- *Ventilation* must be assessed by seeing chest walls and lungs.
- Tension pneumothorax, flail chest, massive hemothorax, and open pneumothorax are all clinical diagnosis and not radiological diagnosis and need immediate treatment.

Circulation

- Circulation is assessed based on three clinical criteria:
  1. Conscious level (implies cerebral perfusion)
  2. Skin color
  3. Rapid thready pulse is more reliable warning sign than blood pressure
- Indicators of shock in the injured patient
  - Agitation or confusion
  - Tachycardia, tachypnea, and diaphoresis
  - Cool mottled extremities
  - Weak distal pulses
  - Decreased pulse pressure and urine output
  - Hypotension
- Emergency resuscitation with *1–2 liters of warm crystalloid solution* through two large bore, short, peripheral intravenous (IV) catheters

Permissive hypotension:
- Maintain good blood supply to vital organs such as brain, heart, and kidney

Target systemic pressure: 70–90 mm Hg
- If head injury suspected, have pressure > 90 mm Hg
- Fluids such as 250 mL of O negative blood or normal saline are infused
- Excessive crystalloids and colloids are avoided as they cause hemodilution and increase coagulopathy and acute respiratory distress syndrome (ARDS)
- Severely injured hypovolemic patients must receive massive transfusion protocol (1 packed red cells: 1 fresh frozen plasma: 1 platelets)

Tranexamic acid:
- 1 gm IV over 10 minutes followed by 1 gm for 8 hours
- It should be given to all trauma patients suspected to have significant hemorrhage with pulse rate (PR) >110 beats per-minute or blood pressure (BP) < 110 mm Hg systolic
- It must be administered in 3 hours of injury and even given by paramedics in prehospital environment

Identification and management of hemorrhage:
- *Gold standard investigation: Whole body computed tomography scan (WBCT)* from head to pelvis with IV contrast for severely injured adult blunt trauma patient
- WBCT is done as early as possible with resuscitation being on the go
- Provisional hot report is issued in minutes for WBCT and definitive report is obtained after 30–60 minutes
- All patients who undergo immediate laparotomy [e.g., abdominal injuries or pelvic bleeding after focused assessment with sonography for trauma (FAST)] must have a pelvic binder until pelvic fracture is excluded by WBCT

Disability and Exposure

- *Glasgow coma scale* is the score used in trauma setting to measure the disability.
- Fully expose the patient and examine front and back.

- Log roll should not be performed until pelvic fracture is excluded.
- If you want to move the patient during primary survey, for example, to CT scan, *20 degrees roll with inline spinal stabilization must be used.*
- *Springing the pelvis to look for pelvic fracture is not performed nowadays. Diagnose pelvic fracture only by radiological method.*

Radiographs in Trauma

- Lateral cervical spine
- Anteroposterior chest
- Anteroposterior pelvis

Damage control surgery in orthopedics (DCO): Temporary stabilization of long bone fractures with external fixators and planning for intramedullary nailing after 4 days.

Early total care (ETC): Early fracture fixation of all fractures.

But DCO and ETC are not competition for each other and must complement each other at needed places

- *Example:* If you are planning ETC of intramuscular (IM) nailing of a femur fracture and on table patient becomes unstable due to chest trauma or head trauma, we must convert ETC to DCO by just external fixation

Criteria for DCO/damage control surgery (DCS)	*Criteria for ETC*
• Hypothermia <34° • Acidosis <7.2 • Serum lactate >5 mmol/L • Coagulopathy • Blood pressure (BP) <70 mm Hg • Transfusion approaching around 15 units • Injury severity score >36	• Hemodynamically stable • No inotropes needed • No hypoxia • No hypercapnia • Lactate level <2 mmol/L • Normal coagulation/ • Normothermia • Urine output >1 mL/kg/h

Resuscitation in Trauma

Resuscitative Thoracotomy

- Open pericardium to relieve cardiac tamponade.
- Perform internal cardiac massage.
- Cross clamp the distal thoracic aorta.
- Manage intrathoracic bleeding.

Criteria for Selection:

- Patients with penetrating thoracic trauma who have signs of life on reaching emergency department are selected. Survival rate of this procedure in penetrating trauma is 35%.
- Blunt trauma patients usually have poor outcomes with survival rates as low as 1%.

Emergency Department Thoracotomy (Table 2)

TABLE 2: Indications and contraindications for emergency intervention.

Indications	*Contraindications*
Salvageable postinjury cardiac arrest: • Penetrating trauma to torso within 15 minutes of prehospital CPR • Blunt trauma within 10 minutes of prehospital CPR • Penetrating neck trauma or extremity trauma in 5 minutes *Severe postinjury hypotension (<60 mm Hg):* • Cardiac tamponade • Intrathoracic hemorrhage, intraabdominal bleed, and neck injury bleeding • Air embolism	• *Penetrating trauma:* CPR > 15 minute and no signs of life (pupillary reflex, respiratory effort, or motor activity nil) • *Blunt trauma:* CPR > 10 minutes with no signs of life or asystole without cardiac tamponade

(CPR: cardiopulmonary resuscitation)

Recent advance:

Resuscitative endovascular balloon occlusion of the aorta (REBOA): Quicker, less invasive method of achieving aortic occlusion during initial resuscitation, providing another tool to combat early exsanguinating blood loss.

Goals of Resuscitation

- Optimizing tissue perfusion
- Ensuring normothermia
- Restoring coagulation
- Judicious use of crystalloids and transfusion
- Maintain oxygen delivery index >500 mL/min per square meter and cardiac index >3.8L/min per square meter

Extra Edge

- *Norepinephrine* is the agent of choice in increasing systemic vascular resistance
- Goal to normalize lactate is within 24 hours
- Acute coagulopathy of trauma (ACOT)
- Activated protein C is a key element in ACOT
- Thromboelastography (TEG) and rotational thromboelastometry (ROTEM) viscoelastic hemostatic assays—helps in goal directed hemostasis
- *Massive transfusion [10 units of packed red blood cells (PRBC) in 6 hours] Protocol:* 1:2 red cell: plasma ratio used

Venous lactate level—uses in resuscitation:
- Useful marker of resuscitation and physiological state of the patient
- *Values:* <2 mmol/L—fully resuscitate and give early total care (ETC) is possible
- *2–3 mmol/L:* Observe whether improving or deteriorating on resuscitation
- *>3 mmol/L:* Under resuscitated, resuscitate further or do damage control surgery (DCS) if surgery is urgent
- *>5 mmol/L:* No doubt, DCS is the management

Injury Scoring Systems (Box 1)

- *Abbreviated injury scale (AIS):* Anatomic system of injury classification
- Injury severity score (ISS)
- Glassgow coma scale (GCS) scoring
- Revised trauma scoring (RTS)
- Trauma and injury severity score (TRISS)
- Mangled extremity severity score (MESS)

Abbreviated Injury Scale

- It tells the probability of threat to life scale based on individual injury.
- It has a seven-digit code and is represented as 123456.7.
- Post dot code (7th digit) describes the severity code and ranges from 1 to 6 as follows

1 Minor	4 Severe
2 Moderate	5 Critical
3 Serious	6 Maximum (fatal)

- Pre dot codes represent the anatomic region, structure, specific structure, and level of injury as follows"
  1 Anatomic body region
  2 Type of anatomic structure
  3/4 Specific anatomic structure
  5/6 Level of injury
- Pre dot code for Body region (first digit) is as follows
  1 Head
  2 Face
  3 Neck
  4 Thorax
  5 Abdomen and Pelvis
  6 Spine
  7 Upper extremities
  8 Lower extremities
  9 Burns and other trauma

Abbreviated injury scale severity code and its probability of death is as follows:

AIS severity code	*Probability of death %*
1	0
2	1–2
3	8–10
4–5	50
6	100

BOX 1: Various injury scoring systems.

Revised trauma score (RTS):
- R—respiratory rate
- T—tie and see Blood pressure (BP)
- S—scale (Glasgow coma scale)

Trauma injury and severity score (TRISS):
- R—RTS
- I—injury severity score
- S—seen Age
- S—specific mechanism (blunt or penetrating)

Mangled extremity severity score (MESS):
- M—main energy that caused injury
- E—extremity ischemia
- S—seen Age
- S—shock

Secondary Survey

- Head-to-toe examination
- Further evaluation with imaging and other diagnostic modalities
- More detailed neurologic evaluation
- Torso examination, seat belt marks, and superficial injury to neck and abdomen
- Assessment of pelvis and pulse rate (PR) to assess position of prostate and for any bleeding
- Perfusion of the extremities

AMPLE Assessment

- A—allergy
- M—medications
- P—past medical history
- L—last meal
- E—events of incident

DAMAGE CONTROL SURGERY (ABBREVIATED LAPAROTOMY)

The surgery is restricted to two goals only:
- Stop any active bleed.
- Control any contamination.

TABLE 3: Phases of trauma management.

Phase 1: ***Initial exploration***	***Phase 2:*** ***Secondary resuscitation***	***Phase 3:*** ***Definitive treatment***
• Control active hemorrhage and contamination • *Midline incision:* Four quadrant packing done • Gastrointestinal tract (GIT) perforations closed with sutures or staples • External drains kept for pancreatic/bile duct injuries • Temporary closure of abdomen using plastic sheet known as Opsite • This technique of closure is known as "VACPAC or Opsite sandwich"	• Transfer to intensive care unit (ICU) • Ventilatory support • *Correct the deadly triad:* Hypothermia, acidosis, and coagulopathy	• Planned re-exploration and definite surgery • Done 48–72 hours after secondary phase • Complex reconstruction must be avoided

TABLE 4: Stages and indications of damage control surgery.

Stage	*Procedure*
I	Select the patient
II	Control hemorrhage and contamination
III	Intensive care unit (ICU) resuscitation
IV	Definitive repairs
V	Closure of abdomen

Indications of damage control surgery:

- *Anatomical:*
  - Difficult to achieve hemostasis
  - Complex injury such as liver, pancreas, etc.
  - Combined solid, hollow, and vascular injuries
  - Inaccessible major venous like retrohepatic inferior vena cava (IVC) injury
  - Nonoperative control of other injuries is in more demand such as in pelvic fracture
  - Time consuming procedure anticipated
- *Physiological:*
  - Temperature <34°C
  - pH <7.2
  - Serum lactate >5 mmol/L (n = 2.5)
  - Prothrombin time (PT) >16 seconds
  - Partial thromboplastin time (PTT) >60 seconds
  - >10 units transfused
  - Systolic BP <90 mm Hg for > 60 seconds
- *Environmental:*
  - Operating time >60 minutes
  - Inability to approximate abdominal incision
  - Relook of abdomen needed

The aim is to resuscitate the patient and plan for definite surgeries after the patient becomes stable.

Indications for Damage Control Surgery

- Refractory hypothermia (temperature <35°C)
- Profound acidosis (arterial pH <7.2 and base deficit <15 mmol/L)
- Refractory coagulopathy

TABLE 5: Management strategies for various traumatic injuries.

Arterial injuries	Interposition polytetrafluoroethylene (PTFE) graft
Venous injuries	Preferentially ligated
Hepatic injuries	Perihepatic packing
Translobar gunshot wounds of liver	Balloon catheter tamponade
Bleeding pulmonary injuries	Wedge resection using stapler
Penetrating pulmonary injuries	Pulmonary tractotomy
Cardiac injuries	Pledgeted repair
Pancreatic injuries	Packed and evaluation of ductal integrity later
Urologic injuries	Catheter diversion
Small gastrointestinal (GI) injuries	Rapid whipstitch using prolene and temporary closure of abdomen

Note: Corresponding traumas are discussed in concerned chapters by specialists.

DEADLY TRIAD

Following a trauma and protracted surgery in physiologically unstable patient, the three factors that carry high mortality are:

- Hypothermia
- Acidosis
- Coagulopathy

Hence, originated a phenomenon—Damage Control Surgery.

Phases of DCS ***(Tables 3 and 4)****:*

- *Phase 1:* Initial exploration
- *Phase 2:* Secondary resuscitation
- *Phase 3:* Definitive operation

Procedures in Damage Control Surgery

Procedures in DCS are given in **Table 5**.

Burns and its Effects (Based on Advanced Trauma Life Support, 10th Edition)

R Rajamahendran

METABOLIC PROBLEMS FOLLOWING BURNS

Burns produce an inflammatory reaction:

- This leads to vastly increased vascular permeability.
- Water, solutes, and proteins move from the intra to the extravascular space.
- The volume of fluid lost is directly proportional to the area of the burn.
- *Above 15% of surface area, the loss of fluid produces shock.*

MAJOR DETERMINANTS OF OUTCOME OF BURN

- Percentage surface area involved
- Depth of burns
- Presence of an inhalational injury

Criteria for admission to a burns unit:
- Partial-thickness and full-thickness burns totaling greater than 10% total body surface area (TBSA) under 10 years age
- Partial-thickness and full-thickness burns totaling greater than 20% TBSA in other age group
- Full-thickness burns greater than 5% TBSA in any age group
- Any burns in face, hands, feet, genitalia, perineum, and major joints

ASSESSING AREA OF BURN

- The patient's whole hand is 1% total body surface area (TBSA) and is a useful guide in small burns (Palm rule).
- The Lund and Browder chart is useful in larger burns.
- The rule of nines is adequate for first approximation only.

Rule of Nine (Alexander Wallace Rule) (Figs. 1 and 2)

- *Each upper limb:* 9% TBSA
- *Each lower leg:* 18% TBSA
- *Anterior or posterior trunk:* 18% TBSA
- *Head and neck:* 9% TBSA
- *Perineum:* 1% TBSA

Recent advance:
- In children, head and neck is relatively large and may account for 18–21%.
- *Infants:* 21% TBSA.
- The *Berkow formula* is used to determine burn size accurately in children.

Lund and Browder Chart

- Most accurate method for calculating the burns percentage.
- *Percentage of burns for head at birth:* 18%
- *Percentage of burns for head at 1 year:* 16%
- *Percentage of burns for head at adult age:* 6%

DEGREES OF BURNS (FIGS. 3 TO 6)

- *First degree:* Involves only epidermis.
- *Second degree:* Involves epidermis and some part of dermis (also known as partial-thickness burns); further divided into.
- *Superficial second degree or superficial partial thickness:* Involves upper part of dermis.
- *Deep second degree or deep partial thickness:* Extends up to reticular layer of dermis.
- *Third degree or full-thickness burns:* Involves full thickness of dermis.
- *Fourth degree burns:* Involves subcutaneous fat and deep structures.

Degrees of burns depend on time of burns, temperature of burns, and material causing burns **(Table 1)**.

- Burning of human skin at 44°C takes 6 hours for irreversible damage **(Flowchart 1)**.
- Burning of human skin at 70°C takes only 1 second for epidermal destruction.

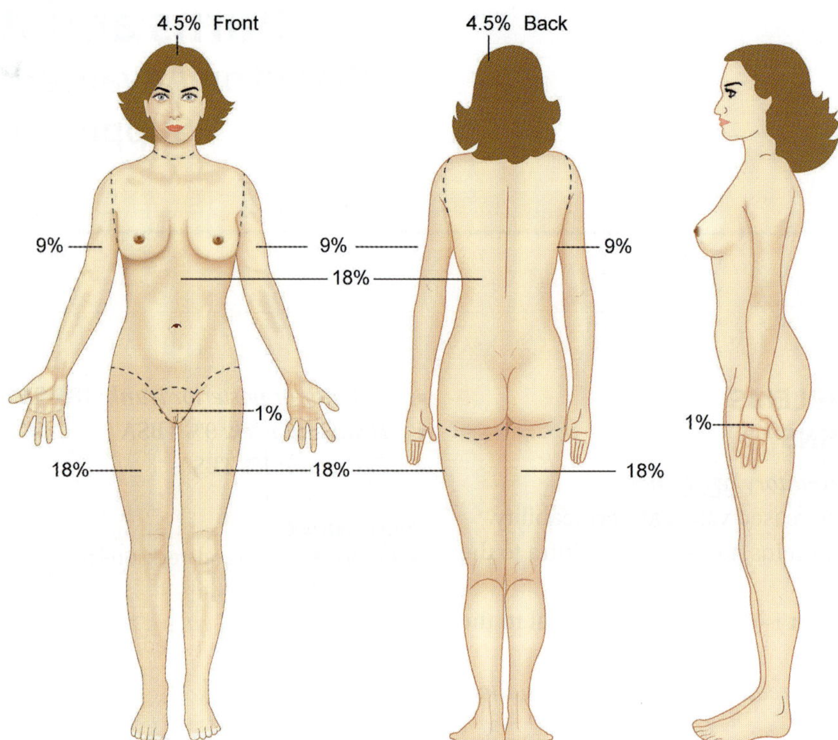

Fig. 1: Rule of nine.

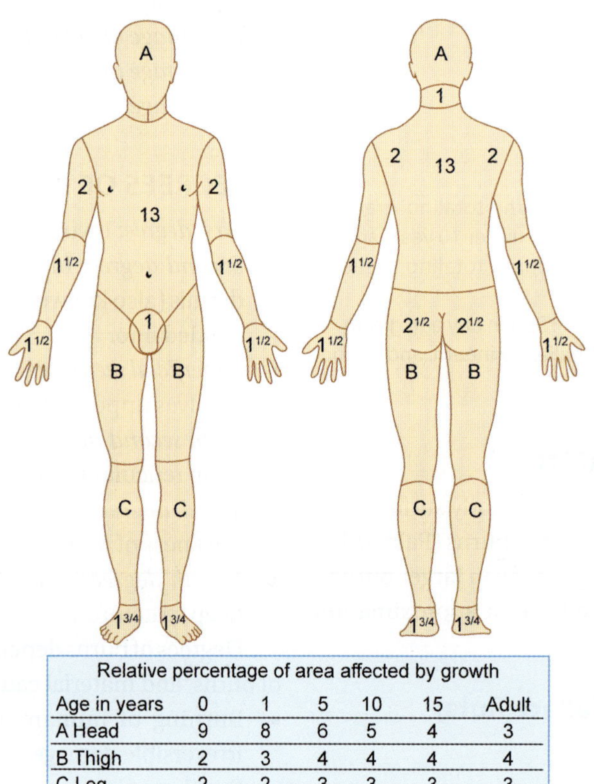

Relative percentage of area affected by growth						
Age in years	0	1	5	10	15	Adult
A Head	9	8	6	5	4	3
B Thigh	2	3	4	4	4	4
C Leg	2	2	3	3	3	3

Fig. 2: The Lund and Browder chart.

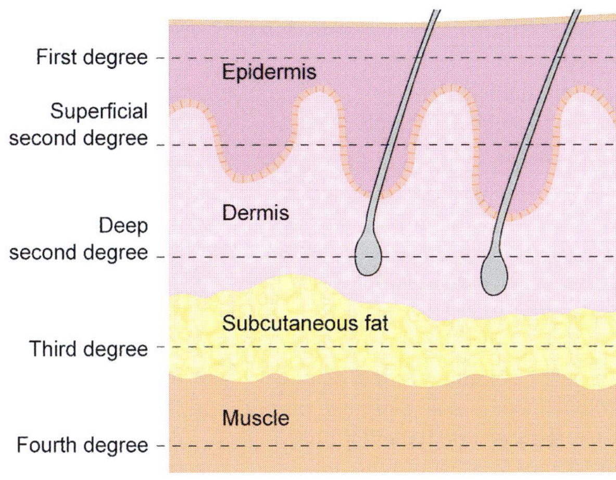

Fig. 3: Degree of burns.

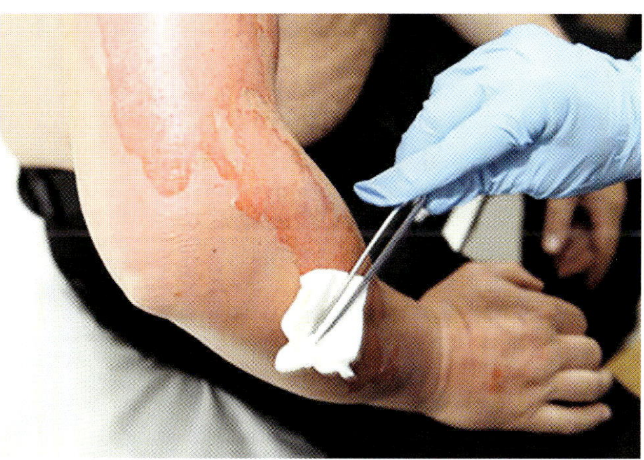

Fig. 4: First-degree burns.

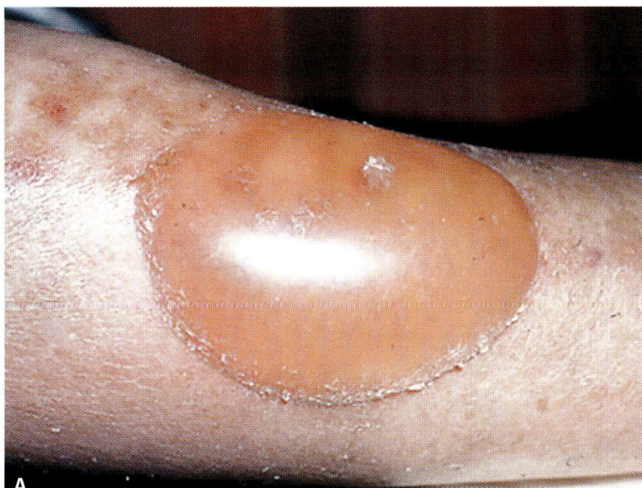

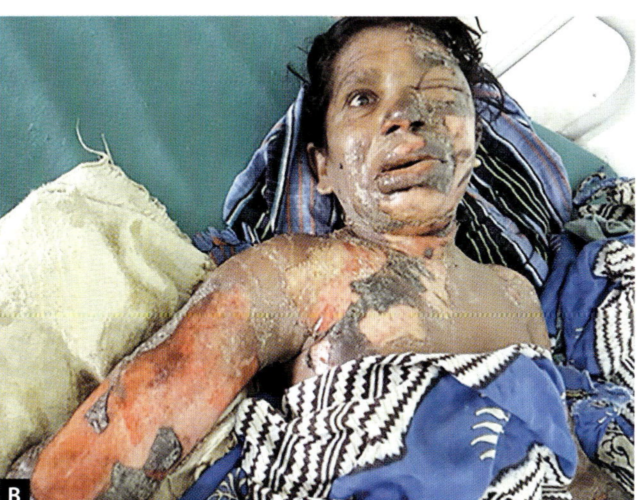

Figs. 5A and B: Second-degree burns.

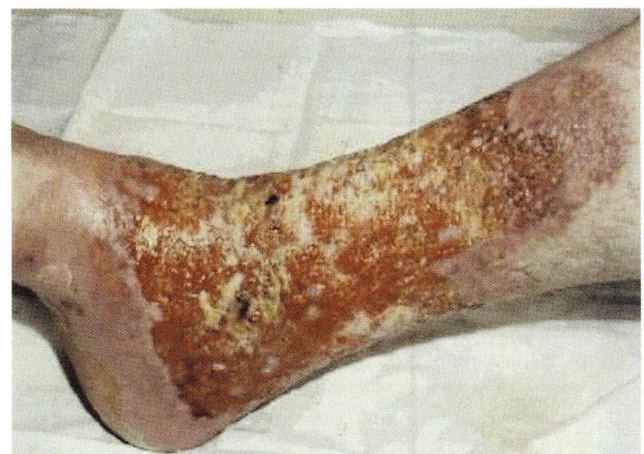

Fig. 6: Third-degree burns.

- Similarly cause of burns decides the depth of burns such as:
  - *Scalds:* Superficial
  - *Fat burns:* Deep dermal
  - *Flame burns:* Mixed deep dermal and full thickness
  - *Alkali burns:* Deep dermis and full thickness
  - *Acid burns:* Weak one, superficial; strong one, deep dermal
  - *Electrical:* Full thickness

  Wound management is given in **Table 2.**

MANAGEMENT OF BURNS

- *Immediate care:*
  - Sedation
  - Analgesics and antibiotics

TABLE 1: Degrees of burns.

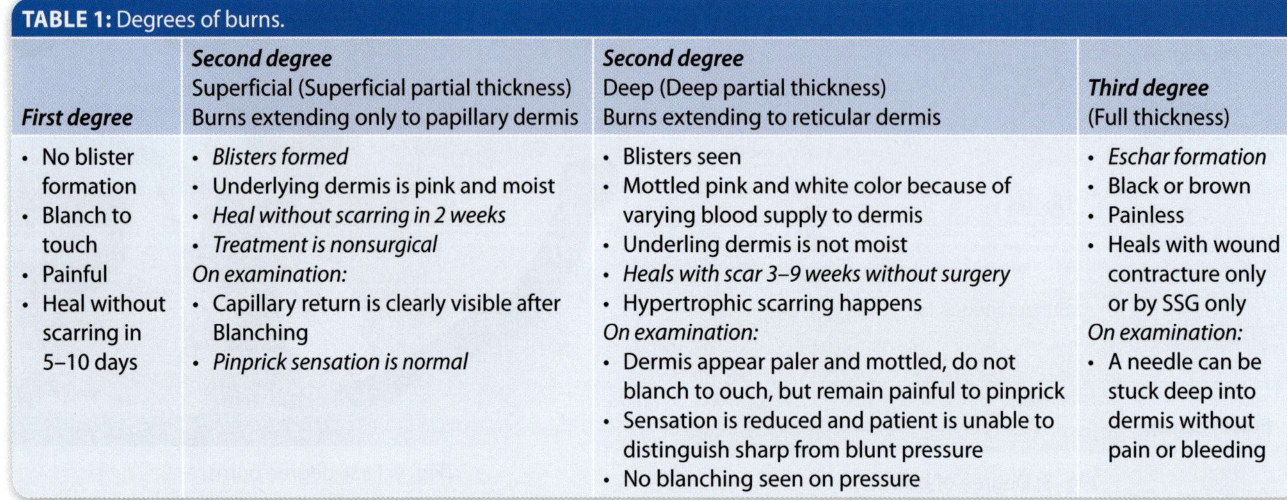

First degree	*Second degree* Superficial (Superficial partial thickness) Burns extending only to papillary dermis	*Second degree* Deep (Deep partial thickness) Burns extending to reticular dermis	*Third degree* (Full thickness)
• No blister formation • Blanch to touch • Painful • Heal without scarring in 5–10 days	• *Blisters formed* • Underlying dermis is pink and moist • *Heal without scarring in 2 weeks* • *Treatment is nonsurgical* *On examination:* • Capillary return is clearly visible after Blanching • *Pinprick sensation is normal*	• Blisters seen • Mottled pink and white color because of varying blood supply to dermis • Underling dermis is not moist • *Heals with scar 3–9 weeks without surgery* • Hypertrophic scarring happens *On examination:* • Dermis appear paler and mottled, do not blanch to ouch, but remain painful to pinprick • Sensation is reduced and patient is unable to distinguish sharp from blunt pressure • No blanching seen on pressure	• *Eschar formation* • Black or brown • Painless • Heals with wound contracture only or by SSG only *On examination:* • A needle can be stuck deep into dermis without pain or bleeding

Flowchart 1: Burns degrees and management according to the depths.

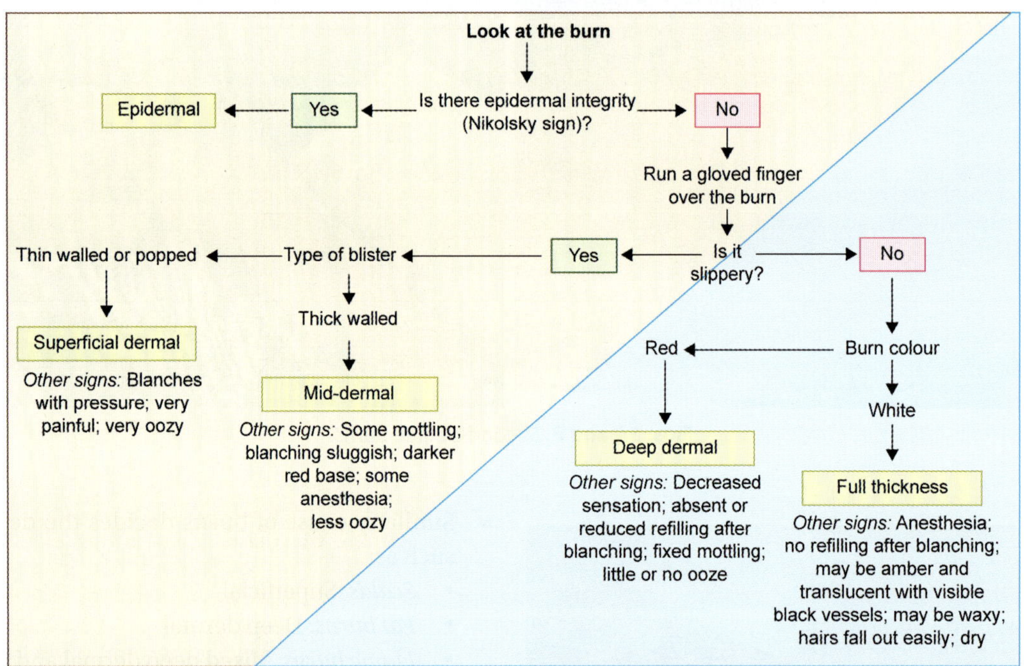

TABLE 2: Wound management.

Group A	*Group B*
Good wound management and supportive care are enough for them; they heal in 14 days, cosmetically good looking • Ointments • Exposure treatment • Collagens • Natural membranes such as amniotic membrane	• May take weeks to months to heal • Forms eschar, granulation tissue, and wound contraction • The course of healing by secondary intention must not be allowed and must be treated by primary intention—healing with direct closure, skin graft, and substitutes

   - Fluid resuscitation
   - Escharotomy
- *Follow up care:*
   - Dressing
   - Wound cover
   - *Late care:*
      - Skin grafting
      - Contracture release

Fluids for Resuscitation

- *In children with burns over 10% TBSA and adults with burns over 15% TBSA,* consider the need for intravenous fluid resuscitation.
- If oral fluids are to be used, salt must be added.
- Fluids needed can be calculated from a standard formula.
- The key is to monitor urine output.

Ideal Fluid

There are three types of fluid used. The most common are crystalloids

1. *Crystalloids:* Ringer's lactate or Hartmann's solution
2. *Colloids:* Human albumin solution or fresh frozen plasma
3. Some centers use hypertonic saline.

Extra Edge

- Ringer's lactate (RL) is the preferred agent for resuscitation for initial for 24 hours.
- Nasogastric intubation is done to decrease the risk of emesis and possible aspiration due to paralytic ileus.
- Dextran is a colloid and can be used after 24 hours; however, albumin is the preferred and most widely used colloid.

- *About crystalloids:*
   - Ringer's lactate is the most commonly used crystalloid. Crystalloids are said to be as effective as colloids for maintaining intravascular volume.
   - They are also significantly less expensive.
   - Another reason for the use of crystalloids is that even large protein molecules leak out of capillaries following burn injury; however, nonburnt capillaries continue to sieve proteins virtually normally.
- *Hypertonic saline:*
   - Hypertonic saline has been effective in treating burns shock for many years. It produces hyperosmolarity and hypernatremia.
   - This reduces the shift of intracellular water to extracellular space.
   - Advantages include less tissue edema and a resultant decrease in escharotomies and intubations.
- *Colloids:*
   - Plasma proteins are responsible for the inward oncotic pressure that counteracts the outward capillary hydrostatic pressure.
   - Without proteins, plasma volumes would not be maintained as there would be edema.
   - *Proteins should be given after the first 24 hours of burn* because, before this time, the massive fluid shifts cause proteins to leak out of the cells.

Modified Parkland Formula

- *TBSA% × weight (kg) × 4 = volume (mL) needed*
- Half this volume is given in the first 8 hours, and the second half is given in the subsequent 16 hours
- The volume replacement is by crystalloids.

Muir and Barclay Formula

- The most common *colloid-based formula* is the Muir and Barclay formula:
- 0.5 × percentage body surface area burnt × weight = one portion; periods of 4/4/4, 6/6, and 12 hours respectively
- One portion to be given in each period

Recent advance:

- Formula for fluid calculation in children:
- *The Galveston formula* uses 5,000 mL/TBSA burned (in metre square) + 2.000 mL/m^2 total for maintenance in the first 24 hours. This formula accounts for maintenance needs and the increased fluid requirements of a child with a burn.

Other formula used:

- *Brooke formula:* Uses both crystalloids and colloids

Maintenance

- The key to monitoring of resuscitation is urine output.
- It should be between 0.5 and 1.0 mL/kg body weight per hour.
- If the urine output is below this, the infusion rate should be increased by 50%.

Advanced Trauma Life Support (ATLS) 10th edition guidelines of resuscitation:

- Superficial burns or scalds (1st degree and 2nd degree)

Above 14 years:

- Fluid input = 2 mL Ringer lactate × weight in kg × total body surface area (TBSA)
- Maintain urine output 0.5 mL/kg/h

Below 14 years:
- Fluid input = 3 mL RLX weight in kg × TBSA (<14 years)
- Maintain urine output 1 mL/Kg/h

Electrical injury (all ages):
- Fluid input = 4 mL RL × weight in kg × TBSA
- Maintain urine output 1–1.5 mL/kg/h

Escharotomy

- Circumferential full-thickness burns to the limbs require emergency surgery to avoid compartmental syndrome.
- The tourniquet effect of this injury is easily treated by incising the whole length of full-thickness burns.
- This should be done in the mid-axial line, avoiding major nerves.

Level of Escharotomies

- *Upper limb:* Mid-axial, anterior to the elbow medially to avoid the ulnar nerve.
- *Hand:* Midline in the digits.
- *Lower limb mid-axial:* Posterior to the ankle medially to avoid the saphenous vein.
- *Chest:* Down the chest lateral to the nipples, across the chest below the clavicle and across the chest at the level of the xiphisternum **(Fig. 7)**.

Topical Antimicrobials

- *Silver sulphadiazine 1%:* Effective against *Pseudomonas* and methicillin-resistant *Staphylococcus aureus* (MRSA).
- Silver nitrate solution *0.5%:* Highly effective against *Pseudomonas*. It produces black staining of surroundings.
- *Mafenide acetate 5%:* Painful to apply; produces metabolic acidosis.
- *Silver sulphadiazine and cerium nitrate:* Cerium nitrate forms sterile eschar and boosts cell-mediated immunity.

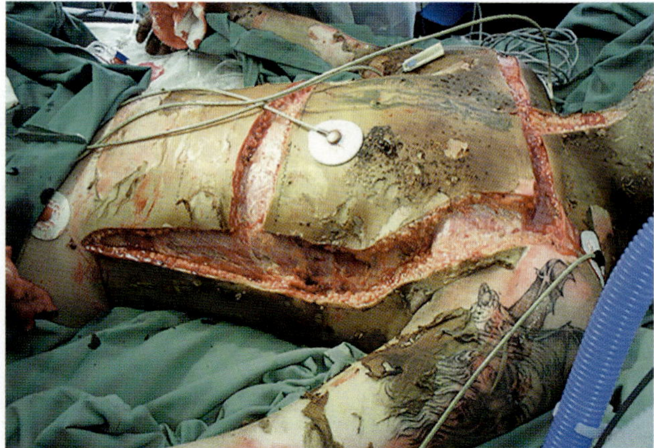

Fig. 7: Escharatomies to avoid respiratory problem.

Management of Burns Wound

- *Closed method:* Occlusive dressing with antimicrobials is applied over the wound.
- *Exposure method:* It is used for face and head. No dressing is made and wound is left open after applying the agent **(Table 3)**.

Topical Treatment

- *Hydrocolloid dressings:* Hydrocolloid dressings need to be changed every 3–5 days. They are particularly useful in mixed-depth burn as the high protease levels under the occlusive dressings aid with the debridement of the deeper areas of burn. They also provide a moist environment, which is good for epithelialization.
- *Biological, synthetic (e.g., Biobrane), and natural (e.g. amniotic membranes) dressings* also provide good healing; they will become detached if applied to deep dermal wounds as the eschar needs to separate. They are therefore not as useful in mixed-depth wounds and better only for superficial burns as one-stop management.

Healing of Third-Degree Burns

- Collagen dressing
- Grafting
- Early debridement and grafting are the key to effectively treating deep partial- and full-thickness burns in a majority of cases.
- Meshed grafts

TABLE 3: Management of burns wound.

Exposure method	*Closed method*
Advantage: • Easy dressing method *Disadvantages:* • Increased pain and heat loss • Risk of cross contamination	*Advantages:* • Less pain and less heat loss • Less risk of cross contamination *Disadvantage:* • Increased bacterial growth is seen if dressing not changed daily twice

Management of Deep Burns

- Deep dermal burns need tangential shaving and split-skin grafting.
- All but the smallest full-thickness burns need surgery.
- The anesthetist needs to be ready for significant blood loss.
- Topical adrenaline reduces bleeding.
- All burnt tissue needs to be exercised.
- Stable cover, permanent or temporary, should be applied at once to reduce burn load.

Delayed Reconstruction of Burns

- Eyelids must be treated before exposure keratitis arises.
- Transposition flaps and Z-plasties with or without tissue expansion are useful.
- Full-thickness grafts and free flaps may be needed for large or difficult areas.
- Hypertrophy is treated with pressure garments.
- Pharmacological treatment of itch is important.

Nutrition in burns:
- Burns patients need extra feeding.
- Burns above 15% needs feeding by nasogastric tube method.
- Rapid excision of burns and stable coverage of the wound are most significant factors in reversing the catabolic state.
- *Commonly used formulas for nutrition are:*
  - Curreri formula
  - Sutherland formula
  - Davies formula

Extra Edge

Feeding formulas: Calories needed:
- *Curreri formula:*
  - Age 16–59 years = 25 (weight) + 40 (TBSA burns)
  - Age 60+ = 20 (weight)+ 65 (TBSA)
- *Sutherland formula:*
  - Children: 60 Kcal/kg + 35 Kcal% TBSA
  - Adults 20 Kcal/Kg + 70 Kcal% TBSA

ELECTRICAL BURNS

- Low voltage injuries
- High voltage injuries (1,000 V)

Low Tension (Domestic Injuries) (Fig. 8A)

- Contact point develops small deep burns and the damage may go to nerves and tendons but very little.
- The alternating current causes tetany and some patients are unable to release the device until the power is switched off.
- Alternating current can interfere with normal cardiac pacing and can cause cardiac arrest. The cardiac arrest is not due to myocardial damage, and hence, resuscitation is successful.

High-Tension Injuries (Fig. 8B)

- High-tension injuries can be caused by flash, flames, and current itself from high-voltage current that travels from line to earth via patient.
- Flash burn can ignite patient clothes.
- The entry and exit points are damaged and patient can have underlying muscle damages, which cause compartment syndromes.
- Myoglobin damage can cause myoglobinuria and renal dysfunction.

Other complications in high-voltage burns:
- Severe metabolic acidosis
- Direct myocardial damage and cardiac arrest with raised cardiac enzymes
- Gangrene of the limb leading to amputation

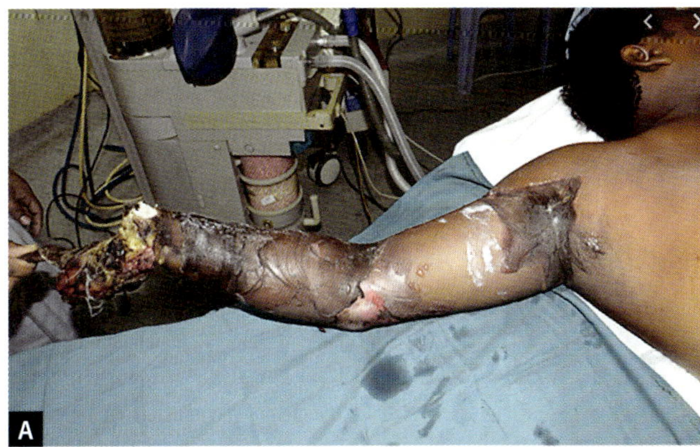

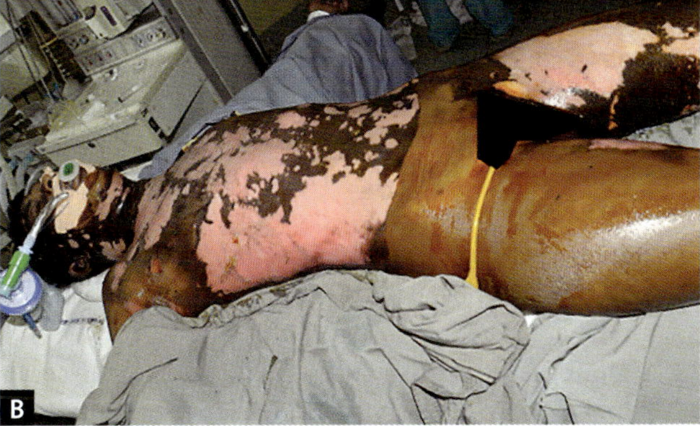

Figs. 8A and B: (A) Low-tension injuries; (B) High-tension injuries.

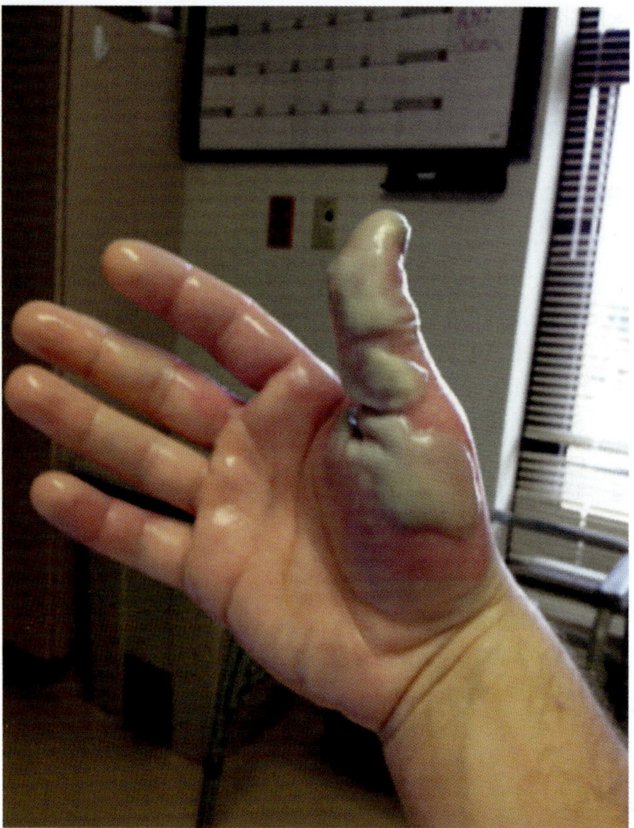

Fig. 9: Chemical burns.

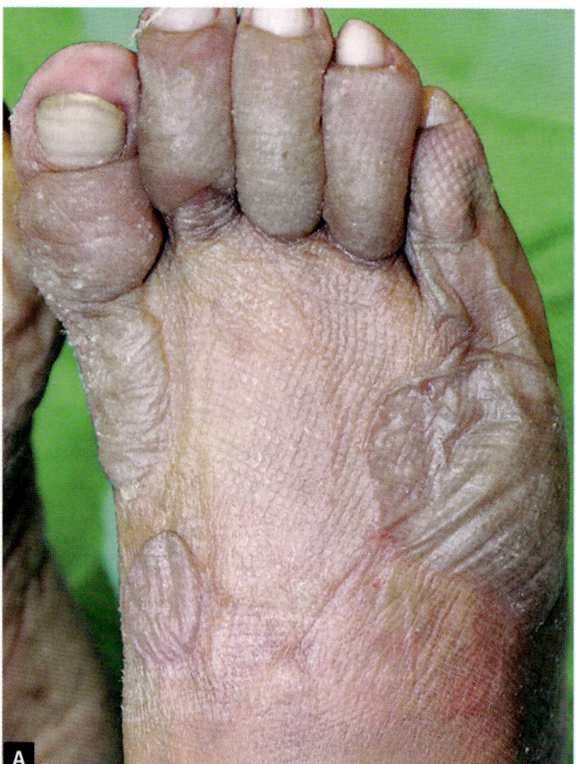

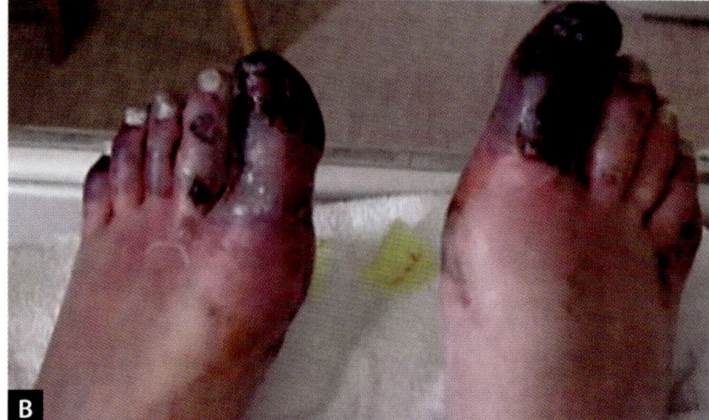

Figs. 10A and B: Frost bite.

CHEMICAL BURNS

- *Two types of damages:* One due to skin contact and other due to systemic absorption **(Fig. 9)**.
- Copious irrigation with water is initially used, but please remember powder forms of contact must not be washed with water as it causes more damage (example, phosphorous powder—it must be removed with forceps and not with water).
- Alkali burns cause more destructive damage than acids, especially if contact with eyes.
- Most common acid injury is hydrofluoric acid, it is generally a weak acid but chelated with calcium and magnesium. Hence, hypocalcemia is a serious issue with acid.
- Initial management includes calcium gluconate topical gel; if severe, must used Bier's block using 10% calcium gluconate gel.
- If concentration of acid is >50%, high chances of hypocalcemia and arrythmia and hence must undergo early excision.

FROST BITE

- Frost bite is a cold burn in which a part of the body freezes and cells get disrupted and tissue dies **(Figs. 10A and B)**.
- Other mechanisms of injury are vasoconstriction and reperfusion injury on rewarming releasing free radicles.
- It commonly involves the fingers, toes, cheeks, the tip of the nose, and the ears.
- It has 4 stages like burns.

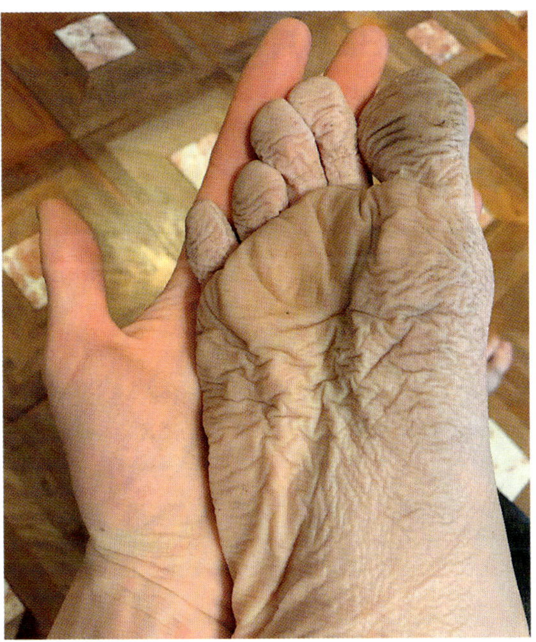

Fig. 11: Trench foot.

- *Stage 1:* Hyperemia and no necrosis
- *Stage 2:* Vesicles, painful, and skin loss+
- *Stage 3:* Hemorrhagic vesicles and skin loss+
- *Stage 4:* Muscle/bone involved

Treatment

- *Gentle rewarming is the correct method.*
- *Nonsteroidal anti-inflammatory drugs (NSAIDs)*
- Wait for demarcation to occur
- Injured areas kept clean and dry
- Prevent infection
- *Excision of dead tissues can be done even after months*
- Tissue plasminogen activators and nerve blocks in 24 hours of injury can prevent amputations.

TRENCH FOOT

- Prolonged immersion in cold water (no freezing as in frost bite)
- Stasis and occlusion occur **(Fig. 11)**.

Wound Healing and Wound Infections

R Rajamahendran

CLASSIFICATION OF WOUND CLOSURE AND HEALING

- *Primary intention:*
  - Edges are approximated in cut
  - Normal healing is seen with minimal scar
- *Secondary intention:*
  - Wound left open to heal by granulation
  - Contraction and epithelialization occurs
  - Increased inflammation and proliferation with poor scar
- *Tertiary intention:*
  - It is also known as delayed primary intention.
  - Initially left open wounds are later approximated when healing becomes favorable.

WOUND HEALING

Factors that inhibit wound healing:

Risk factors of increased risk of wound infection are given in **Table 1**.

Type of surgery and infection rates—Bailey and Love 27th Edition Update are given in **Table 2**.

TABLE 1: Factors influencing wound healing—local versus systemic.

Local factors	*Systemic factors*
• Infection • Ischemia • Foreign body • Hematoma • Persistent movement • Mechanical stress • Necrotic tissues	• Diabetes • Radiation • Extremes of age • *Hypothermia* • *Hypoxemia* • *Hypocholesterolemia* • *Hyperglycemia (even if transit)* • Malnutrition • Vitamin C and A deficiency • Zinc and iron deficiency • *Drugs:* Steroids and doxorubicin • Jaundice, uremia, and malignancy

TABLE 2: Surgical types and infection rates with and without prophylaxis.

Type of surgery	*Examples of surgeries*	*Infection rate with prophylaxis*	*Infection rate without prophylaxis*
Clean surgery (no viscus opened)	• Heart, brain, joint, and transplant surgeries • Herniorrhaphy • Swelling excision	1–2%	1–2%
Clean contaminated surgery (Viscus opened and minimal spillage)	• Wound of bowel, biliary, and pancreatic surgery • Uncomplicated appendicitis • Gastrojejunostomy	3%	6–9%
Contaminated surgery (open viscus with spillage or inflammatory diseases)	• Appendiceal abscess • Perirectal abscess drainage • Infected laceration • Fecal peritonitis	6%	13–20%
Dirty surgery (pus, perforation, or incision through abscess)	• Worst wound • Acute cholecystitis with spillage of pus from gallbladder • Traumatic wound • Bowel obstruction with enterotomy and spillage of content	7%	40%

TYPES OF WOUND SUTURING

- *Primary suturing:* Done for clean wound within 6 hour
- *Delayed primary suturing:* Done for lacerated wound within 48 hours.
- *Secondary suturing:* Done for infected wound in 10–14 days.

High-yield facts in wounds:
- *Degloving injury:* Avulsion injury involving skin and subcutaneous tissue with intact fascia
- Limb salvage primarily depends on vascular injury
- If suture mark is to be avoided, skin suture should be removed by 1 week.
- Best scar is seen in very old people
- Worst position for scars is sternum
- Best skin graft for open wound is autograft

PRESSURE SORES

- Pressure sores are tissue necrosis with prolonged pressure.
- There are also known as bed sores, pressure ulcers, and decubitus ulcers **(Fig. 1)**.
- Incidence is 5% in hospitalized patients.
- Pressure sore is *most common in ischium* > greater trochanter > sacrum in the gluteal region.
- After gluteal region, the sites in order are heel > lateral malleoli > occipital region.
- Pressure sore occurs if external pressure exceeds 30 mm Hg of capillary occlusive pressure.
- *Prevention is the best treatment:*
  - Bedridden patients turned every 2 hours once.
  - Wheelchair patients must lift themselves every 10 minutes for 10 seconds.
- *Treatment:*
  - Debridement
  - Vacuum-assisted closure (VAC) devices at negative *-125 mm Hg suction pressures*
  - Flaps

Classification of pressure sores:
- *Stage 1:* Non blanchable erythema (no breech in epidermis).
- *Stage 2: Partial-thickness skin loss extending to epidermis and dermis.*
- *Stage 3:* Full-thickness skin loss extending to subcutaneous tissue (not to fascia).
- *Stage 4:* Skin loss extends to fascia + muscles + bone or tendon or joint.

Recent concept (NBE 2017)—dressing in pressure sore:
- During dressing for pressure ulcers, keep the ulcer tissue moist and surrounding skin dry

NECROTIZING FASCIITIS

- Necrotizing fasciitis is the rapid progressive bacterial infection characterized by involvement and necrosis of the subcutaneous tissue and fascia, *with typical sparing of underlying muscle.*
- Most common site of infection is *lower extremity*
- It may involve trunk and perineum (Fournier's gangrene) **(Fig. 2)**, abdominal wall (Meleney's gangrene), head and neck, and any other site.

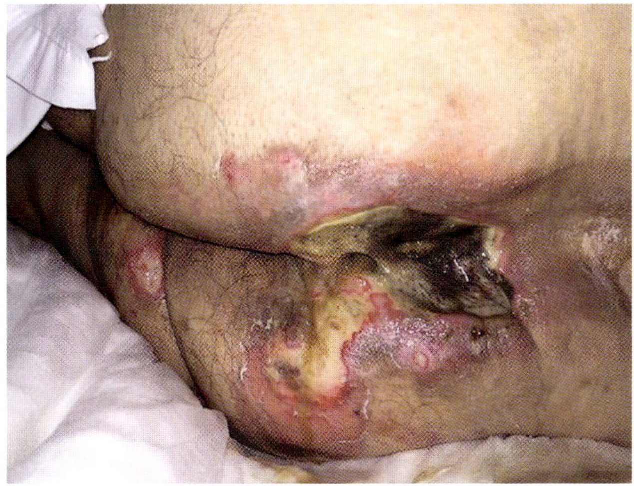

Fig. 1: Stage-3 bedsore.

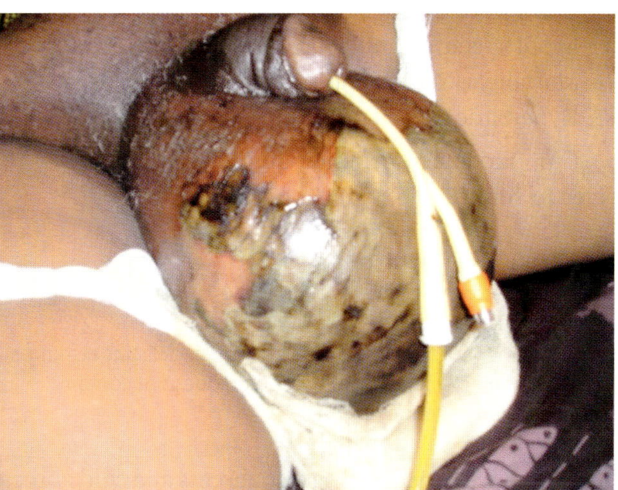

Fig. 2: Fournier's gangrene.

TABLE 3: Comparison of cellulitis and erysipelas features.

Cellulitis (Fig. 3)	*Erysipelas (Fig. 4)*
Spreading nonsuppurative inflammation of *subcutaneous tissue and fascial* planes	Spreading inflammation of *skin and subcutaneous tissue*
Most common due to *Streptococcus pyogenes*	Most common due to *Streptococcal pyogenes*
Sequelae: Abscess, bacteremia, pyemia, and local gangrene	Toxemia is always a feature
• Red shiny stretched warm skin. Pitting edema • Surrounding lymph vessels may be involved and result in red streaks due to lymphangitis • There is no sharp demarcation between the involved and uninvolved area	• Always associated with cutaneous lymphangitis Vesicles form • Sharply demarcated infection
• Discharge is purulent	Serous
Elevation of limb and antibiotics	Penicillins
Milian's ear sign: Cellulitis not involved because skin is closely adherent to subcutaneous tissue	Positive in ear lobule

- *Most common single etiological agent: Group A beta Hemolytic streptococci* (usually caused by polymicrobial organisms).
- *Risk factors:* Diabetes, immunocompromised, smoking, penetrating trauma, obesity, intravenous (IV) drug abuse, and skin infection (abrasions, bites, and boils).
- *Pain is the most common presenting symptom* and pain is disproportionately high.
- Wood hard texture in subcutaneous tissue.
- *Systemic features:* Fever, hypotension, tachycardia, progression to septic shock, disseminated intravascular coagulation (DIC) and multiple organ dysfunction syndrome (MODS).
- *Treatment:* Urgent surgical debridement + IV fluids + broad spectrum antibiotics + supportive treatment
- Mortality is 100% without debridement.
- Hyperbaric oxygen therapy.

Comparison of cellulitis and erysipelas features is given in **Table 3**.

Erysipelas:
- Classic descriptions of erysipelas show "butterfly" involvement of the face
- Involvement of the ear (Milian's ear sign) is a distinguishing feature for erysipelas, since this region does not contain deeper dermis tissue **(Fig. 5)**

Difference between pyogenic abscess and cold abscess is given in **Table 4**.

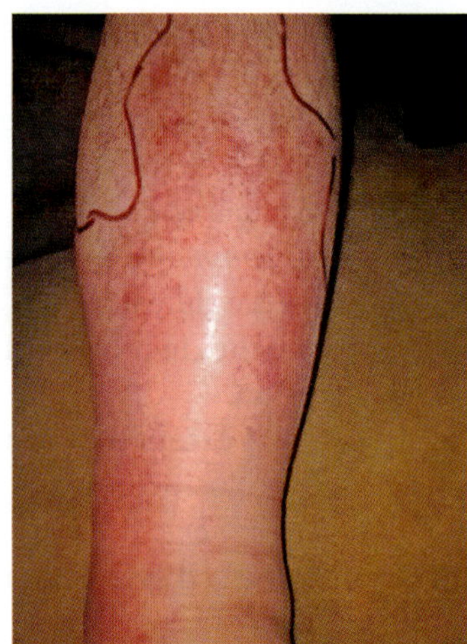

Fig. 3: Cellulitis having no sharp demarcation.

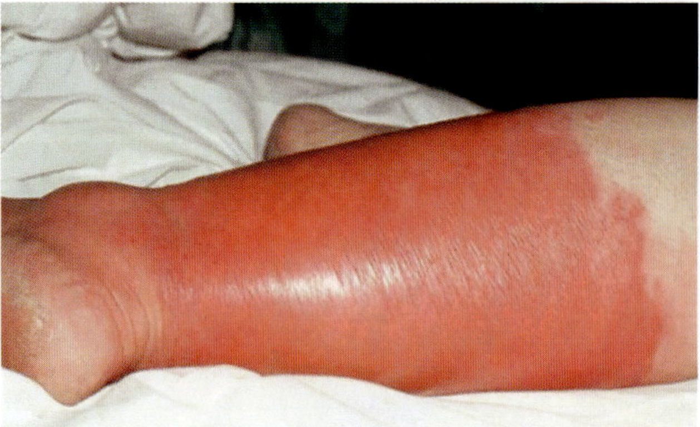

Fig. 4: Erysipelas showing clear demarcation of border.

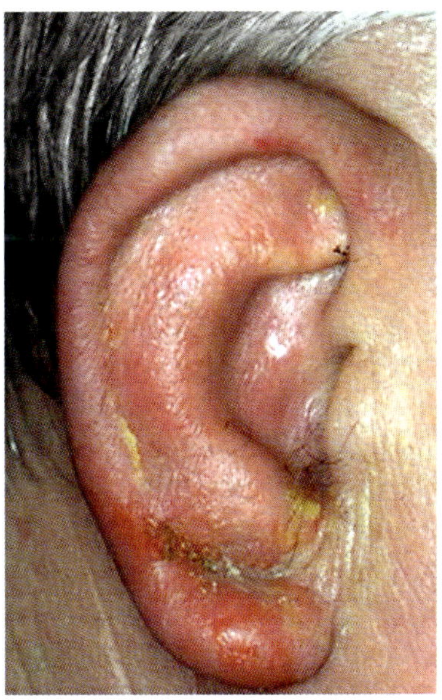

Fig. 5: Milian's ear sign.

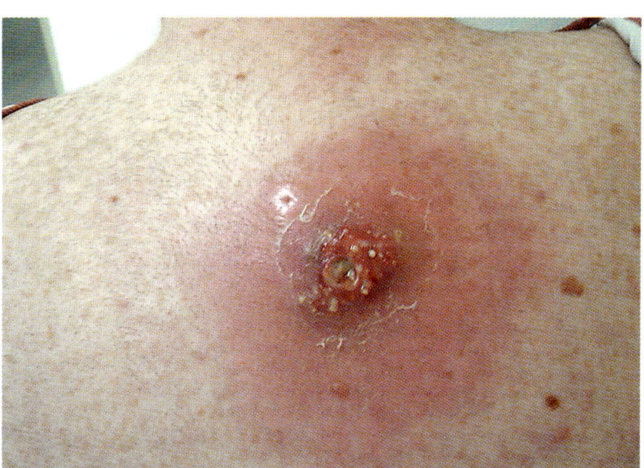

Fig. 6: Pyogenic abscess.

TABLE 4: Difference between pyogenic abscess and cold abscess.

Pyogenic abscess (Fig. 6)	*Cold abscess*
Pyogenic bacteria: Staphylococcus and *Streptococcus*	Tuberculosis
Red warm with inflammatory signs	No signs of inflammation
Dependent drainage: By cruciate incision	Nondependent drainage is done
Drain placed	No need of drain

Hilton's Method of Drainage of Abscess

- Abscess in neck, axilla, and parotid are drained by means of using Lister sinus forceps **(Fig. 7)**.
- We will not do incision and drainage using cruciate incision in these places because of the presence of *neurovascular structures* seen underneath in these places.

Infections in the hand:
- *Acute paronychia:* Subcuticular infection caused by *Staphylococcal aureus*
- *Chronic paronychia:* Chronic nail infection caused by *Candida*
- *Felon:* Terminal pulp space infection
- *Deep palmar abscess*: Abscess beneath flexor tendons (frog hand)
- *Herpetic whitlow:* Caused by Herpes simplex; small vesicles and crusts in Dental workers; Self-limiting

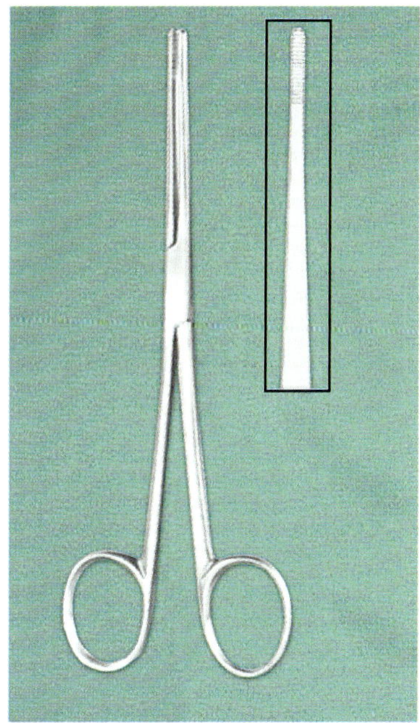

Fig. 7: Lister sinus forceps for abscess drainage in neck, axilla and parotid.

ACUTE PARONYCHIA

- Most common infection of hand.
- *Most common organism: Staphylococcus aureus*
- Infection burrows under nail bed and causes severe pain.
- Early antibiotics are advised (penicillin combinations)
- Incision may not be necessary. Freer elevator is used to lift the nail and abscess is drained.
- Incision drainage may also be done as shown in **Figure 8**.

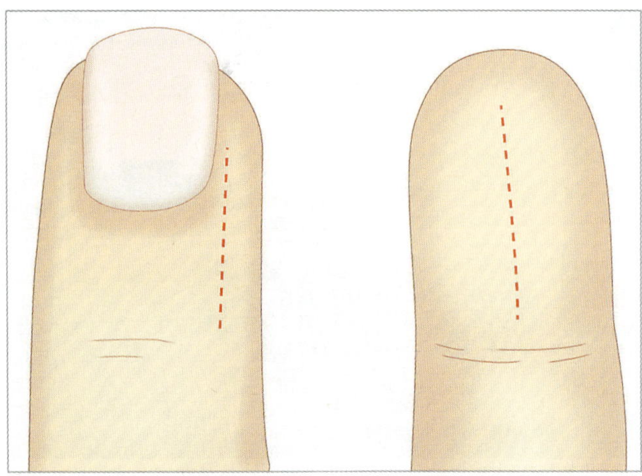

Fig. 8: Incisions for paronychia.

INTERMEDIATE DEPTH INFECTIONS

- Felon
- Deep web space infection

Felon

- Pulp space infection of terminal or middle phalanx
- Tension in the distal digital segment can become so great that the arteries to the bone are compressed, resulting in *gangrene of the fingertip and necrosis* of the distal 75% of the terminal phalanx.
- With infection of the digital pulp space, one must not wait for fluctuance before making the decision for surgery because of the danger of ischemic necrosis of the skin and bone.
- A single volar or unilateral longitudinal incision may be used as shown in **Figure 8**.
- Similar to a paronychia, *S. aureus is the most common causative agent.*
- More proximally, a pulp space infection at the base of the finger can travel through the lumbrical canal into the palm to create a deep palmar space infection.

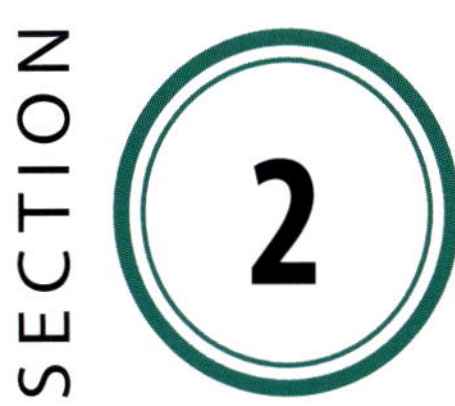

Section 2 Gastrointestinal Tract Emergencies

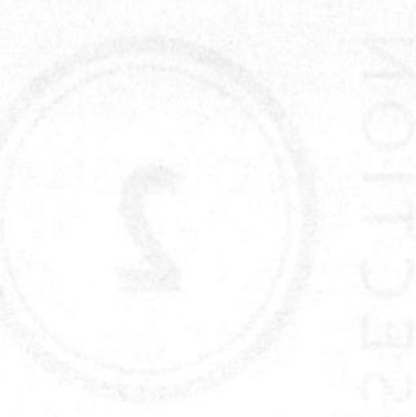

CHAPTER 6

Abdominal Trauma

R Rajamahendran

INTRODUCTION

- The most common injured organ in penetrating trauma—liver > stomach.
- The most common organ injured in blunt trauma—spleen > liver.

The two initial procedures for Abdominal injury are:

1. Diagnostic peritoneal lavage (DPL).
2. Extended focused assessment with sonogram for trauma (eFAST).

DIAGNOSTIC PERITONEAL LAVAGE

- Insert a cannula below the umbilicus. About 1,000 mL of warmed ringer lactate is instilled into the abdomen and is then drained out and analyzed **(Fig. 1)**.
- *Results in blunt trauma:*
  - Presence of >1 lakh red cells/μL
  - >500 white cells/μL is positive (It is equivalent to 20 mL of blood in peritoneal cavity)
  - Frank aspiration of >10 mL on cannula insertion is also positive

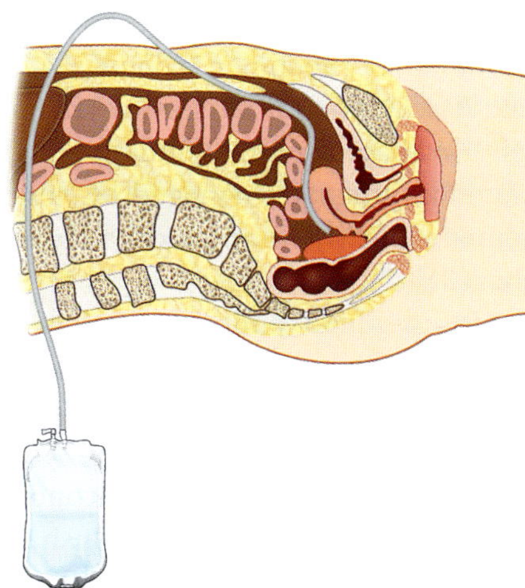

Fig. 1: Diagnostic peritoneal lavage.

In penetrating trauma, one-tenth of above value is positive.

- Diagnostic peritoneal lavage has sensitivity about 97–98%.
- Since it is invasive and so many false positive results resulted in negative laparotomies, this is gradually replaced by eFAST in practice.
- Diagnostic peritoneal lavage is especially useful in the hypotensive, unstable patient with multiple injuries as a means of excluding intra-abdominal bleeding **(Table 1)**.

FOCUSED ASSESSMENT WITH SONOGRAM FOR TRAUMA

- Focused assessment with sonogram for trauma is used in all abdominal trauma patients whether hemodynamically *stable or unstable (but not much helpful in penetrating trauma).*
- It is a rapid bedside diagnostic procedure to identify any free fluid in abdomen (could not tell blood or ascitic fluid).
- It is not 100% sensitive.
- Noninvasive and repetitive.
- *Traditional four views:*
  1. *Subxiphoid transverse view:* Assess pericardial fluid.

TABLE 1: Positive finding on diagnostic peritoneal lavage (DPL).

Criteria for positive finding on DPL		
	Abdominal trauma	*Thoracoabdominal stabs*
RBC count	>100,000 cells/mL	>10,000 cells/mL
WBC count	>500 cells/mL	>500 cells/mL
Amylase level	>19 IU/L	>19 IU/L
Alkaline phosphatase	>2 IU/L	>2 IU/L
Bilirubin level	>0.01 mg/dL	>0.01 mg/dL

(RBC: red blood cell; WBC: white blood cell)

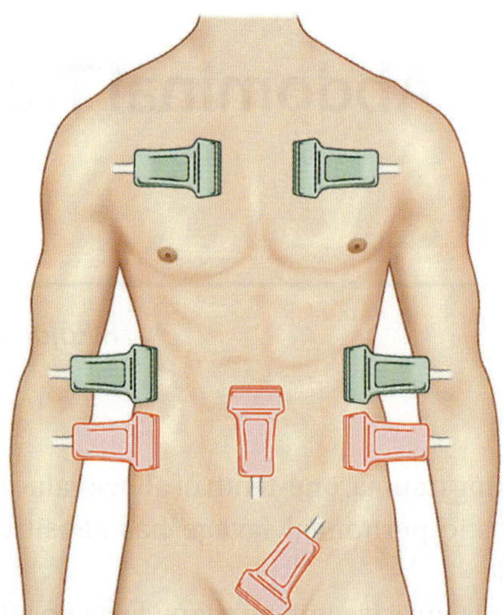

Fig. 2: Red probes are traditional FAST; Green probes are extended FAST. (FAST: focused assessment with sonogram for trauma)

2. *Right upper quadrant longitudinal view:* Collection in Morrison pouch or any liver/renal injuries.
3. *Left upper quadrant longitudinal view:* Collection in perisplenic region or any splenic injuries.
4. *Suprapubic longitudinal and transverse view:* Collection in pelvis; assess bladder and pouch of Douglas (POD).

- *Extended Fast or eFAST* has two additional right and left thoracic views to rule out pneumothorax *(stratosphere sign)* or hemothorax **(Fig. 2)**.
- *Limitations:*
  - Can detect only when intraperitoneal fluid >100 mL
  - Not helpful in detecting bowel injury
  - Not useful for retroperitoneal injuries
  - Cannot reliably determine source of hemorrhage nor grade the injury
  - FAST positive, i.e., free fluid does not decide upon operative intervention.

In case of stable abdominal injuries, CECT abdomen is the gold standard for detecting abdominal injuries.

PROTOCOLS IN MANAGEMENT OF ABDOMINAL TRAUMA

Protocols in management of abdominal trauma are given in **Flowcharts 1 and 2.**

SPLENIC TRAUMA

- It is most commonly injured organ following blunt trauma (23.8%) versus penetrating (8.5%).

Flowchart 1: Algorithm for the evaluation and management of blunt abdominal trauma.

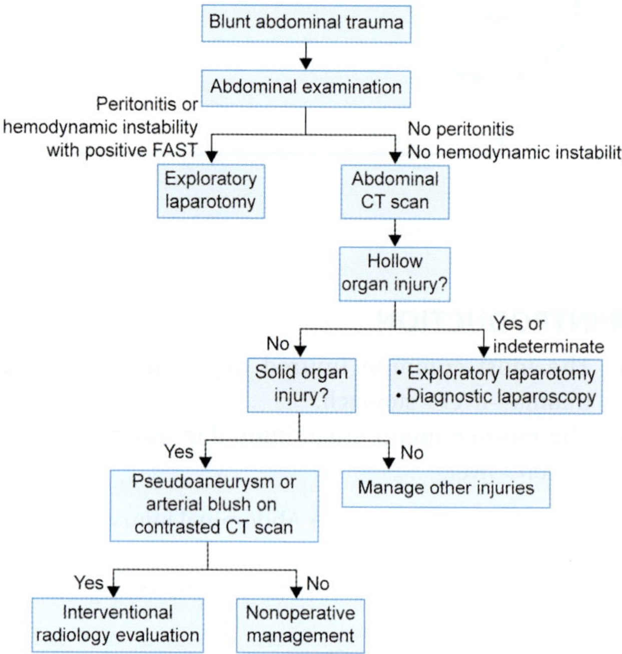

(CT: computed tomography; FAST: focused abdominal sonography in trauma)

- Presentation varies depending on the grade of injury; higher-grade injuries are associated with greater hemodynamic instability **(Table 2)**.
- In low grade injuries, there will be initial bleeding and then it stops. But there will be delayed initiation of hemorrhage, which can occur up to weeks after injury (Latent Period of Baudet).
- The rate of rebleeding is 10.6%.
- In stable patients, contrast-enhanced computed tomography (CECT) abdomen is done.
- American Association for Surgery of Trauma (AAST) grading is used based on CECT finding.
- The splenic injuries are managed by nonoperative management (NOM) in approximately 90% cases **(Flowchart 3)**.
- Due to increasing interventional radiologist management by angiography and embolization, even grade 3, 4, 5 are now managed by NOM within 24 hours **(Fig. 3)**. Splenorrhaphy is shown in **Figure 4**.

Patients who are managed by NOM must undergo CECT before discharge. Appearance of tumor blush in CECT is an indication of angioembolization as it corresponds to false aneurysm in the splenic artery **(Fig. 5)**.

Flowchart 2: Algorithm for the evaluation and management of anterior abdominal stab wounds.

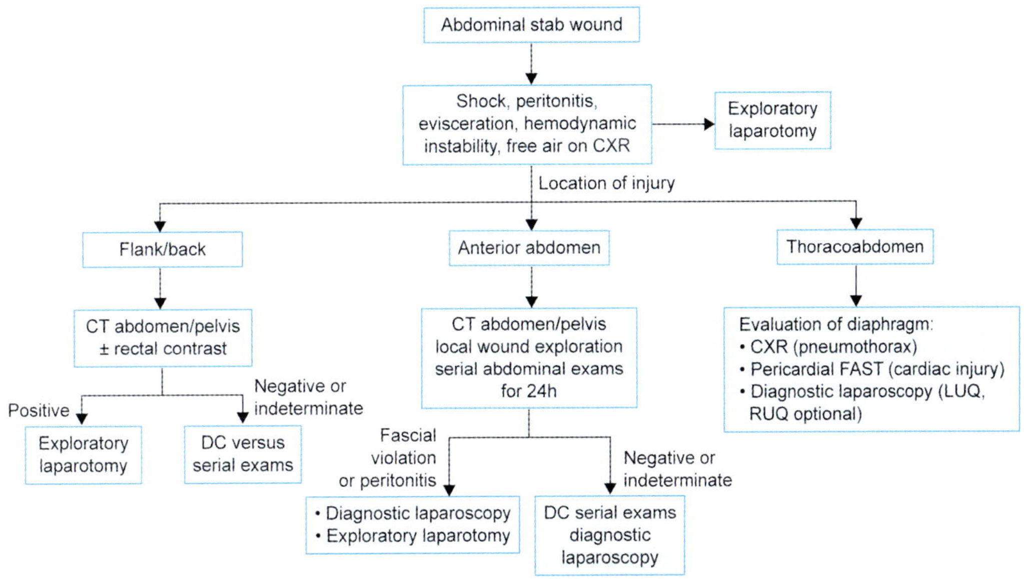

(CT: computed tomography; CXR: chest x-ray; DC: discharge; FAST: focused abdominal sonography in trauma; LUQ: left upper quadrant; RUQ: right upper quadrant)

Source: Adapted from Martin MJ, Brown CVR, Shatz DV, Alam HB, Brasel KJ, Hauser CJ, et al. Evaluation and management of abdominal stab wounds: A Western Trauma Association critical decisions algorithm. J Trauma Acute Care Surg. 2018;85(5):1007-15.

TABLE 2: Criteria for grading of splenic injury based on computed tomography.

Grade	*Description*
Grade 1	Subcapsular hematoma involving <10% of surface area, parenchymal laceration <1 cm depth, or capsular tear
Grade 2	Subcapsular hematoma involving 10–50% of surface area, intraparenchymal hematoma le<5 cm, or parenchymal laceration measuring 1–3 cm
Grade 3	Subcapsular hematoma involving >50% of surface area, ruptured subcapsular or intraparenchymal hematoma 5 cm or larger, or parenchymal laceration greater than 3 cm depth
Grade 4	Any injury associated with a splenic vascular injury or active bleeding confined within the splenic capsule and parenchymal laceration involving segmental or hilar vessels resulting in >25% devascularization
Grade 5	Any injury with splenic vascular injury* and active bleeding extending beyond the spleen into the peritoneum and shattered spleen

*Vascular injury is defined as a pseudoaneurysm or arteriovenous fistula and appears as a focal collection of vascular contrast that decreases in attenuation with delayed imaging. Active bleeding from a vascular injury presents as vascular contrast, focal or diffuse, that increases in size or attenuation in the delayed phase.

HEPATIC TRAUMA

- Liver is the most common organ injured by penetrating mechanisms in abdomen (26.1%) versus blunt (22.2%).
- Mortality rates are 22% and 12.5%, respectively

Management of Blunt Liver Trauma

- Management purely depends on hemodynamic stability.
- If stable, CECT abdomen is done to grade the liver injury and admitted in intensive care unit (ICU) for monitoring with serial examinations, vital signs, and laboratory investigations such as hematocrit and arterial blood gas (ABG) analysis.
- AAST grading is done based on CECT **(Table 3)**.

Additional points:

- Advance one grade for multiple injuries up to grade III.

Flowchart 3: Splenic trauma management.

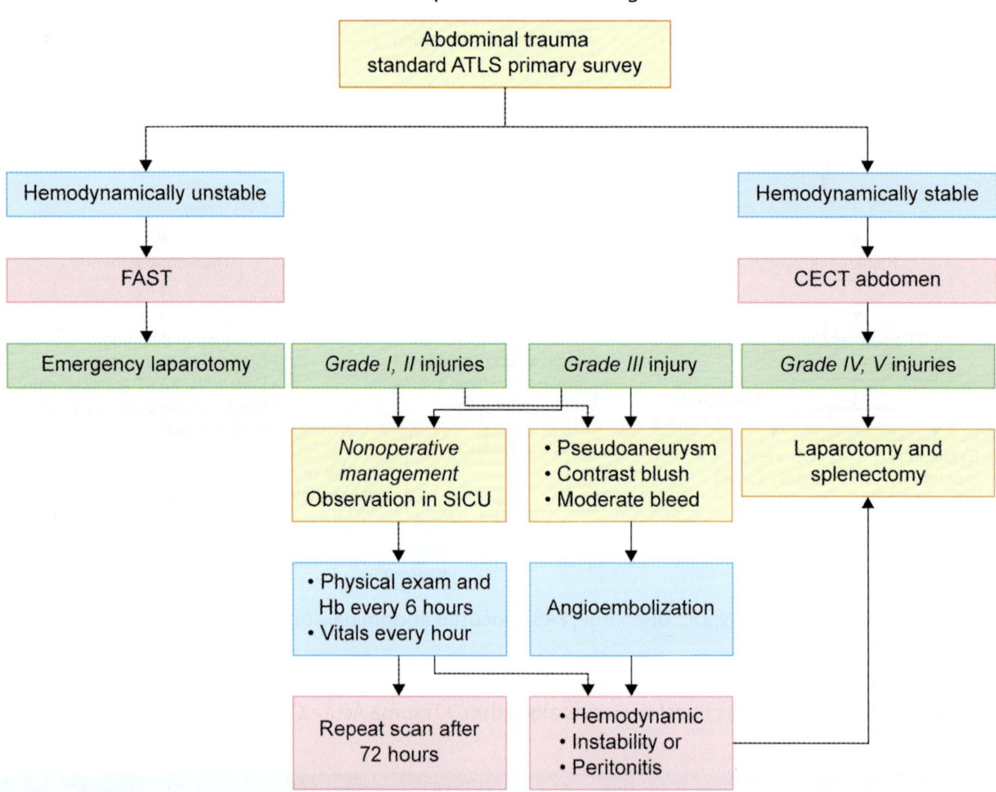

(ATLS: advanced trauma life support; CECT: contrast-enhanced computed tomography; FAST: focused abdominal sonography in trauma; Hb: hemoglobin; SICU: surgical intensive care unit)

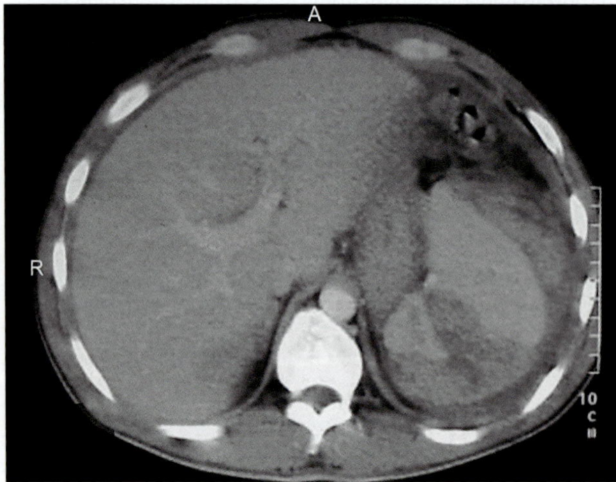

Fig. 3: Splenic trauma contrast-enhanced computed tomography (CECT) abdomen.

- Vascular injury (i.e., pseudoaneurysm or arteriovenous fistula): Appears as a focal collection of vascular contrast that decreases in attenuation on delayed images.
- *Active bleeding:* Focal or diffuse collection of vascular contrast that increases in size or attenuation on a delayed phase.
- Patients with bleeding hepatic trauma (unstable) should be explored.
  - Perihepatic packing and manual compression over bleeding site
  - Pringle maneuver (occlusion of portal triad by digital/clamp)
  - Minor bleeding requires topical hemostatic agents such as fibrin glue, bioglue, thrombin-soaked gelatin foam sponge; electrocautery; argon plasma coagulation or *suture hepatorrhaphy with 0 chromic catgut suture.*
  - Major bleeding requires *perihepatic packing* and shift to ICU **(Fig. 6)**.

In case of hemodynamic unstable patient—4 P's

- *Pressure*
- *Pringle*
- *Plug*
- *Pack*

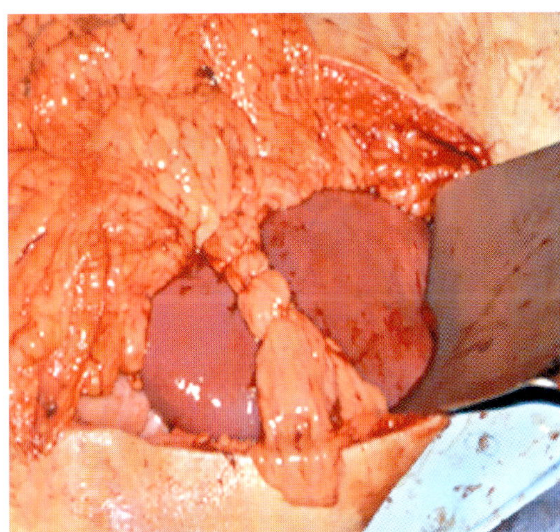

Fig. 4: Splenorrhaphy.

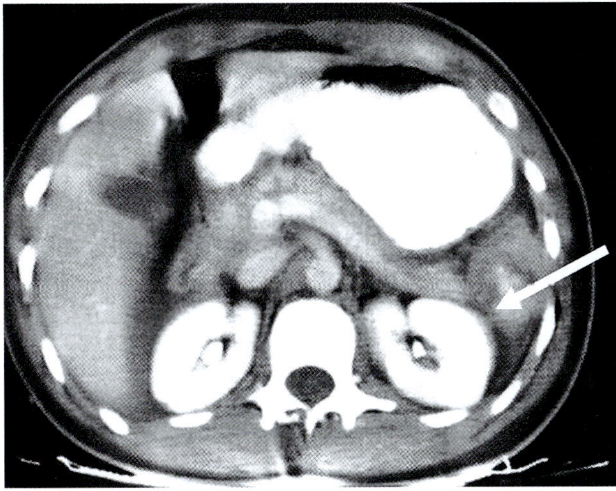

Fig. 5: Tumor blush in spleen.

After 24–48 hours, patient is shifted to elective operation theatre (OT) for unpacking and definite repairs.

- Remove the pack, look for bleeding.
- Consider angioembolization
- Hepatic artery injuries should be repaired; if right hepatic artery ligated, cholecystectomy to be done.
- *The hepatic artery can be ligated but not the portal vein (PV) during surgery PV must be stented and not ligated.*
- *Closed suction drain is kept.*

- Management of penetrating liver trauma needs exploration and the techniques employed are the same as for blunt trauma.

TABLE 3: Grading of liver injuries (according to American Association for the Surgery of Trauma).

Grade	Findings
Grade 1	• *Hematoma:* Subcapsular, <10% surface area • *Laceration:* Capsular tear, <1 cm parenchymal depth
Grade 2	• *Hematoma:* Subcapsular, 10–50% surface area • *Hematoma:* Intraparenchymal, <10 cm diameter • *Laceration:* Capsular tear 1–3 cm parenchymal depth, <10 cm length
Grade 3	• *Hematoma:* Subcapsular, >50% surface area or ruptured subcapsular or parenchymal hematoma • *Hematoma:* Intraparenchymal, >10 cm • *Laceration:* Capsular tear, >3 cm parenchymal depth • Vascular injury with active bleeding contained within liver parenchyma
Grade 4	• *Laceration:* Parenchymal disruption involving 25–75% hepatic lobe or involves 1–3 Couinaud segments • Vascular injury with active bleeding breaching the liver parenchyma into the peritoneum
Grade 5	• *Laceration:* Parenchymal disruption involving >75% of hepatic lobe • *Vascular:* Juxtahepatic venous injuries (retrohepatic vena cava/central major hepatic veins)

- Late complications such as abscess, bilioma, and hemobilia needs treatment in the form of percutaneous drain, endoscopic retrograde cholangiopancreatography (ERCP), and stenting, respectively.

OTHER INDIVIDUAL ORGAN INJURIES

Pancreas

- Most common mechanism is blunt trauma.
- Investigation of choice (IOC) is CT scan.
- Amylase and lipase are insensitive.
- In penetrating trauma, the injury is diagnosed only by laparotomy **(Fig. 7)**.

Management:

- Distal body and tail to the left of superior mesenteric vessels managed by closed suction drainage.
- If duct is involved, distal pancreatectomy is done.
- Proximal injuries [right of superior mesenteric artery (SMA)] manage conservatively; rarely, Whipple procedure (pancreaticoduodenectomy)may be needed **(Fig. 8)**.

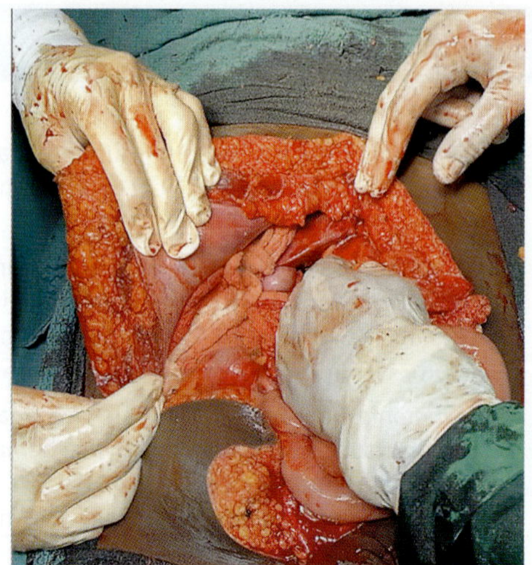

Fig. 6: Packing for liver injury.

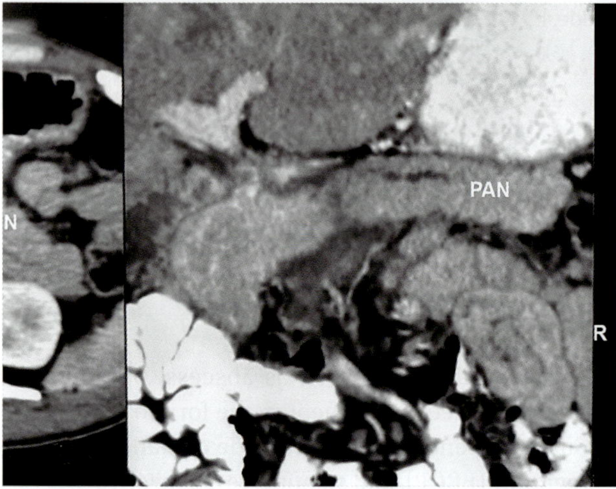

Fig. 7: Pancreatic transection injury.

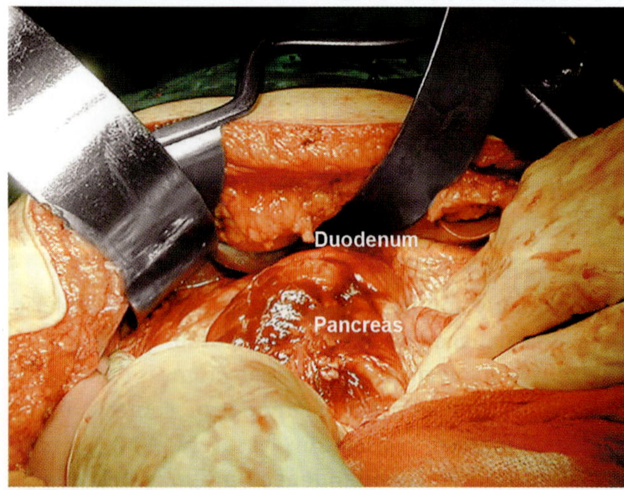

Fig. 8: Duodenopancreatic injury.

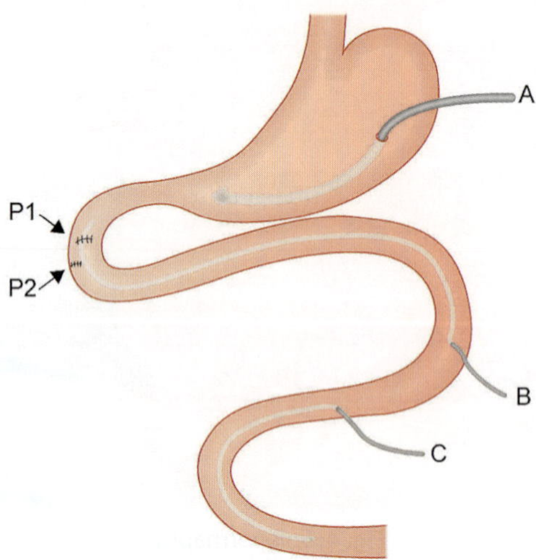

A. Venting decompressive gastrostomy
B. Decompressive duodenostomy
C. Feeding jejunostomy

Fig. 9: Triple tube ostomy for pancreaticoduodenal injuries.

- Pylorus exclusion procedure (closure of pylorus) to minimize pancreatic enzyme stimulation is done.
- Damage control surgery with packing and drainage tube or triple tube ostomy **(Fig. 9)** and referral to definite surgery is done.

Stomach

- Most common mechanism is penetrating trauma.
- Nasogastric tube showing blood may indicate gastric injury.
- Surgical repair is always done.
- Do not miss the exit injuries in stomach while repairing.

Duodenum

- It is usually associated with pancreas injuries.
- CT is the IOC.
- Only sign is gas or fluid collection in retroperitoneum and leakage of oral contrast.
- First, third, and fourth part can be repaired like a small bowel by sutures.
- Second part needs damage control surgery.
- Triple tube ostomy is done —(A) decompressive gastrostomy, (B) decompressive duodenostomy, and (C) feeding jejunostomy is done after repair of second part injury **(Fig. 9)**

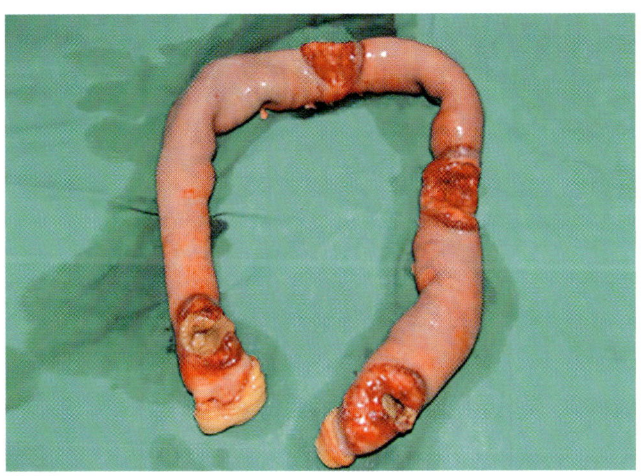

Fig. 10: Colon.

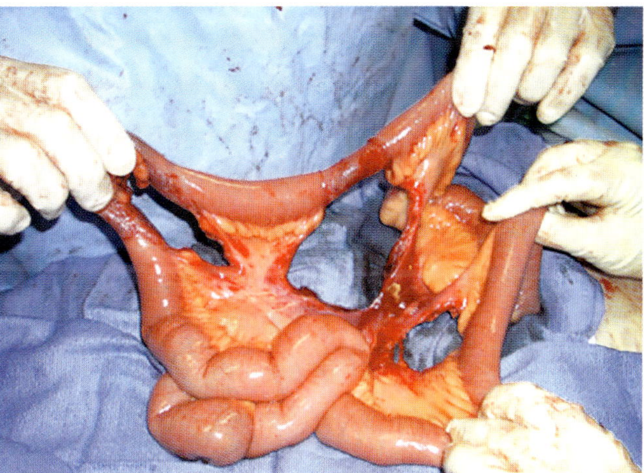

Fig. 11: Devascularization of bowel segments.

Small Bowel

- The most common mechanism of injury is blunt trauma > penetrating trauma.
- Urgent repair is indicated.
- Bowel ischemia due to mesenteric injury and needs resection of bowel.
- Hematomas at mesenteric border must be explored to rulc out perforations.
- Damage control involving "clip and drop" of damaged or resected bowel may be necessary. Apply titanium clips to cut ends and re explore after 48 hours.

Colon

- Most common mechanism is penetrating >blunt injury **(Fig. 10)**.
- Less contamination can be repaired primarily.
- For extensive contamination, unstable patients, doubtful viability of bowel, CLIP and DROP technique is used.
- Defunctioning colostomy or definitive repair is done after 48 hours.

Rectum

- 5% colon injuries involve rectum—mostly, penetrating injury
- Per rectum (PR) examination shows blood in rectum.
- It may be associated with pelvic injuries associated with bladder and proximal urethral injury.
- Intraperitoneal rectal injury is managed like colon injuries.
- Extraperitoneal full-thickness injury needs diverting end colostomy such as Hartman with distal closure or loop colostomy.
- Presacral drainage is no longer used.

Mesenteric injuries:

- These are seen in seat belt injury.
- *Two types of tears:*
  1. Longitudinal
  2. Transverse
- For longitudinal tears, only repair is done.
- *Transverse tear is dangerous.* Bowel is devascularized **(Fig. 11)** and hence, resection and anastomosis are done.

EMERGENCY ABDOMINAL OPERATIONS

- Rapid midline laparotomy incision and enter into peritoneum and localize the source of bleeding.
- Liver—pringle maneuver and digital occlusion of aorta at the diaphragmatic hiatus.
- Spleen—clamping of the hilum of spleen.
- *Left medial visceral rotation (Mattox maneuver)*—needed for supracolic injuries (aorta, celiac axis, proximal SMA, and left renal arteries) **(Fig. 12)**.
- *Right medial visceral rotation (Cattel-Braasch Maneuver)* —for IVC injuries **(Fig. 13)**.

ZONES OF RETROPERITONEUM

In retroperitoneum, 4 zones are explained and based on the hematoma, in each zone, management differs **(Table 4 and Fig. 14)**.

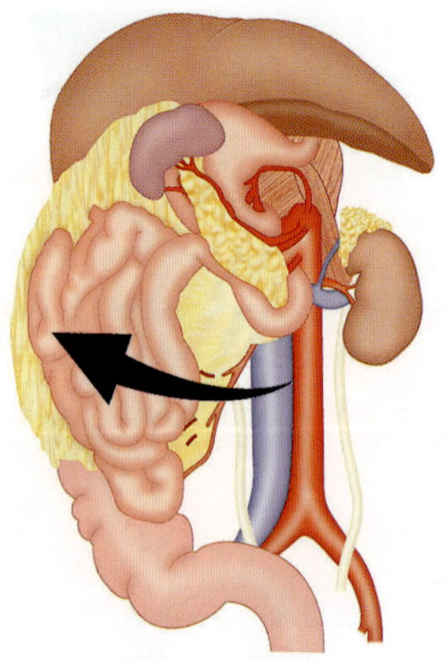

Fig. 12: Mattox maneuver.

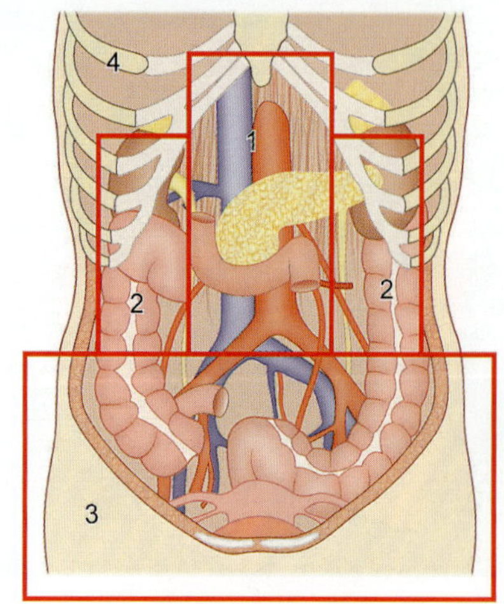

Fig. 14: Zones of retroperitoneal hematoma.

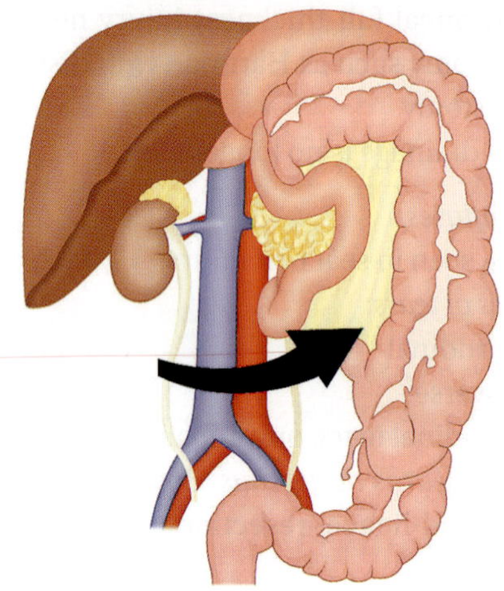

Fig. 13: Cattell maneuver.

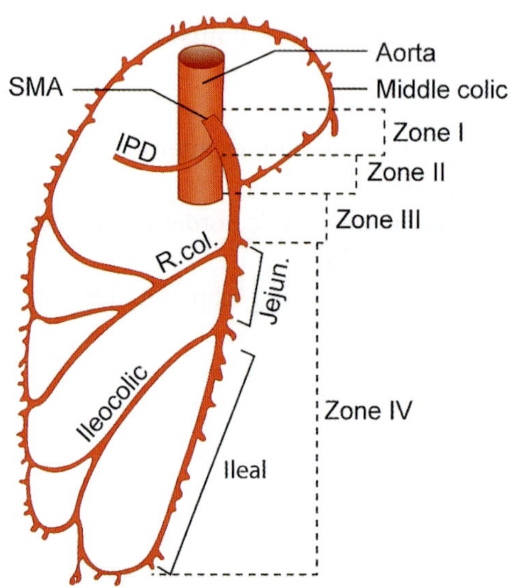

Fig. 15: Superior mesenteric artery injuries—Fullen zones. (R. col.: right colic artery; IPD: inferior pancreaticoduodenal artery; SMA: superior mesenteric artery)

TABLE 4: The classification of retroperitoneal zones and the corresponding management based on the location of the hematoma.

Zones	*Contents*	*Management*
Zone I	Central vascular structures such as aorta and IVC	Needs exploration
Zone II	Kidneys and adrenal glands	Observed
Zone III	Retroperitoneum associated with pelvic vasculature	External pelvic compression and fixation
Zone IV	Retro hepatic IVC and hematoma behind portal vein	Observation

(IVC: inferior vena cava)

Fullen zone classification of SMA injuries **(Fig. 15)**:

- Zone I—located posterior to pancreas; exposed by Mattox maneuver.
- Zone II—from pancreatic edge to middle colic branch, approached via lesser sac.
- Zone III and IV—distal SMA injuries; approached directly within mesentery.

CHAPTER 7

Esophagus

R Rajamahendran

PERFORATIONS IN ESOPHAGUS

- Most common cause of perforation in esophagus is iatrogenic (endoscopy induced).
- *Instrumental perforations*: Conservative treatment is enough because septic load is less.
- *Most common site of perforation in the era of flexible scopy is in the thoracic esophagus during some procedures.*
- *Initial test used is X-ray chest, which may show mediastinal air* —Naclerio V sign **(Figs. 1A and B)**.

"Naclerio V sign": Presence of air at the cardiophrenic angle **(Figs. 1A and B)**

- *Investigation of choice to detect perforation of esophagus is by contrast-enhanced computed tomography (CECT) thorax with oral contrasts.*
- Contrast material of choice to diagnose esophageal perforation is thin dilute *barium.*
- But we practically *first use Gastrograffin* to see for perforation in esophagus.
- If Gastrograffin swallow is negative and if we have a doubt, we confirm further there by doing barium swallow *(barium contrast is the most sensitive test).*
- *Perforation management principles are:*
  - Treatment of contamination
  - Wide local drainage
  - Source control
  - Enteral feeding access **(Box 1)**
- *Gold standard in treatment of perforations is surgery in <24 hours:*
  - Cervical esophageal perforations approached via neck incision
  - Mid esophageal perforations approached via right thoracotomy
  - Lower esophageal perforation approached via left thoracotomy or laparotomy
- Selected cases can be treated by stenting or conservative treatment.

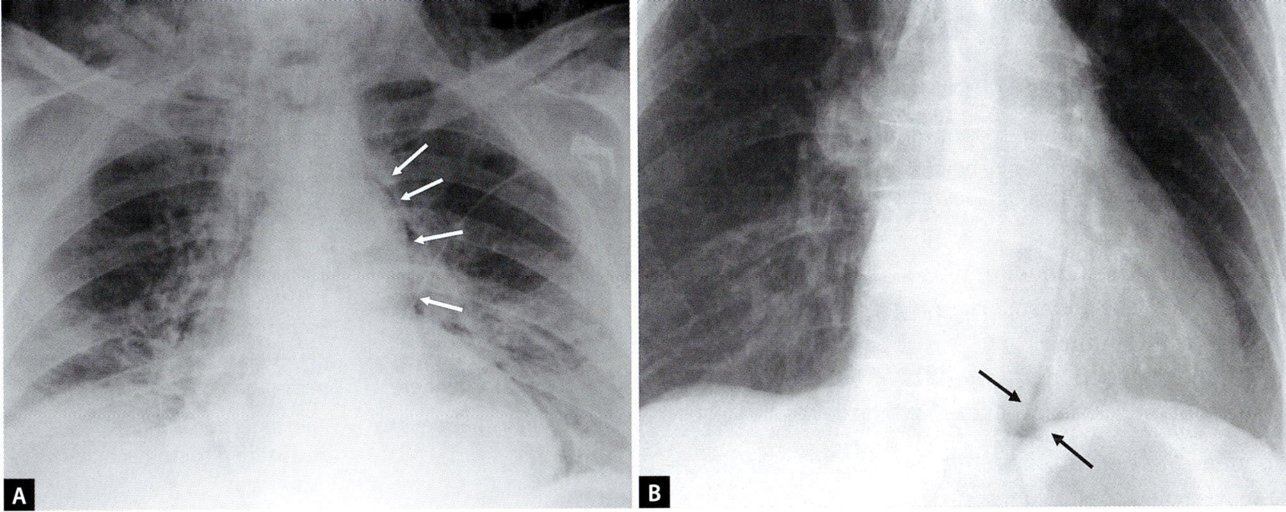

Figs. 1A and B: (A) X-ray chest showing pneumomediastinum; (B) Naclerio V Sign.

BOX 1: Management protocols.

- *Nonoperative management can be tried in following situations:*
  - Small septic load with minimal cardiovascular upset
  - Perforation made by scope
  - Confined collection in mediastinum
  - Cervical esophagus perforation
- *Operative management is a must in following situations:*
  - Large septic load and septic shock
  - Spontaneous perforations
  - Pleural breaching++
  - Abdominal esophagus perforation

Mallory–Weiss Tear

- Mucosal tear of esophagogastric (EG) junction following a bout of sudden vomiting after a heavy drinking.
- The tear occurs because of the *unrelaxed cardia.*
- Tear is *90% located at cardia (most common on lesser curve side and less common on greater curve side)* <10% in lower esophagus.
- Tear is limited to submucosa and mucosa only *(no perforations).*

Clinical Features

- It is most common in age group *60 years with 80% are men*—alcoholics.
- Presents with hematemesis, 90% bleeding stops spontaneously.
- Initial treatment is conservative.
- Persistent bleeding needs *endoscopic electrocoagulation*, angiographic embolization, and laparoscopic oversewing of tear.

Boerhaave Syndrome (Barotrauma)

- Boerhaave syndrome is spontaneous perforation due to vomiting against a closed glottis.
- Most common site is *lower third toward posterior and left side.*
- Second most common site is mid esophagus.
- Complete tear with spillage of highly infective contents into mediastinum.
- The tear occurs due to *failure of opening of glottis* (Mallory-Wiess tear is due to un relaxed cardia).

Complications: Hydropneumothorax, pneumomediastinum, and pleural effusion.

Clinical Features of Boerhaave Syndrome

Mackler's triad:

- Vomiting
- Chest pain
- Subcutaneous emphysema

Treatment

Surgery is must.

- *Perforation <24 hours:* Primary closure and external drainage
- *Perforation >24 hours:* Primary closure not possible; surgical resection is must followed by proximal esophagostomy, distal end closure, and feeding jejunostomy along with external drainage. Colonic interposition in a later date maybe done.

CORROSIVE INJURY OF ESOPHAGUS

- Most cases of corrosive injury of esophagus are accidental consumption **(Table 1)**.
- Sometimes, suicidal attempts may be a cause.

Management

- Endoscopy must be performed by skilled endoscopist in early phase (< 24 hours) to know the extent of injury.
- Zargar grading is made based on endoscopy findings.

Zargar's Grading (Figs. 2A to E)

- *Grade 1:* Erythema
- *Grade 2a:* Superficial ulcers

TABLE 1: Alkali versus acid ingestion—comparative effects.

Alkali ingestion	*Acid ingestion*
More common	Less common
More devastating	Less devastating in the esophagus
Long term dysfunction seen	–
Liquefactive necrosis	*Coagulative necrosis*
Because of liquefactive necrosis, the penetration is deep. 3 phases are there	Eschar forms and limits the penetration; hence, esophageal perforation is rare
Chronic injury happens to esophagus	Acid ingestion is more devastating to stomach than esophagus

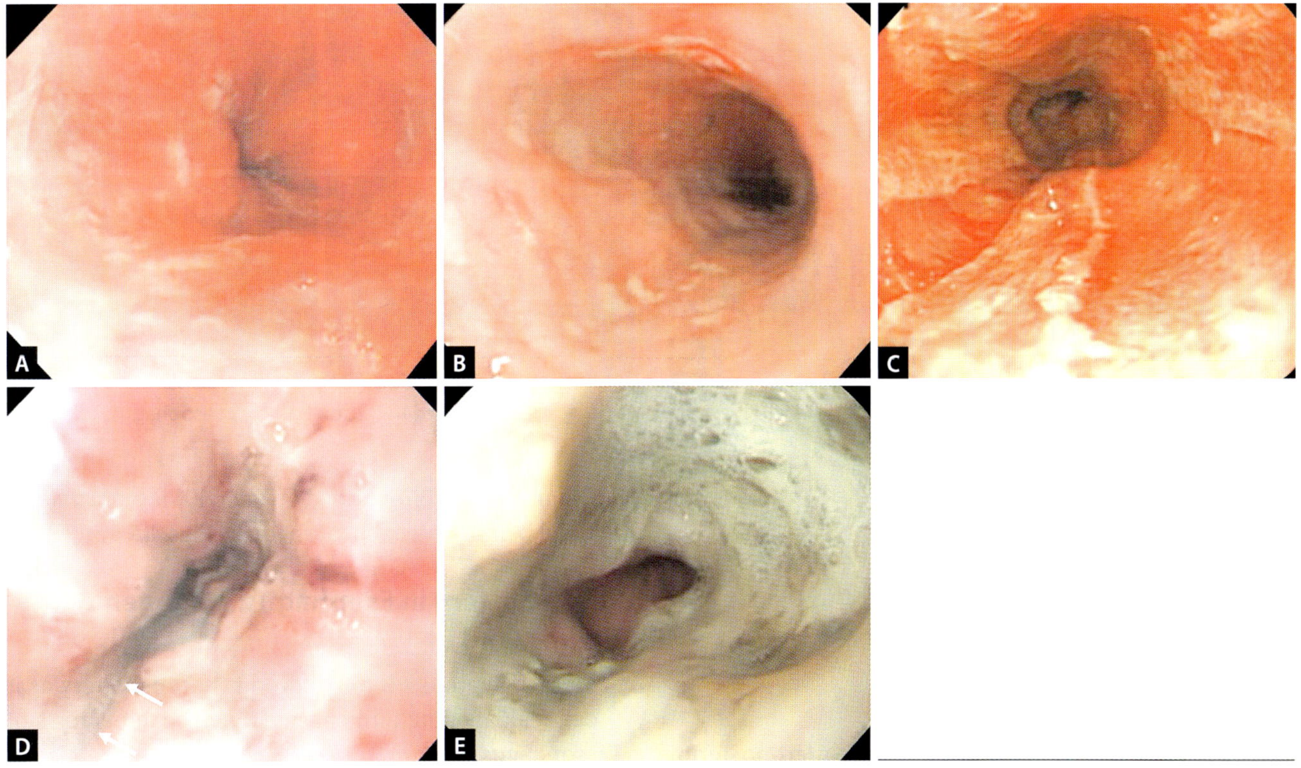

Figs. 2A to E: Zargar grading.

- *Grade 2b:* Deep ulcers
- *Grade 3a:* Scattered necrosis
- *Grade 3b:* Severe necrosis, diffusely+
- *Grade 4:* Perforation of esophagus

Recent Updates in Treatment

- Ryles tube insertion or wash is contraindicated.
- Neutralizing agents that were commonly used once upon a time is no more used as they may hide the endoscopic findings and grading.
- If patient is having difficulty to swallow in the initial phase, we can do feeding jejunostomy for nutrition (feeding gastrostomy is avoided as we will be using the stomach as conduit).
- Antibiotics and intravenous (IV) fluids are started.
- Management depends on the grade.
- Grade 1 and 2a can take oral diet and can be discharged.
- Grade 2b and 3a need surgical intensive care and close monitoring.
- Grade 3b and 4 need emergency thoracotomy and repair.

Long-term Outcome of Corrosive Cases

- They develop strictures after 6 months and result in dysphagia and undergo serial dilatations or resections.
- Corrosive injury esophagus has 1,000-fold risk of squamous cell carcinoma.

Management of corrosive stricture:

- Single strictures can be dilated using balloon or Savary–Gillard dilators.
- Multiple strictures in esophagus will need colonic replacement conduit.

FOREIGN BODIES IN ESOPHAGUS

Most common foreign body (FB) in children: Coin

Most common FB in adults: Food bolus (may be fish bone and mutton bone)

- If an adult is coming with food bolus as obstruction, we must rule out underlying stricture or cancer.

In children, the most common site of FB is at the level of cricopharynx and we must plan and remove it earliest with endoscopy as there is risk of the coin entering the trachea and causing stridor.

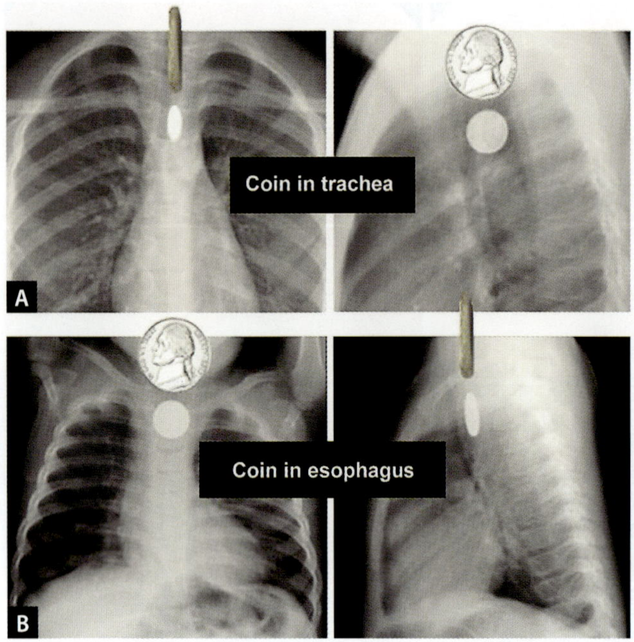

Figs. 3A and B: Esophageal coin.

X-ray is taken immediately in both anteroposterior (AP) and lateral views to locate the coin.

Nowadays, flexible scopy is used using graspers available.

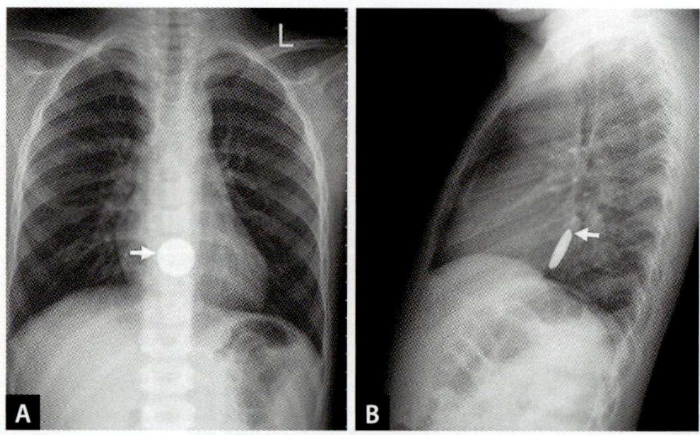

Figs. 4A and B: Button battery in esophagus.

Esophageal FB is identified on lateral X-ray looking like a slit and behind the tracheal shadow **(Figs. 3A and B)**.

Button Battery in Esophagus: Management (Figs. 4A and B)

- Most dangerous FB in children is button battery as it can leak alkaline and causes liquefactive necrosis of esophagus.
- Even if the button battery has passed into stomach or small bowel, endoscopy is mandatory to look for any damage in the esophagus.

CHAPTER 8

Stomach

R Rajamahendran

PEPTIC ULCER PERFORATION

Peptic ulcer is most common in duodenum first part.

Anteriorly located ulcers can go for perforation.

In stomach, incisura at lesser curve is the common site of perforation.

Clinical Features of Perforation

- A patient with perforation leaks the bowel contents into the peritoneum resulting in severe peritonitis and lands up in sepsis.
- *On examination:*
  - Patient has severe abdominal pain, low blood pressure (BP), and tachycardia.
  - Board-like rigidity is seen on palpation.
  - Diffuse guarding is noted.
  - On percussion, liver dullness will be obliterated due to leaked out air from perforation.

Investigations

- Immediate X-ray chest is done with diaphragm as shown in **Figure 1**.
- Air under diaphragm is seen in 50–60% of the cases of perforation and it is confirmatory if present.
- If air under diaphragm is not seen, we must take contrast-enhanced computed tomography (CECT) abdomen, which is >95% sensitive.

Management

- Intravenous (IV) fluids started and resuscitation is the key for survival.
- Antibiotics are started.
- Ryles tube aspiration done.
- Patient shifted to operation theatre at the earliest possible.
- In the operation theater (OT), midline laparotomy is done and thorough lavage with normal saline is done.
- Lavage is done until the peritoneal cavity is free of any debris.
- Perforation is identified and closure is done using modified Graham's patch of omental pedicle as shown in **Figure 2**.

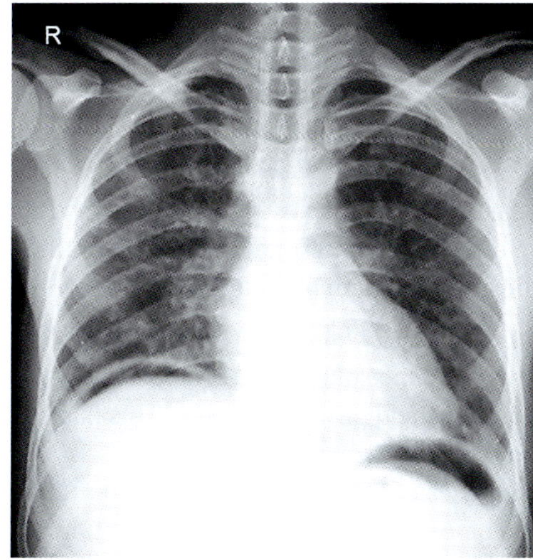

Fig. 1: X-ray shows air under diaphragm.

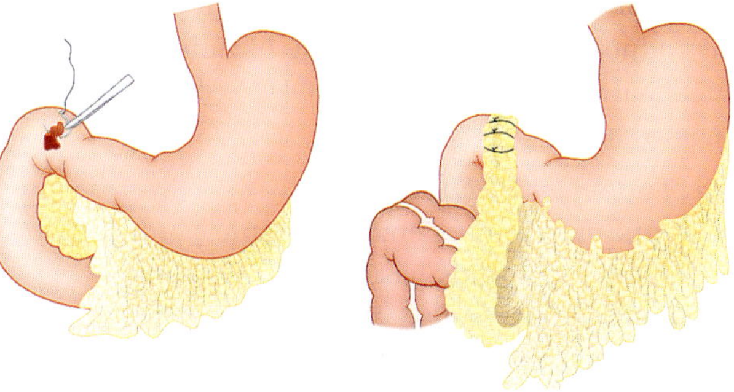

Fig. 2: Modified Graham's patch.

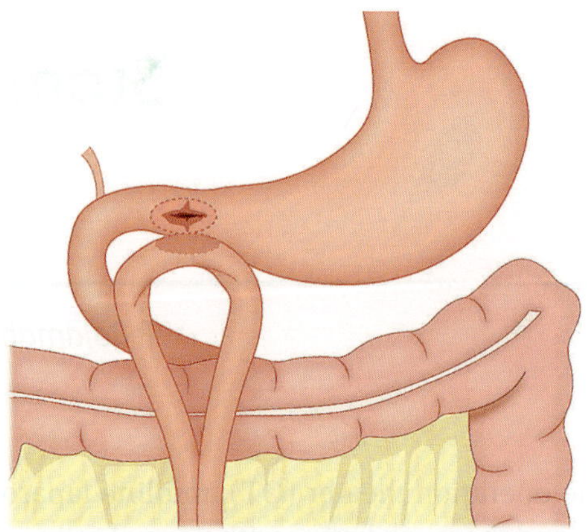

Fig. 3: Thal patch.

- If the ulcer is >3 cm, it is called giant ulcer, which may need jejunal serosal patch (Thal patch) with pyloric exclusion and anterior gastrojejunostomy (GJ) as shown in **Figure 3**.

In cases of gastric ulcer, if patient is stable, we can do distal gastrectomy and Billroth 2 reconstruction. But if patient is unstable, only omental patch repair done.

UPPER GASTROINTESTINAL BLEEDING

Upper gastrointestinal (UGI) bleeding is defined as bleeding in the gastrointestinal tract (GIT) until duodenal jejunal flexure (ligament of Treitz).

Presentations of UGI bleeding:

- *Melena:* Presence of black tarry stools, due to digestion of blood by the digestive enzymes. This happens when blood loss is <60 mL.
- *Hematochezia:* When blood loss is >60 mL, the undigested blood comes along with stools as hematochezia.
- *Hematemesis:* Blood vomiting is the most common presentation of duodenal ulcer bleeding.

Most common cause is duodenal ulcer bleeding. Posterior wall duodenal ulcers usually penetrate into gastroduodenal artery and cause bleeding from gastroduodenal artery (GDA). Hence, GDA is called as artery of hemorrhage.

List of causes for UGI bleeding:

- Peptic ulcers—duodenal and gastric
- Erosive esophagitis, gastritis, and duodenitis
- Mallory-Weiss tear
- Esophagogastric varices
- Cancer
- Dieulafoy lesion

Protocol in Upper Gastrointestinal Bleeding due to Duodenal Ulcer

- *Step 1:* The patient is admitted, Ryles tube is inserted, IV fluids are started, blood is sent for cross matching, and injection proton pump inhibitors are started in nonvariceal bleed cases.
- *Step 2:* Refer for early UGI endoscopy within 12 hours for endoscopic diagnosis of the etiology.
- *Step 3:* If there is bleeding is from duodenal ulcer, Forrest classification is used.

Forrest classification:
- *Grade 1:* Actively bleeding vessel
- *Grade 2a:* Visible vessel (no active bleed)
- *Grade 2b:* Clot in the posterior ulcer
- *Grade 2c:* Black spot
- *Grade 3:* Healed ulcer

- *Step 4:*
  - Grade 1, 2a, and 2b are taken for endotherapies, such as adrenaline injection combined with endoscopic coagulation and clipping of the bleeding vessel.
  - Grade 2c and 3 can be discharged giving medical treatment.
- *Step 5:* If the bleeding is persisting; based on the following criteria- Surgery is planned

Indications of Surgery in Bleeding Duodenal Ulcer

- Failed endoscopy >2 times
- Rare blood group
- Hemodynamically unstable
- >6 units of blood transfused
- >3 units transfused per day

Surgical Management

- Emergency laparotomy done via midline incision.
- Duodenum opened and three-point "U" suture done on the posterior wall of duodenum to arrest the bleeding.
- If patient is stable, truncal vagotomy can be added along with previous surgery **(Fig. 4)**.

Scoring Systems in Upper Gastrointestinal Bleeding

- *Blatchford score:* Nonendoscopy score based on clinical variables only (score varies from 0 to 23):
  - Hemoglobin

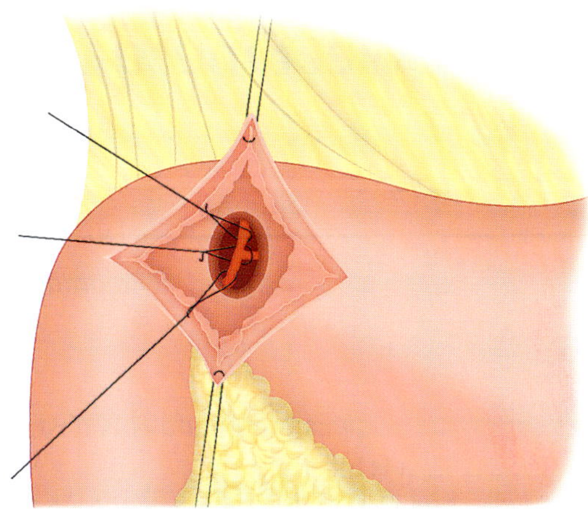

Fig. 4: 3-point U suture.

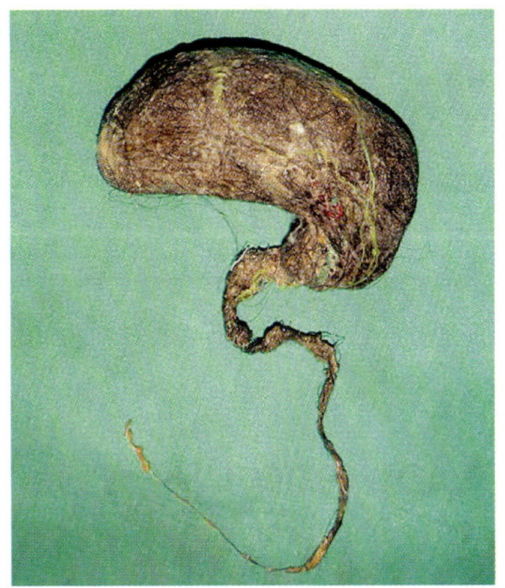

Fig. 5: Trichobezoar with Rapunzel syndrome.

- Urea
- Systolic BP
- Pulse rate
- Melena
- Syncope
- Liver or cardiac diseases
- *Rockall score (score varies from 0 to 11):* Based on:
  - Age
  - Shock
  - Comorbid diseases
  - Endoscopic findings
  - Endoscopic grading

BEZOARS

- *Trichobezoars:* Hair balls in stomach, exclusively seen in psychiatric young, female patients. Hair balls can lead to perforation, obstruction, and GI bleeding. Diagnosis is made on endoscopy. It is treated by surgical removal of Bezoars **(Fig. 5)**.
- *Rapunzel syndrome:* Long hair of trichobezoar extending from stomach up to ileum.

GASTRIC VOLVULUS

- Stomach can rotate and go for volvulus either in organo axial (longitudinal axis) or mesentrico axial (vertical axis) **(Figs. 6A and B)**.

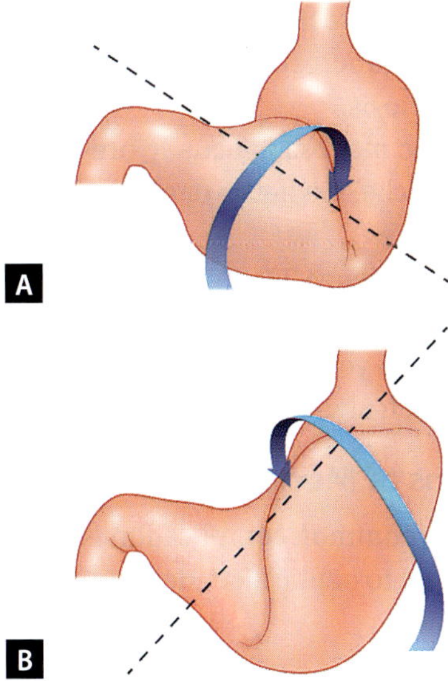

Figs. 6A and B: (A) Mesentrico axial; (B) Organoaxial volvulus.

- Most common type of volvulus is *organo axial volvulus* and this associated with diaphragmatic hernia
- *Borchardt's triad:* Sudden onset of constant retching epigastric pain + inability to vomit + inability to pass the Ryles tube.
- *Urgent surgery must be done:* Gastropexy and closure of diaphragm defects.

CHAPTER 9

Small Bowel Emergencies

R Rajamahendran

MECKEL'S DIVERTICULUM

Meckel's diverticulum is the most common congenital anomaly of gastrointestinal tract (GIT).

- Meckel's is true diverticulum, located in antimesenteric border **(Fig. 1)**.
- It is equal in male and female.
- it is most common ectopic mucosa—most common is gastric (60%), pancreatic, colonic, Brunner's glands, and endometriosis.
- Ectopic gastric mucosa is usually present adjacent to the base of Meckel's in ileum or opposite to Meckel's in small intestine.
- Rule of 2—prevalence 2%, *2-inch length*, located 2 feet proximal to Ileocaecal (IC) valve, and presents most commonly in <2 years age. The length varies with age and not is 2 inch always.

Complications of Meckel's

- Overall, most common complication is bleeding (most commonly due to peptic ulcer developing from ectopic gastric mucosa).
- Most common complication in adults is obstruction, and in children, it is bleeding.
- Obstruction is due to volvulus around the band and intussusception or Littre hernia.
- *Littre's hernia:* Meckel's as content in the sac (Amyand's hernia—appendix)
- *Diverticulitis in* 10–20% cases.
- *Most common malignancy in Meckel's is neuroendocrine tumor (carcinoid tumor)*

Diagnosis of Meckel's

- Meckel can be detected preoperatively by Tc 99m pertechnetate scan, which concentrates in ectopic mucosa **(Fig. 2)**.
- Sensitivity of scan decreases with age as ectopic mucosa disappears as age advances.
- The sensitivity and specificity of the scan can be increased by pentagastrin or glucagon or cimetidine.
- In adults, Meckel's is detected by enteroclysis but usually has no emergency presentation in adults.

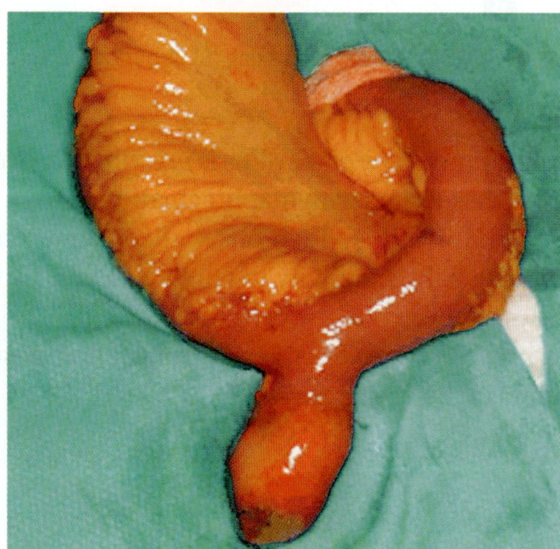

Fig. 1: Meckel's diverticulum.

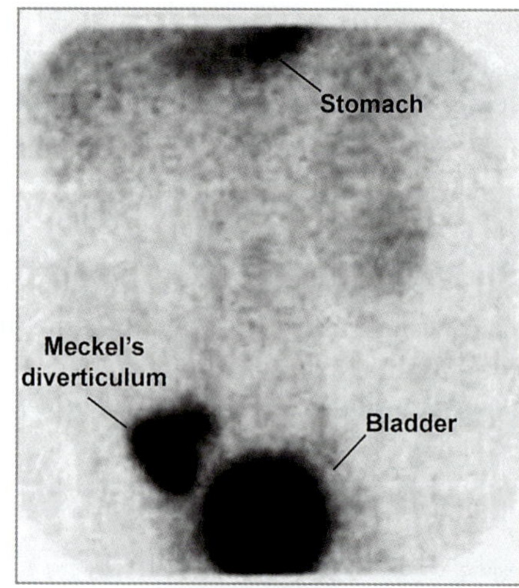

Fig. 2: Tc 99m scan showing Meckel's.

Treatment

- Resection of ileum with anastomosis is done if peptic ulcer is in ileum, gangrene is affecting base, and rarely, if malignancy is associated.
- Please remember, segmental resection is the treatment whenever you do surgery for bleeding because bleeding is usually from adjacent ileum having ectopic mucosa.

RADIATION ENTERITIS

- At radiation dosage >5,000 cGy, the rapidly dividing small intestine enterocytes gets damaged more.
- Most radiation damage is self-limiting.
- Late effects are damage to submucosal vessels, obliterative endarteritis, and submucosal fibrosis.
- *Predisposing factors:*
    - Previous surgery in abdomen
    - Pre-existing vascular disease and diabetes/hypertension
    - *Adjuvant radiosensitizing drugs:* 5FU, doxorubicin, and methotrexate
- *Clinical features: Strictures in small intestine and obstruction/fistula*
- *Radioprotectant: Most effective is amifostine.*
- Radiation exposure of bowels can be reduced intraoperatively by retro peritonealization, omental transposition, and absorbable mesh slings.
- *Diarrhea in radiation enteritis is treated by sucralfate.*
- *Superoxide Dismutase reduces complications.*
- *Most common indication for surgery is obstruction.*

ENTEROCUTANEOUS FISTULA

- Most common cause of enterocutaneous (EC) fistula is iatrogenic **(Fig. 3)**.
- Other causes are Crohn's disease, diverticulitis, and carcinoma Colon.
- High fistulas drain >500 mL/day, intermediate 200–500 mL, and Low <200 mL.

Complications of Fistula

- Fluid and electrolyte disturbance
- Malnutrition
- Necrosis of skin
- Sepsis leading to multiple organ failure and death

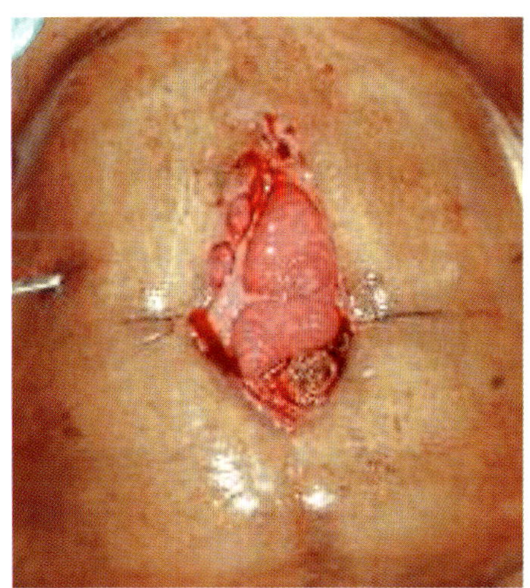

Fig. 3: Enterocutaneous (EC) fistula.

Factors preventing spontaneous closure of fistula:
- *F:* Foreign body in tract
- *R:* Radiation enteritis
- *I:* Inflammatory bowel disease
- *E:* Epithelialization of tract
- *N:* Neoplasm
- *D:* Distal obstruction
- *S:* Short tract

Treatment

- Correction of fluid and electrolyte imbalance
- Antibiotics
- Skin protection
- Total parenteral nutrition (TPN)
- Surgery indicated if fistula fails to heal after 4–6 weeks.
    - Fistulous tract excision along with involved segment and reanastomosis.

Principles in management of enterocutaneous fistula (SNAP):
- *S:* Sepsis elimination
- *N:* Nutrition—a period of total parenteral nutrition (TPN)
- *A:* Anatomical assessment
- *P:* Planned surgery

STOMAS

- Stoma is the process of bringing the colon to abdominal wall for defunctioning the colon or as a permanent procedure.
- Stomas are very important procedures in emergency where the anastomosis is felt unsafe due to poor general condition of the patient.
- Stomas can be ileostomy or colostomy **(Table 1)**.

TABLE 1: Comparison between ileostomy and colostomy based on anatomical location, type, appearance, and nature of contents.

Ileostomy	*Colostomy*
Created in right iliac fossa	Created in transverse colon or sigmoid colon
Types: End or loop	*Types:* End or loop
Ileostomy is sprouted to surface	Colostomy is flushed
Content is liquid	Content is solid stools

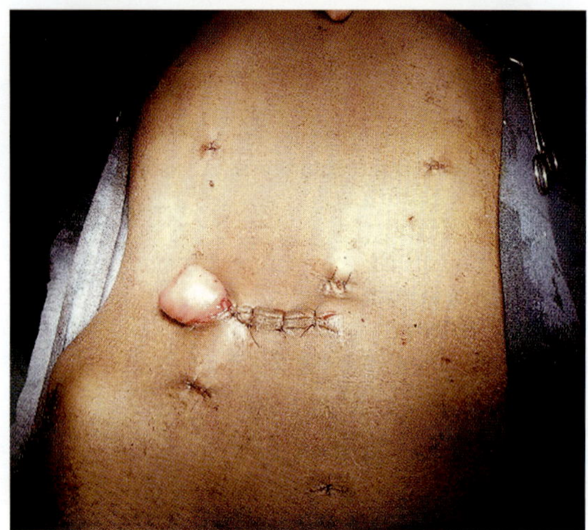

Fig. 4: End ileostomy.

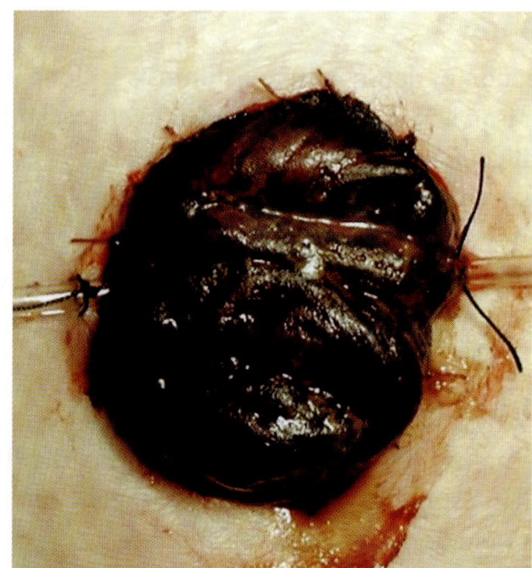

Fig. 5: Ileostomy necrosis.

Ileostomy

Temporary:

- Loop ileostomy is used for allowing the distal anastomosis to heal (e.g., following low anterior resection in cancer rectum or in post radiotherapy/immunocompromised cases) **(Fig. 4)**.
- Advantage with loop ileostomy is that it is easy to reclose without doing a laparotomy.

Permanent:

- It is usually an end ileostomy, which is sprouting.
- Brooke type is commonly used sprouting one.
- Kock's Ileostomy is continent type having a valve.
- It is done following total proctocolectomy in ulcerative colitis.

Complications of Ileostomy

- Most common early complication is *stoma ischemic necrosis* **(Fig. 5)**.
- Most common complication of ileostomy is *skin irritation.*

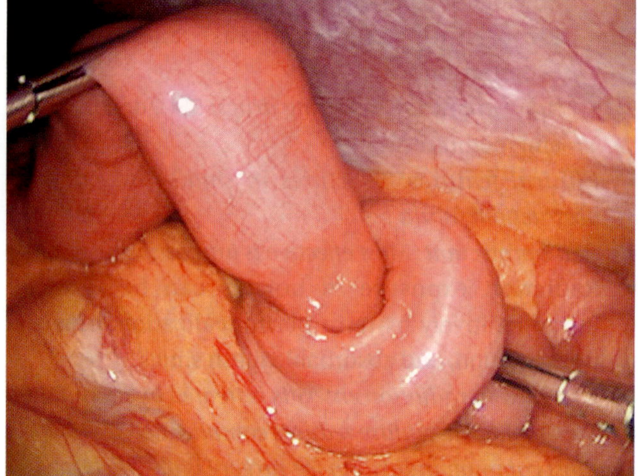

Fig. 6: Intussusception.

- Stoma retraction may be early or late complication (most common in obese patients)
- Fluid and electrolyte loss (Ileostomy output must be <1,500 mL)
- Parastomal hernia (less common than after colostomy)
- Stomal prolapse is a late complication.

SMALL BOWEL INTESTINAL OBSTRUCTION

Pediatric Causes

Intussusception

- Telescoping of one portion of intestine into the other is intussusception **(Fig. 6)**.

- Most common cause of intestinal obstruction in age <3 years.
- Most common type is ileocolic.
- In old age, most common type is colocolic.

Etiology

- *Pediatric:* Idiopathic (70–90%) is thought to be due to rotaviral infection, which causes hypertrophied Peyer's patches.
- *Older infants:* Meckel's diverticulum (Most common in older children)
- *Adults:* Tumors, polyps, and submucosal lipomas

Clinical Features

- Characterized by severe crampy abdominal pain and vomiting
- *Red currant jelly stool*
- *Per Abdomen (P/A):* Sausage-shaped mass
- *Le dance sign:* Empty right iliac fossa
- *Per Rectal (P/R):* Apex may be seen protruding.

Investigation:

- *Barium enema: Claw sign* ***(Fig. 7)*** *and Coiled-spring sign*
- *Ultrasound: Target sign, pseudo kidney sign, and Bulls eye sign*
- *CT scan shows target sign* ***(Fig. 8)***
- *X-ray plain:* Target sign, meniscus sign, and features of step-ladder pattern.

Treatment

- Hydrostatic reduction by contrast agent or air enema under USG guidance is diagnostic and therapeutic for children.
- *Adults and old age:* Direct surgery is taken up as there is high chance for lead point.
- Such procedure is contraindicated in peritonitis and hemodynamic instability.
- While reducing the intussusception, always push from distal part (milk from distal) and never try to pull the inner tube.

Meconium Ileus

- Meconium ileus is the neonatal manifest of cystic fibrosis.
- Pancreatic enzyme deficiency and abnormal chloride secretion results in viscous water poor meconium.
- Failure of passage of meconium in 48 hours with features of obstruction—think of meconium ileus.
- Meconium ileus is associated with Hirschsprung disease, hypothyroidism, and maternal diabetes.
- *Obstruction of thick meconium occurs in ileum.*
- Presents *immediately after birth* with progressive abdominal distension and intermittent bilious vomiting.

Investigations

- *Air fluid levels do not form in spite of complete small bowel obstruction because enteric contents are viscous and thick.*

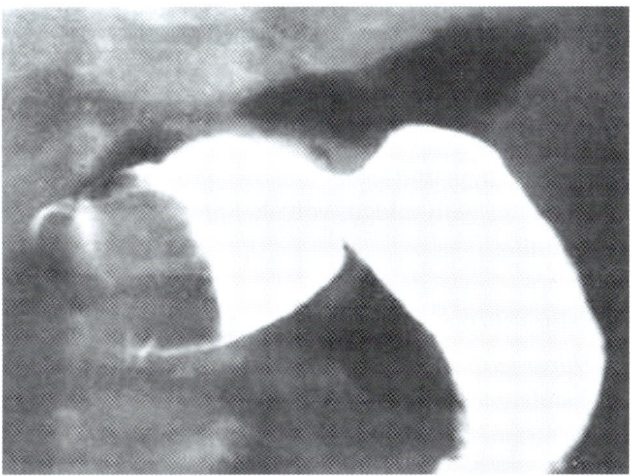

Fig. 7: Claw sign in barium swallow.

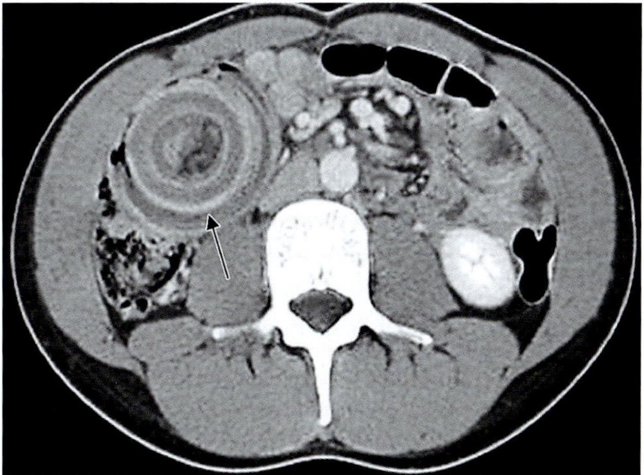

Fig. 8: Target sign in CT scan

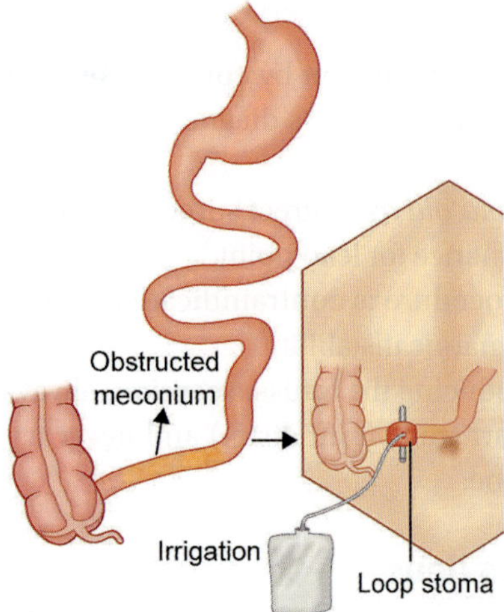

Fig. 9: Bishop–Koop operation.

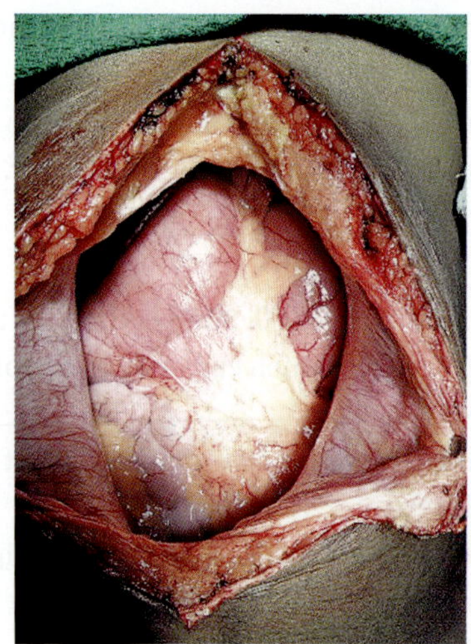

Fig. 10: Ladd's band.

- Dilated loops of small intestine.
- In case of meconium ileus in which perforation has occurred, intra peritoneal *egg shell calcifications* are noted.
- Investigation of choice (IOC) and treatment of choice is water soluble contrast enema.

Management

- *Conservative:* Gastrografin or Mypaque enema when given will easily pass to ileum and may disperse the obstruction due to its high osmolarity and detergent action.
- If this method, fails surgery indicated.
- *Bishop-Koop operation: Resection* of most dilated segment with an end to side anastomosis of colon to ileum. The distal ileal opening is formed into an ileostomy through which the meconium is irrigated post operatively **(Fig. 9)**.

Malrotation of Gut and Midgut Volvulus

- *Incidence:* 1 in 6,000 live births
- *Embryology:* Midgut normally herniates the umbilical ring at about 4th week intrauterine life and returns to abdominal cavity at about 10th week of intrauterine (IU) life, rotates around the axis of superior mesenteric artery (SMA) for 270° in counter clockwise direction.

Types:

- *Incomplete malrotation is the most common malrotation* resulting due to Ladd's band.
- Nonrotation abnormality is the most common anomaly.
- Reverse rotation
- Hyper rotation
- Malrotation with midgut volvulus

Pathology

- The duodenal C loop does not form and the duodenum lies on right side of abdomen as whole whereas the cecum lies on left side.
- The proximal jejunum and ascending colon are fused together and lie on one side and with one pedicle (SMA). This pedicle forms the base for volvulus of midgut.
- *Ladd's band* extends from ascending colon across the duodenum **(Fig. 10)**.
- Duodenal obstruction from Ladd's bands causes bilious vomiting.

Clinical Features

- 90% develop symptoms before 1 year.
- Malrotation without volvulus may present with chronic abdominal pain and failure to thrive and present in adolescent period also.
- Neonates with midgut volvulus present with bilious vomiting.

Investigations

- *Upper gastrointestinal (GI) contrast series* are the gold standard to diagnose the volvulus.
- "Whirlpool sign" is seen in patients with malrotation of gut in contrast-enhanced computed tomography (CECT) abdomen **(Fig. 11)**.

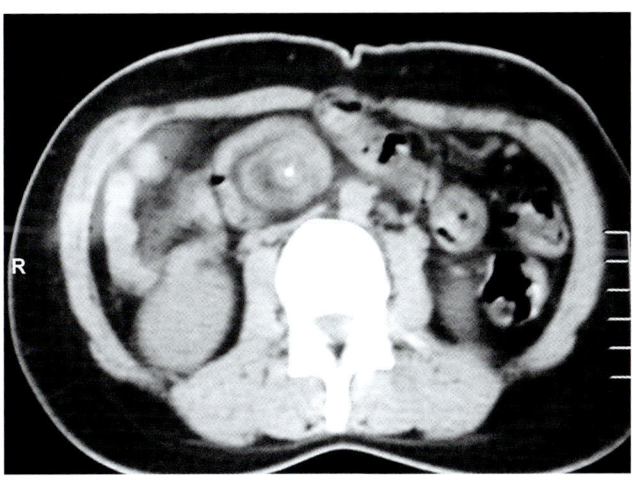

Fig. 11: Whirlpool sign.

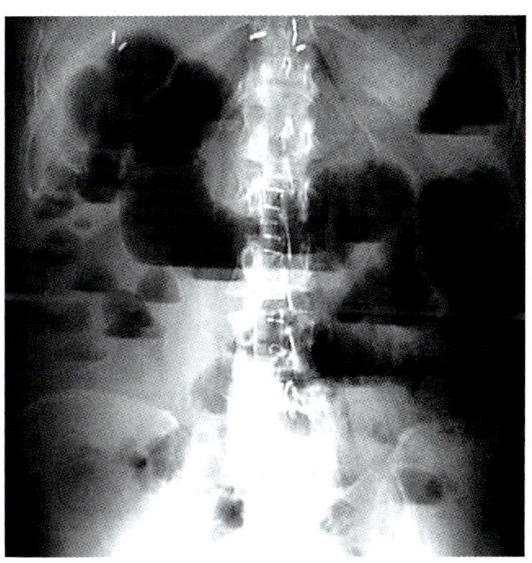

Fig. 12: Step ladder pattern.

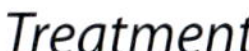

Treatment

"Emergency laparotomy and Ladd's procedure"

- This is not a procedure to correct the malrotation, but it only helps in broadening of the mesenteric pedicle so that it would not go for torsion later.
- The volvulus is *usually clockwise*, hence, rotates the bowel in anticlockwise direction.
- At the end of the procedure, the cecum and large bowel lie on the left side and small bowels on the right side.
- Appendix removed

Adult Causes of Small Bowel Obstructions

Etiology

- *Adhesions (60%):* Most common cause and follows appendicitis or other pelvic operations.
- *Malignancy (20%):* Most common metastasis
- Hernias (10%)
- Crohn's disease (5%)

Clinical features	*Four causes of distension*
• Abdominal crampy pain, when the bowel is strangulated; pain becomes steady and more localized without a colicky component • Vomiting (follows onset of pain) • Obstipation (absolute constipation) • Abdominal distension • Fever • Blood in stool (intussusception	1. Swallowed gas (most common) 2. Fermentation gas by bacteria 3. Extracellular fluid loss 4. Gastrointestinal (GI) secretions • Normal fluid levels; 3–5 each <2.5 cm is normal • Fluid levels >5 indicates small bowel obstruction • *Step ladder pattern:* Small bowel obstruction **(Fig. 12)**

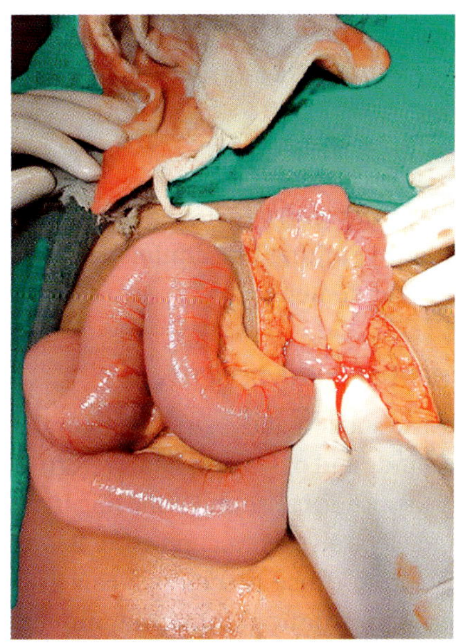

Fig. 13: Adhesive obstruction due to a band.

Management of Acute Small Bowel Obstruction

- *Fluid resuscitation:* Ringer lactate is fluid of choice.
- Monitor urine output.
- Nasogastric decompression.
- With conservative management, 70% cases get relieved.

Treatment as per cause:

- *Adhesive obstruction:* Conservative management is advised for 24–48 hours; maximum only for 48 hours. If obstruction is not relieved, laparoscopic or open adhesiolysis can be done **(Fig. 13)**.

- *Hernia/malignancy obstruction:* Immediate surgery must be done.

Paralytic Ileus (Inorganic Cause)

- *Failure of transmission of peristaltic waves secondary to neuromuscular failure*
    - Most common cause is postoperative
    - Infections
    - Electrolyte abnormalities
        - Uremia
        - Hypokalemia
        - Hyponatremia
        - Hypomagnesemia
        - Hypermagnesemia
    - Hypothyroidism
    - Myocardial infarction
    - Spinal cord injury
    - Retroperitoneal hemorrhage
    - Drugs
    - Mesenteric ischemia

Clinical features of paralytic ileus: There will be abdominal distension and vomiting but diminished bowel sounds and no pain in abdomen.

Management of Paralytic Ileus

- Nasogastric suction and restriction of oral intake until bowel sounds and passage of flatus return
- Identify the prime cause and removing it
- Fluid and electrolyte correction
- If no dynamic cause is seen, we can use *Catchpole regimen*—stimulating intestine movement with adrenergic blocking agent + cholinergic stimulation using neostigmine.

MESENTERIC ISCHEMIA

Mesenteric ischemia is a vascular disorder affecting the small bowel due to SMA/superior mesenteric vein (SMV) occlusions. Based on the etiology, we have following types:

- Acute mesenteric artery ischemia
- Chronic mesenteric ischemia
- Mesenteric vein thrombosis
- Nonocclusive mesenteric ischemia (NOMI)

Etiology

- Sudden occlusion of superior mesenteric artery (50%)
    - Atherosclerosis (most common cause of chronic mesenteric ischemia)
    - Embolism (most common cause of acute SMA ischemia 90% cases)
    - Vasculitis (polyarteritis nodosa)
    - Fibromuscular dysplasia
- Mesenteric vein occlusion (25%)
    - Thrombosis due to oral contraceptive pills (OCP), polycythemia, and neoplasm infiltrating
- Nonocclusive obstruction (25%)
- Severe shock

Acute Mesenteric Ischemia

Clinical Features

- Sudden severe abdominal pain, vomiting, and abdominal distension
- Central abdominal pain with symptoms out of proportion to signs present *(hallmark feature)*
- Functional obstruction with absent bowel sounds
- Shock and peritonitis are rapid.
- 100% mortality if untreated.
- In emboli cases, the obstruction is in mid to distal SMA, distal to origin of middle colic artery. In such cases, some part of bowel is viable **(Fig. 14)**.
- In thrombosis, cases the obstruction is at origin of SMA. In such cases, the bowel is gangrenous from duodenojejunal (DJ) flexure to right colon.
- Investigation to diagnose *laparotomy*

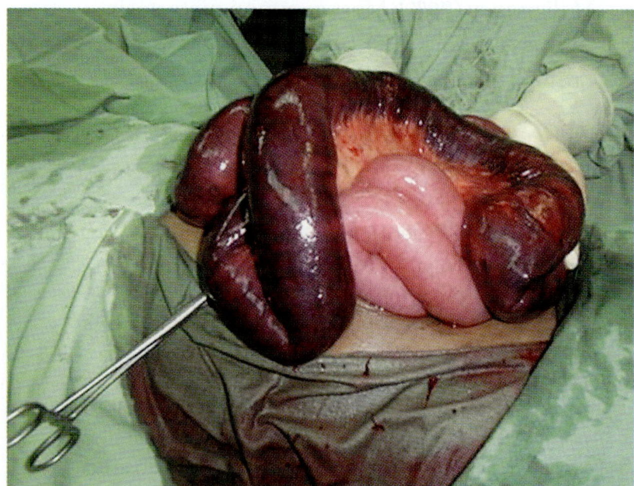

Fig. 14: Acute superior mesenteric artery (SMA) ischemia by embolus.

Treatment

- Resection of nonviable bowel with its mesentery
- Second-look operation

Chronic Mesenteric Ischemia

- Chronic mesenteric ischemia presents with intestinal angina, weight loss, and chronic diarrhea.
- *Gold standard for chronic mesenteric ischemia:* Mesenteric angiography.
- *Atherosclerosis in main splanchnic artery* [celiac, inferior mesenteric artery (IMA), and SMA] is the most common cause of chronic mesenteric ischemia.

Mesenteric Vein Thrombosis

- Mesenteric vein thrombosis is usually due to small peripheral vein thrombosis [SMV OR inferior mesenteric artery (IMV) thrombosis is rare].
- Hence, thrombectomy is not needed (not indicated).
- Fluid resuscitation
- Heparin anticoagulation is sufficient.
- *If peritoneal signs are present,* urgent laparotomy is needed.
- *If peritoneal signs are absent,* heparin (5 days), oral anticoagulation lifelong along with bowel rest, and fluids are enough.

CHAPTER 10

Acute Appendicitis

R Rajamahendran

ACUTE APPENDICITIS

- Acute appendicitis is the most common emergency done worldwide.
- *Murphy's triad:* Migratory pain, vomiting, and fever.

COMMON SIGNS IN APPENDICITIS

- McBurney's point tenderness is tenderness at the point medial two-third and lateral one-third of spinoumbilical line—Mc Burney point.
- *Blumberg sign:* Rebound tenderness.
- *Rovsing's sign:* Palpation of left iliac fossa produces pain in right iliac fossa by shift of bowels.
- *Sherren's triangle hyperesthesia:* Triangle formed by anterior superior iliac spine (ASIS), umbilicus, and pubic symphysis due to irritation of lower abdominal nerves.
- *Cope's psoas sign:* Retrocecal appendicitis on extension of hip produces pain due to irritation over psoas major (muscle that flexes the hip) **(Fig. 1)**.
- *Cope's obturator sign:* Pelvic appendicitis—flexion and medial rotation produces pain **(Fig. 2)**.

COMPLICATIONS OF ACUTE APPENDICITIS

- Spontaneous resolution
- Gangrenous appendicitis
- Free perforation into peritoneal cavity with peritonitis
- *Appendicular mass:* An inflammatory phlegmon formed by greater omentum and small bowel with inflamed appendix.
- Appendicular abscess **(Fig. 3)**

Perforations that happen in <24 hours cause diffuse peritonitis as the omentum has not yet sealed the inflammatory area. Perforations that happen greater than 24 hours cause localized peritonitis or appendicular abscess. In short, delayed perforation is safer than an early perforation.

High-risk factors for perforation of appendix:
- Extremes of age
- Immunocompromised patients
- Fecoliths
- Diabetes
- Pelvic position of appendix
- Previous abdominal surgery will limit the ability of omentum to seal the inflamed appendix.

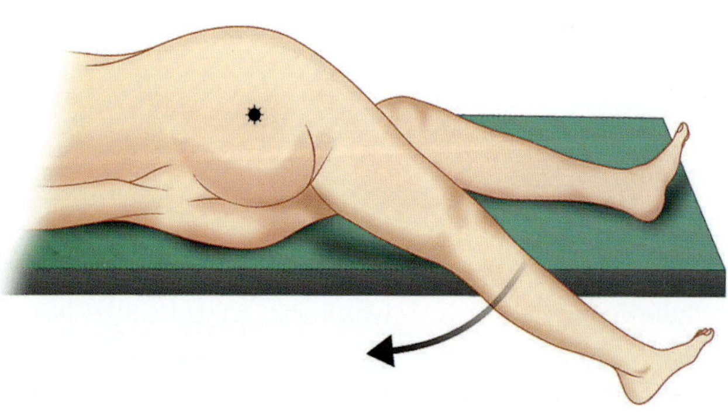

Fig. 1: Cope's psoas test for retrocecal appendicitis.

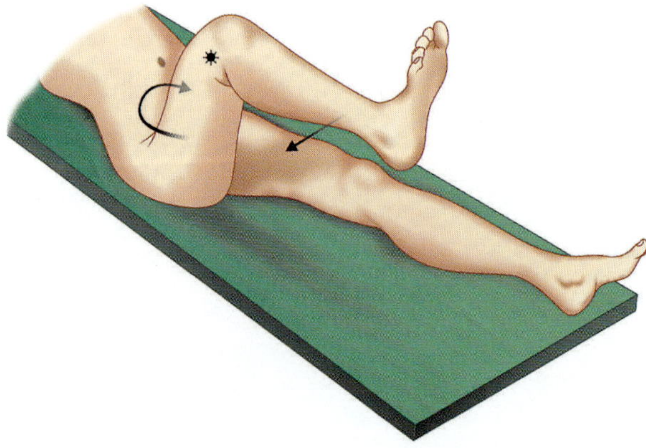

Fig. 2: Cope's obturator test for pelvic position appendicitis.

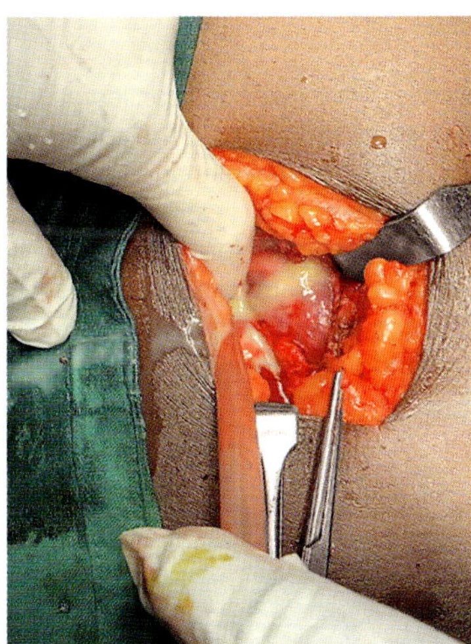

Fig. 3: Appendicular abscess.

INTERESTING FACTS IN APPENDICITIS

- Retrocecal appendicitis can present as silent appendix as the distended cecum will prevent the pressure exerted in right iliac fossa to reach the appendix.
- Early diarrhea can occur if pelvic appendicitis is irritating the rectum.
- Pelvic appendicitis can cause increased frequency of micturition due to bladder irritation.

DIFFERENTIAL DIAGNOSIS OF ACUTE APPENDICITIS

Differential diagnosis of acute appendicitis is given in **Box 1.**

INVESTIGATIONS

With only clinical diagnosis when we operate appendix, there are chances that 15–30% times, it results in normal appendix.

There is a most widely used score known as ALVARDO score to predict the possibility of acute appendicitis:

ALVARDO score:

The mnemonic for this score is MANTRELS

- *M:* Migratory pain
- *A:* Anorexia
- *N:* Nausea
- *T:* Tenderness in right iliac fossa
- *R:* Rebound Tenderness (Blumberg sign)
- *E:* Elevated temperature
- *L:* Leukocytosis
- *S:* Shift of neutrophils to left (more of immature neutrophils)

BOX 1: Differential diagnosis of acute appendicitis.

Children

- Acute gastroenteritis
- Meckel's diverticulitis
- Intussusception
- Mesenteric adenitis

Adults

- Ureteric colicky
- Terminal ileitis
- Perforated peptic ulcers
- Pancreatitis

Adult females

- Pelvic pathology in ovary and uterus
- Ectopic pregnancy
- Mittelschmerz—a midcycle menstrual pain

Elderly

- Diverticulitis
- Cancer
- Torsion of appendices epiploicae
- Mesenteric infarction
- Aortic aneurysm bleeding

The last 2 score is based on laboratory values.

All the variables are given 1 point; tenderness and leukocytosis are given 2 points.

The total score of >7 is strongly predictive of acute appendicitis.

Patients with equivocal score of 5 or 6 will need an ultrasonography (USG) or contrast-enhanced computed tomography (CECT) abdomen.

Ultrasonography is the most useful investigation with a sensitivity of >90%.

Contrast-enhanced computed tomography is most sensitive and specific (>95%) investigation. CECT plays a vital role in very old patients in whom there will be a diagnostic confusion due to cancer and diverticulitis.

TREATMENT OF ACUTE APPENDICITIS

Nonoperative Management

- Surgery remains the gold standard, but in selected cases of acute appendicitis such as absence of appendicolith, perforation, and abscess, we can do nonoperative management.
- Bowel rest, intravenous (IV) antibiotics with third generation cephalosporins and metronidazole are recommmended.
- Success rate is around 85% in such cases, but around one-third of these patients will come for surgery in next 1 year with recurrent symptoms.

BOX 2: Ochsner–Sherren regimen.

Ochsner–Sherren regimen:

Contrast-enhanced computed tomography of the abdomen is performed and the following principles are followed:

- Aspirate (Ryles tube aspiration)
- Bowel rest (nil per oral) and Bladder catheterization
- Charts' maintenance
  - Pulse chart
  - Blood pressure (BP) chart
  - Input/output chart
  - Mass size chart and abdominal girth chart
  - Temperature chart
- Drugs (antibiotics and metronidazole)
- Exploratory laparotomy may be needed in following situations:
  - Increasing perioperative risk (PR)
  - Increasing Ryles Tube aspirate
  - Increasing mass size and abdominal girth chart
  - Increasing temperature
  - Increasing or spreading pain in the abdomen
- Fluids
  - Clinical Improvement is seen in 24–48 hours
  - Failure of the mass to resolve should raise the suspicion of cancer or Crohn's disease
  - Following above protocol, >90% cases resolve well
  - The regimen is usually followed by an interval appendectomy after 6 weeks as per conventional protocols. Some recent studies have confirmed that majority of patients will not develop recurrent appendicitis and were not in favor of interval appendectomy

- When doing such conservative treatment, consent must be obtained of the high failure rates and higher operative risk if the complications occurs.
- Patients above 40 years must be ensured there is no underlying malignancy on follow up.

Appendicular mass: Since the mass is made up of adherent bowel loops, we must avoid surgery at this stage as we can injure the small bowel, and an enterocutaneous fistula can happen. Hence, came a very interesting concept of nonoperative management known as Ochsner-Sherren regimen **(Box 2)** is introduced.

Bailey 28th edition updates are given in **Box 3**.

Operative Management

The conventional open appendectomy is very rarely done nowadays due to laparoscopic facilities in all the places.

Conventional Appendectomy

Under general anesthesia, a grid iron incision is made as shown in the **Figure 4**.

BOX 3: Bailey 28th edition updates.

"Those patients who were managed conservatively; around 29% cases had unexpected tumor in the appendix and especially in patients who were managed with periappendiceal abscess and aged more than 40 years". Hence, careful consideration must be made before sending the patient without operating. At follow up, we must at least ensure there is no residual lesion by doing a magnetic resonance imaging (MRI) or computed tomography (CT) scan

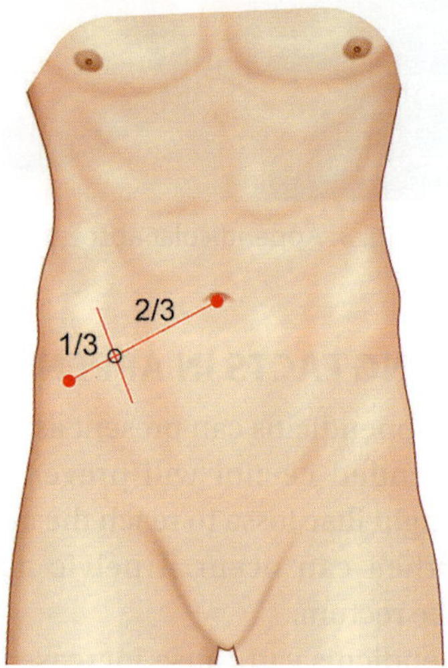

Fig. 4: Grid iron incision.

The other name of this incision is McArthur incision, and it is made perpendicular to the spinoumbilical line at McBurney's point.

The other incision used in girls for cosmetic reasons is Lanz incision, in which a horizontal incision is made 2 cm below umbilicus along the line joining the midclavicular to mi inguinal points. The exposure is better with this incision and can be extended if needed easily **(Fig. 5)**.

When the diagnosis is in doubt, it is better to make an incision in lower midline. The old type of lower paramedian incision known as Battle incision is no more used in practice.

During surgery, appendix must be held with Babcock's forceps or with a Lane's forceps encircling the appendix without damaging the appendix.

Mesoappendix is clamped and cut and ligated with the vessels.

Appendix is clamped at the base and suture ligation done and cut.

Some authors recommend Purse string suture or Z suture of cecal wall invaginating and burying the stump of

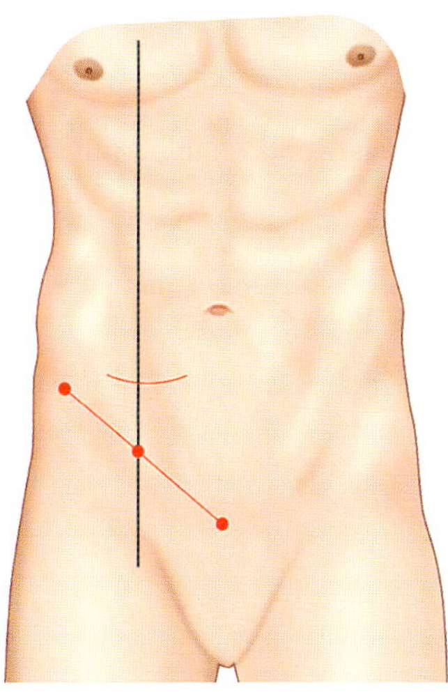

Fig. 5: Lanz incision.

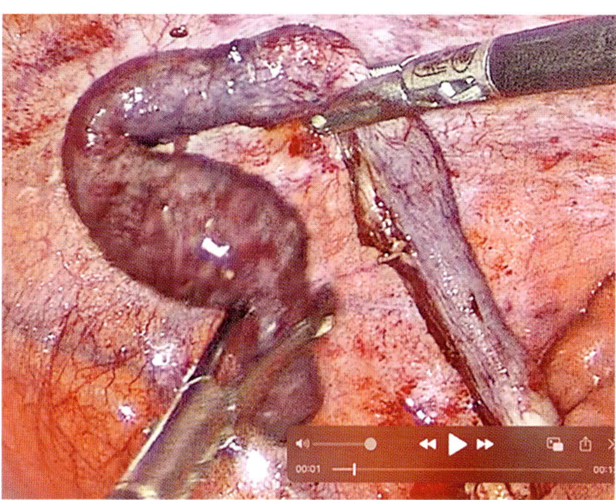

Fig. 6: Laparoscopic appendectomy.

BOX 4: Rutherford morison incision.

Rutherford Morison incision:
- This is not a skin incision
- It is a muscle cutting incision used when there is difficulty in delivering the appendix such as in para or retro cecal position or when it is fixed posteriorly
- It is an oblique incision with lower end in the McBurney's point and extending upward and laterally as necessary
- All the muscles—external oblique, internal oblique, and transversus abdominis—are cut in this incision

appendix. Many surgeons including the author never used to do invagination steps as these are not necessary.

Rutherford Morison incision is given in **Box 4**.

Special Situations

- If the base is gangrenous, we must not ligate the base and just cut the appendix flush to cecum and take two stitches in cecal wall and close the orifice of appendix. Over the above suture, a second layer of Lembert (seromuscular sutures) can be made. Another option is to cut the appendix with a cuff of cecum with a linear stapler.
- In case if a normal appendix is found, we must search for other pathologies such as Meckel's diverticulitis, terminal ileitis, or tuboovarian pathologies. In such case, always remove the normal appendix to avoid future confusions.
- Some situations are there where on tracing the tenia coli, no appendix can be found and branded as *"absent appendix".*
- If appendicular mass is found during surgery, it is safer to abandon the operation and keep a drain and come out.
- If Crohn's disease is associated with appendicitis, it is better to remove the appendix if cecal wall is healthy. But in case if cecal wall is affected by Crohn's along with appendicitis, we must try a course of IV steroids and systemic antibiotics and wait for the inflammation to resolve.

Laparoscopic Appendectomy

By three port technique, one 10 mm camera port in umbilicus and 2 other working ports, (1 in suprapubic and another in left lower quadrant) appendix is removed by using various energy devices and suturing techniques **(Fig. 6)**.

Patient will be kept in Trendelenburg with moderate right elevation of operation theatre (OT) table is used.

COMPLICATIONS OF APPENDECTOMY

- Wound infection—most common postoperative complication
- Intra-abdominal abscess
- Postoperative ileus
- Respiratory complications
- Venous thrombosis and pulmonary embolism
- Portal pylephlebitis leading to intrahepatic abscess
- Fecal fistula
- Adhesive intestinal obstruction

Appendicitis in pregnancy:
- Most common nonobstetric surgical emergency in pregnancy.
- Most common in second trimester.
- Diagnosis is often delayed due to overlapping of some obstetric symptoms such as nausea and vomiting. But lower right quadrant pain is characteristic.
- Magnetic resonance imaging is the most sensitive investigation since USG is not much sensitive.
- Fetal loss occurs in 3–5% of acute appendicitis.
- Laparoscopic appendectomy can be done and better to use open technique for gas insufflation.

Large Bowel Emergencies

R Rajamahendran

LOWER GASTROINTESTINAL BLEEDING

- Bleeding distal to ligament of Trietz is called lower gastrointestinal (GI) bleeding.
- It can be from small bowel or from large bowel.
- Most common presentation is bleeding per rectum **(Table 1)**.
- *Step 1:* Resuscitate the patient and confirm the bleeding is from rectum by doing an initial proctoscopy examination.
- *Step 2:* Even though this is a lower GI bleeding, Ryles tube is inserted first to rule out whether the bleeding is from upper gastrointestinal (UGI) causes presenting as lower GI bleeding.
    - *If Ryle's tube shows clear bile:* UGI causes of bleeding are ruled out.
    - *If Ryle's tube shows blood:* Proceed with UGI protocol.
    - *If Ryle's tube shows greenish gastric aspirate:* We must do UGI scopy before colonoscopy.
- *Step 3:*
    - Investigation of choice (IOC) for lower GI bleeding is colonoscopy.
    - More than 90% time, the lower GI bleed cause is identified and managed accordingly.
- *Step 4:*
    - If UGI and colonoscopy are normal, the bleeding can be from small bowel, and we call this source of bleeding as obscure GI bleeding.
    - The IOC for obscure GI bleed is capsule endoscopy. If capsule scopy identified the source, management is done accordingly.
- *Step 5:*
    - If capsule scopy is normal we must proceed with Technetium 99m labeled red blood cell (RBC) pertechnetate scan, which can detect bleeding as <0.1 mL/minute.
    - The major drawback is it cannot identify the exact location of bleeding, it will give a gross image of the bleeding quadrant.
    - If Tc 99m scan shows active bleeding, immediately, we must do superior mesenteric angiography—it detects bleeding of 0.5 mL/minute.
    - Please remember, we will do angiography only when active bleed is present.
    - During angiography, selective embolization can be done for the bleeding vessel.

TABLE 1: Differential diagnosis of lower gastrointestinal bleeding based on colonic and small bowel causes, categorized by severity of bleeding.

Colonic causes		*Small bowel causes*
Massive bleed	*Minor bleed*	
• Diverticulosis (MC) • Angiodysplasia • Ulcerative colitis • Mesenteric ischemia • Radiation colitis	• Hemorrhoids (MC) • Fissure • Cancer • Solitary rectal ulcer • Polyps	• Angiodysplasia (MC) • Polyps • Tumors • Crohn's disease

(MC: most common)

Angiodysplasia

- Abnormal dilated submucosal vessels are known as angiodysplasia.
- It is most common in cecum and ascending colon >rectum >Small bowel (jejunum).
- Produces troublesome bleeding by rupture of the vessels.
- *Investigation of choice:* Colonoscopy and treated by coagulation in same time.
- *Heyde's syndrome:* It is defined as type 2 von Willebrand disease (VWD) patients having angiodysplasia + valvular aortic stenosis.

SIGMOID COLON DIVERTICULITIS

- Most common site of diverticulum in colon is at sigmoid colon.
- It is usually multiple and found on the mesenteric border.
- It is most common in old age.
- Most common complication is diverticulitis (inflammation and perforation of the diverticulum).

Clinical Features of Diverticulitis

- They present with left iliac fossa pain and fever.
- On examination, localized tenderness and guarding present in left iliac fossa is noticed.

Investigation of Choice

- Contrast-enhanced computed tomography (CECT) abdomen and pelvis with intravenous (IV) contrast **(Fig. 1)**.
- Colonoscopy is not advised in acute stage as there is risk of perforation of the diverticulum during inflammation stage.
- Modified Hinchey classification is used for diverticulitis:
  - *Stage 0:* Clinical diverticulitis
  - *Stage 1:* Pericolic/localized abscess
  - *Stage 2:* Pelvic abscess
  - *Stage 3:* Generalized purulent peritonitis
  - *Stage 4:* Generalized fecal peritonitis.

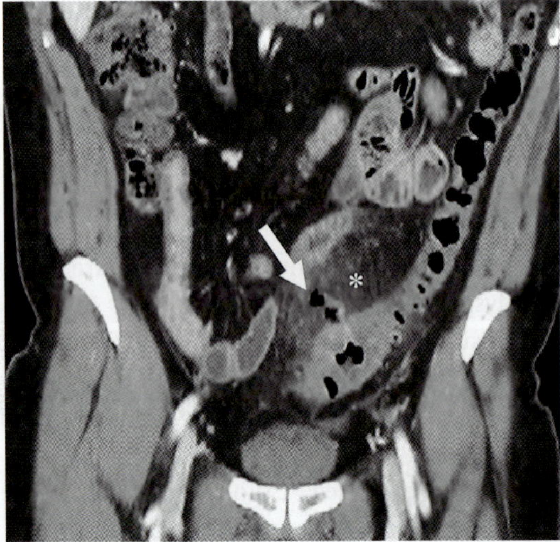

Fig. 1: Contrast-enhanced computed tomography (CECT) abdomen showing diverticulitis with pericolic air leak. Leak is shown by white arrow.

Management

- Hinchey stage 0 is managed by nonoperative management with antibiotics.
- Hinchey stage 1 and 2 are managed by ultrasound (USG)-guided drainage.
- Hinchey stage 3 is managed by laparoscopic lavage and drainage tube in pelvis as per latest protocols.
- Hinchey stage 4 is managed by Hartmann's procedure (proximal end colostomy + resection of diverticulum segment + closure of rectal stump).

TOXIC MEGACOLON

- Megacolon is defined as transverse colon diameter >5.5 cm with loss of haustration.
- *It is caused by:*
  - Ulcerative colitis
  - Crohn's disease
  - Salmonellosis
  - Amoebic colitis
  - Pseudomembranous colitis
  - Ischemic colitis.
- Ulcerative colitis is a common inflammatory bowel disorder usually presents as diarrhea and bleeding.
- If inflammation is confined to the rectum (proctitis), there is usually no systemic upset and extra-alimentary manifestations are rare. The disease often remains confined to the rectum, usually with a benign course.
- Colitis is almost always associated with bloody diarrhea and urgency.
- Severe and/or extensive colitis may result in anemia, hypoproteinemia, and electrolyte disturbances.
- Pain is unusual. Children with poorly controlled colitis may have impaired growth.
- The more extensive the disease, the more likely extraintestinal manifestations are to occur.
- Extensive colitis is also associated with systemic illness, characterized by malaise, loss of appetite, and fever.

Truelove and Witt Score is used to grade the severity of Ulcerative colitis.

- Mild disease is characterized by fewer than four stools daily, with or without bleeding. There are no systemic signs of toxicity.
- Moderate disease corresponds to *more than 4 stools daily*, but with few signs of systemic illness. There may be mild anemia. Abdominal pain may occur. Inflammatory markers, including erythrocyte sedimentation rate and C-reactive protein, are often raised.

- Severe disease corresponds to more than six bloody stools a day and evidence of systemic illness, with fever, tachycardia, anemia, and raised inflammatory markers. Hypoalbuminemia is common and an ominous finding.

Fulminant Type

- Fulminant disease is associated with >10 bowel movements daily, fever, tachycardia, continuous bleeding, anemia, hypoalbuminemia, abdominal tenderness, and distension, the need for blood transfusion and in the most severe cases, progressive colonic dilation (toxic megacolon) is seen on X-ray **(Fig. 2)**.
- This is a very significant finding, suggestive of disintegrative colitis, and an indication for emergency surgery if colonic perforation is to be avoided.

Management

- Emergency colectomy with ileostomy is done as there is high risk of perforation and sepsis **(Fig. 3)**.

LARGE BOWEL OBSTRUCTIONS

- Most common cause of large bowel obstruction is malignancy in the left side colon.
- Second common causc is volvulus.

Sigmoid Volvulus

- Twisting of a segment of the intestine on an axis formed by its mesentery is volvulus.
  - It is the most common site of volvulus—sigmoid colon.
  - Patients are very old-aged male who take more fiber diet with long redundant colon.
  - *Coffee bean appearance* is seen in X-ray **(Fig. 4)**.
  - *Bird Beak appearance* in barium enema of sigmoid volvulus **(Fig. 5)** is seen.
  - *Anticlockwise* > *clockwise* in sigmoid volvulus **(Fig. 6)**

Treatment of Sigmoid Volvulus

- Fluid resuscitation followed by endoscopic decompression using *sigmoidoscope*.
- Rectal tube is inserted to maintain it.
- This procedure is contraindicated in evidence of perforation or strangulation.

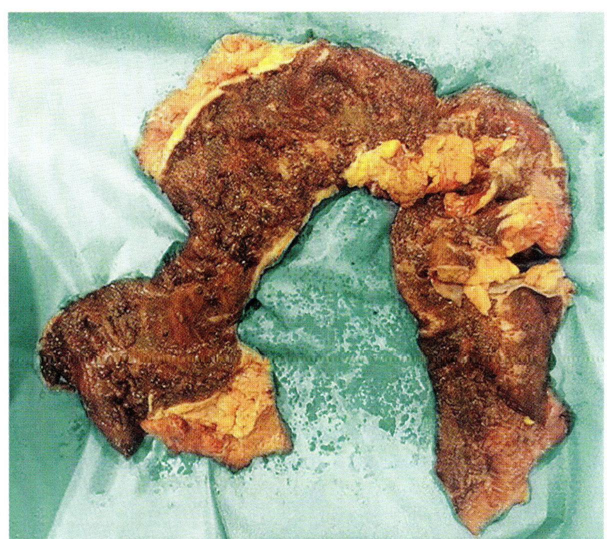

Fig. 3: Toxic megacolon—total colectomy specimen.

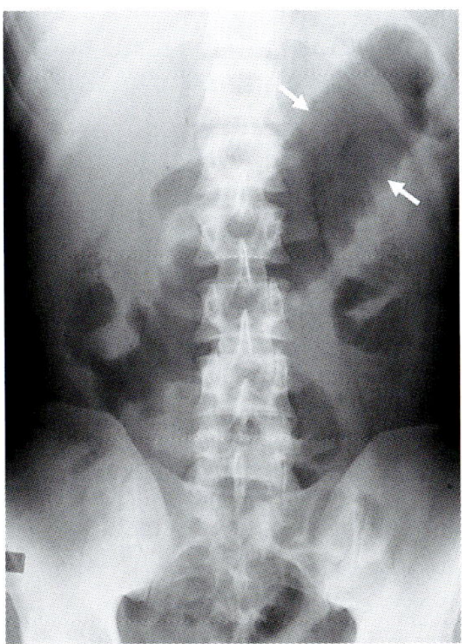

Fig. 2: Toxic megacolon.

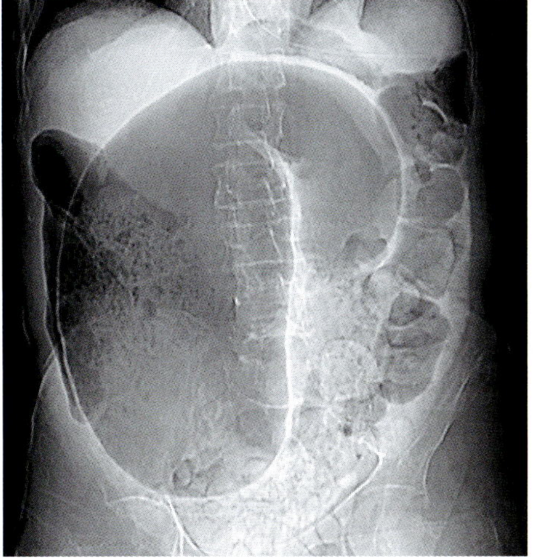

Fig. 4: Coffee bean appearance in Sigmoid volvulus.

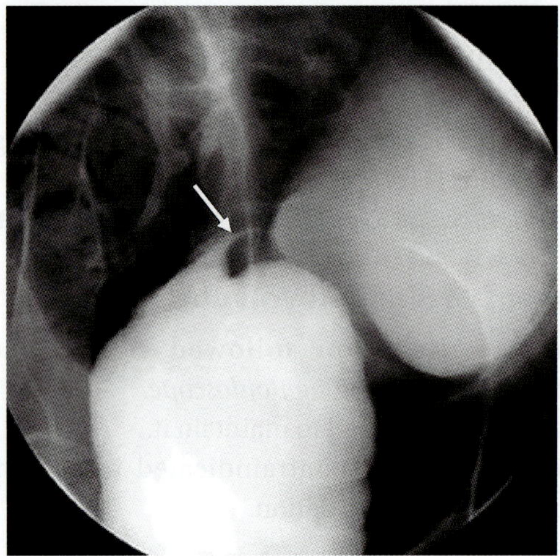

Fig. 5: Barium enema showing bird beak appearance in sigmoid volvulus.

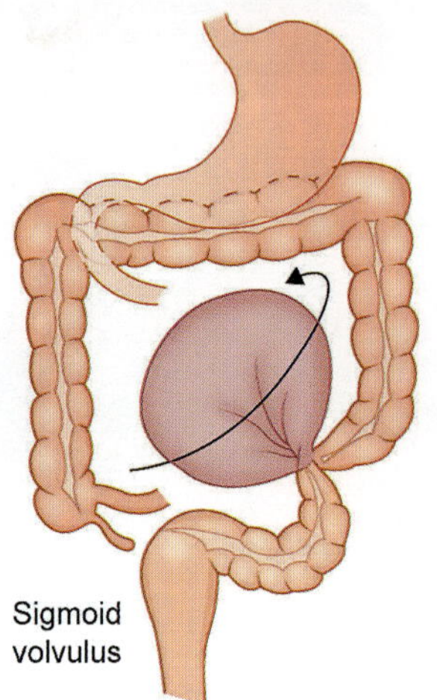

Fig. 6: Sigmoid volvulus.

- Recurrence rate is high.
- *Definitive treatment is sigmoid colectomy.*

Resections in Colon

- *Hartmann's operation:* Proximal end colostomy + resection of pathological bowel + distal stump closure and left inside; reversal will be done after 6 weeks **(Fig. 7)**.
- *Paul–Mikulicz operation:* Proximal colostomy and distal bowel brought out as fistula like double barrel colostomy **(Table 2)**.

INTRA-ABDOMINAL ABSCESS

- The most common site of intraperitoneal abscess is pelvis.

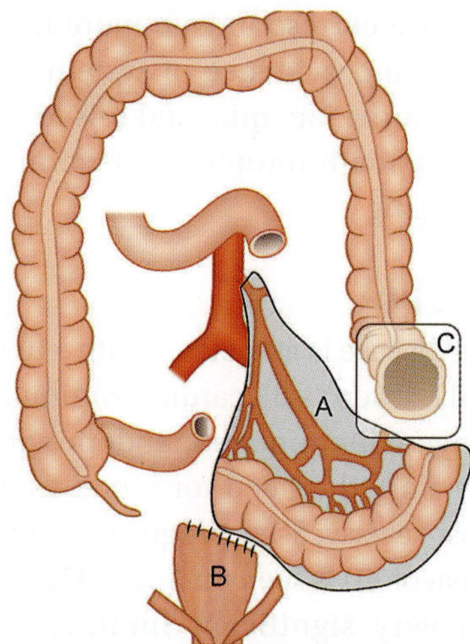

Fig. 7: Hartmann's procedure

TABLE 2: Emergency procedures based on location of obstruction and growth.

Site of obstruction	*Procedure*
Right colon	Right hemicolectomy with ileo transverse anastomosis/terminal ileostomy with distal mucus fistula
Sigmoid colon	• Hartmann's operation • Paul–Mikulicz operation • Sigmoid colectomy with primary colorectal anastomosis
Cancer RECTUM	Loop transverse or sigmoid colostomy

- Right subhepatic space (Rutherford Morison's Pouch) is the most dependent portion of abdominal cavity in recumbent position.
- Pelvic cavity is the most dependent portion of abdominal cavity in upright position.
- Computed tomography (CT) scan is the IOC of intra-abdominal abscess.
- *Treatment of choice:* CECT guided drainage of abscess

Subphrenic spaces:
- Intraperitoneal
  - *Left anterior (left subphrenic space):* Splenic abscess
  - *Left posterior (lesser sac):* Pancreatitis, perforated posterior gastric ulcer
  - *Right anterior (right subphrenic space):* Appendix, gall bladder, and intestinal infections
  - *Right posterior (right subhepatic- Morison's):* The most common site of subphrenic abscess
- *Extraperitoneal spaces:*
  - *Right:* Bare area of liver
  - *Left:* Lies around left suprarenal and kidney—site for perinephric abscess

Left Subhepatic Space (Lesser Sac)

- The most common cause of infection here is complicated acute pancreatitis. In practice, a perforated gastric ulcer rarely causes a collection here because the potential space is obliterated by adhesions.
- When perforated gastric ulcer happens into lesser sac there will be no generalized peritonitis and it will be difficult to diagnose.

Right Subhepatic Space (Rutherford Morison Pouch)

- Common causes of abscess here are perforating cholecystitis, a perforated duodenal ulcer, a duodenal cap "blow-out" following gastrectomy and appendicitis
- Most dependent part of abscess in supine patient.

CHAPTER 12

Rectum and Anus Emergencies

R Rajamahendran

ANORECTAL ABSCESS

- Most common type of anal abscess is perianal abscess.
- Second most common is ischiorectal abscess.
- Most common reason for ischiorectal abscess is poor blood supply.
- Ischiorectal abscess spreads from one side to other in a horseshoe-shaped tract.
- Anorectal abscess is drained by cruciate incision **(Fig. 1)**.

HORSESHOE ABSCESS

- Ischiorectal abscess extending both sides in a horseshoe pattern is called horseshoe abscess **(Fig. 2)**.
- Modified Hanley's technique is used for drainage of this abscess.

PROLAPSED HEMORRHOIDS (GRADE-4 HEMORRHOIDS)

- These patients come to hospital with severe bleeding associated with pain.
- On examination, the pile mass is found outside and not reducible as shown in **Figure 3**.
- These patients are initially treated with glycerine oil + magnesium sulphate powder packs, which may reduce the edema and help in reduction.
- Ideally, open hemorrhoidectomy by Milligan-Morgan operation is done after the edema gets reduced **(Fig. 4)**.

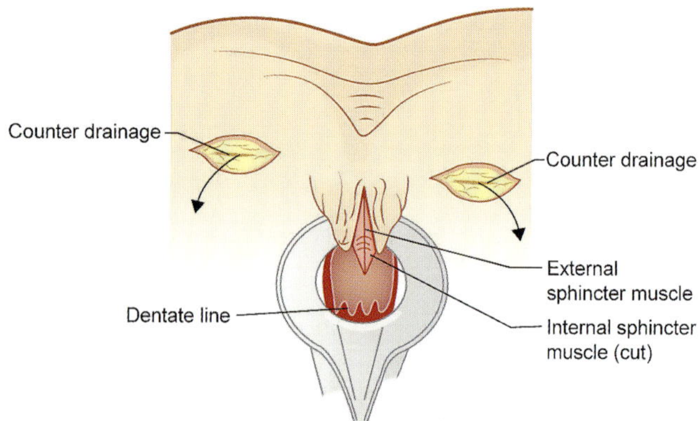

Fig. 2: Horseshoe abscess.

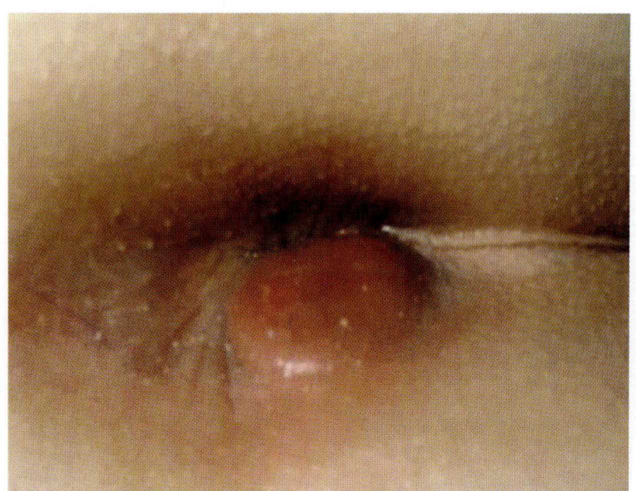

Fig. 1: Perianal abscess.

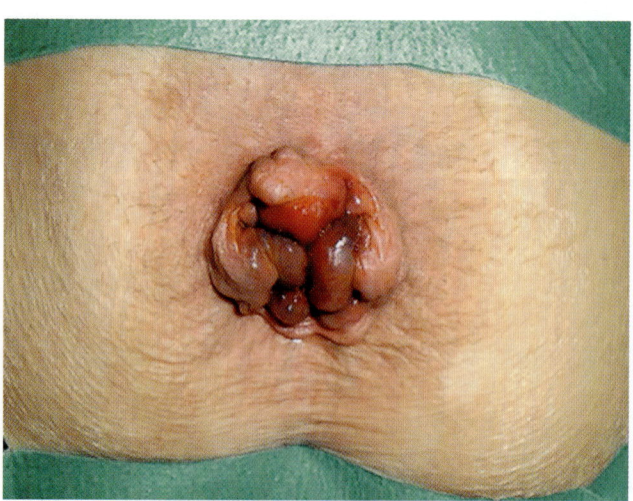

Fig. 3: Hemorrhoids.

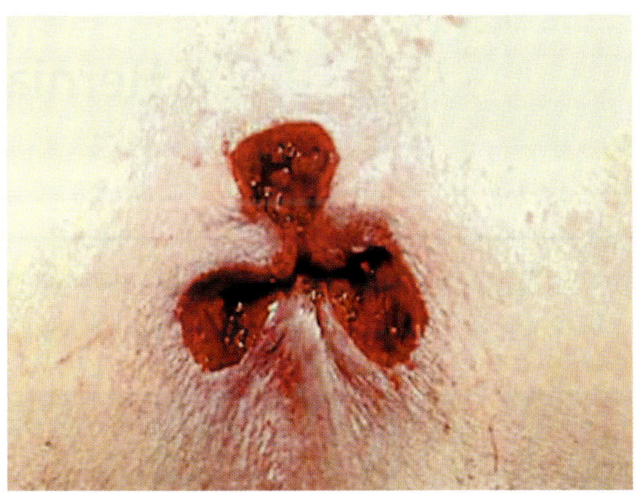

Fig. 4: Open hemorrhoidectomy.

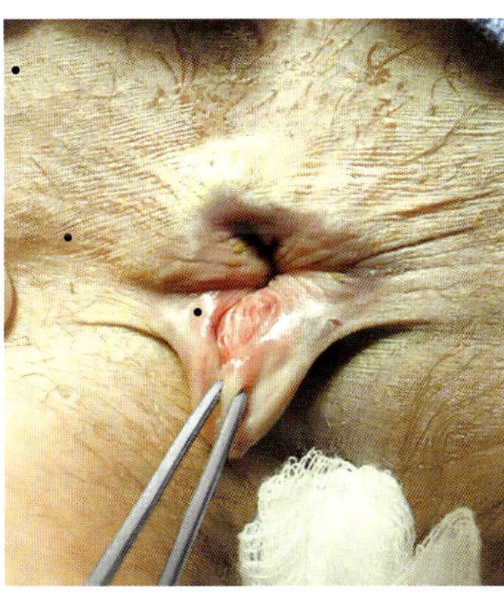

Fig. 5: Posterior fissure in ano.

- Many newer techniques such as stapler, laser are all available now, but not used in emergency settings.

ACUTE FISSURE IN ANO

- It is a tear in anal mucosa that is pain sensitive.
- It is most common in 6 o'clock.
- *In pregnancy:* 12 o'clock
- *In Crohn's:* Lateral positions
- *Clinical features:* Severe painful defecation with spasm and bleeding per rectal examination
- *Sentinel tag:* Protective tag present in chronic fissure **(Fig. 5)**.

Management

- *Conservative:* Laxatives, glyceryl trinitrate ointment local application, diltiazem application, and sitz bath.
- *Surgical treatment of choice:* Lateral sphincterotomy—internal sphincter cut at lateral position (3/9 o'clock position)—Notara's operation.

CHAPTER 13

Hernia

R Rajamahendran

OBSTRUCTED INGUINAL HERNIAS

Management

- *Resuscitation:* Nasal oxygen and intravenous fluids.
- Parenteral antibiotics.
- Delay should not be made for operation.
  - "Danger is in delay not in operation"

Take the patient to operation theatre under general anesthesia.

Steps at operation:

- Paint with povidone iodine from xiphisternum to midthigh (may need laparotomy for nonviable bowel).
- Inguinoscrotal incision made.
- Before separating the sac from cord structures, open the *fundus of sac first* to release the toxic contents.
- If you push the toxic fluid into the abdomen, peritonitis may develop.
- Constriction is usually seen in 50% cases at deep ring and 50% cases at superficial ring.
- Look for the bowel viability and hold the bowel before releasing the constriction with hernia director (grooved hernia director).
- Normal bowel is pinkish red; peristalsis seen, glistening.
- In such cases push the bowel inside and do herniorrhaphy.

If bowel is not viable (gangrenous, lusture less, and no peristalsis) ***(Fig. 1)****:*

- Keep a warm pad over the bowel.
- 100% oxygen given nasal.
- Wait for 10 minutes with oxygen and examine the bowel again.
- If viable, put it back in the abdomen.
- If nonviable, abdomen is opened through midline incision.

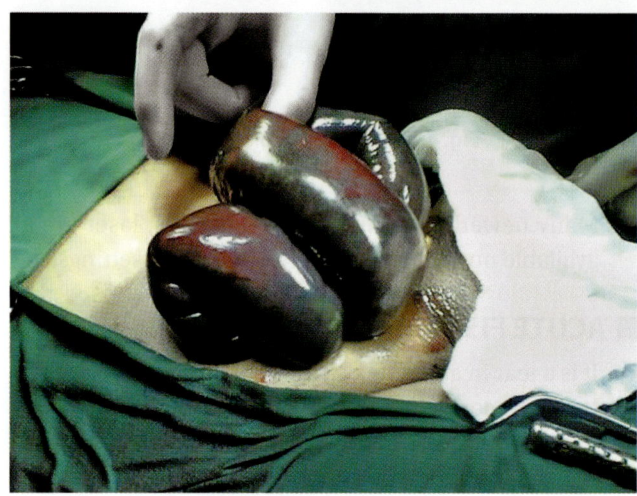

Fig. 1: Strangulated bowel.

What will you do in Gangrene Content?

Nonviable bowel:

- *Small bowel:* End-to-end resection anastomosis.
- *Omentum:* Excise the gangrenous part.

Large bowel:

Patients who are unfit for resection and anastomosis, the following procedure is done in emergency.

- *Hartmann's operation* ***(Figs. 2A and B)****:* Gangrenous colon is excised and the proximal end is brought out as colostomy and distal end is closed and left inside temporarily. 6 weeks later reanastomosis is done.

Strangulation in Maydl's Hernia

- *Maydl's hernia (Retrograde strangulation)* is "W" shaped hernia **(Fig. 3)**.
- Gangrene in the obstructed bowel starts first at the neck of sac, then immediately at the antimesenteric border distally.

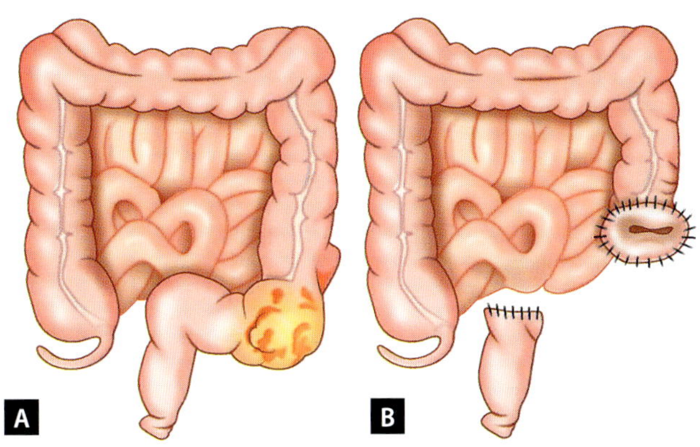

Figs. 2A and B: Hartman's operation.

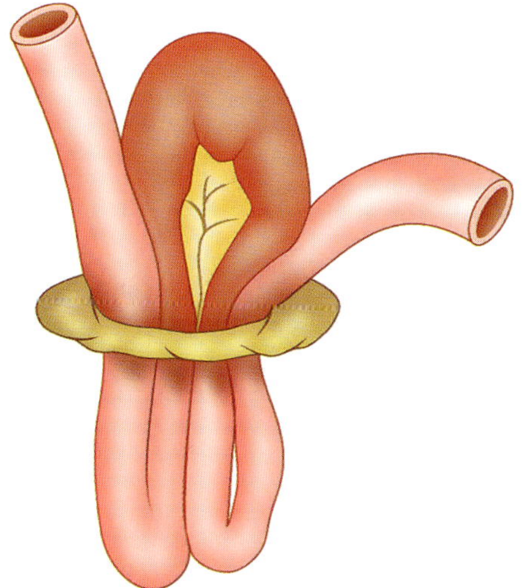

Fig. 3: Maydl's hernia.

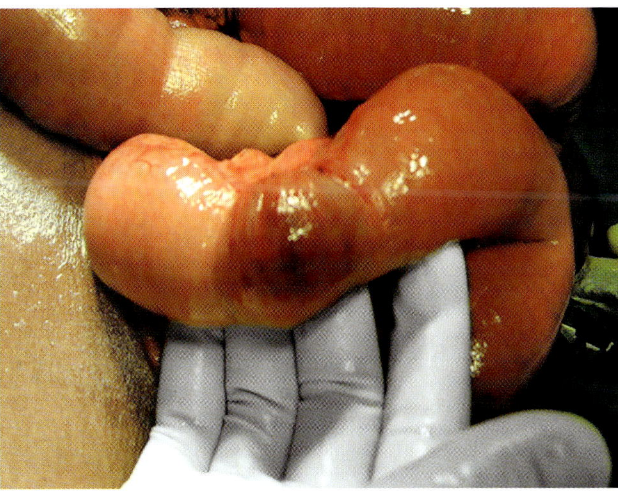

Fig. 4: Richter's hernia.

- Therefore, in Maydl's hernia, the distal antimesenteric border is inside the abdomen, which goes for strangulation first.
- Hence, look for the full length of intestine by pulling out the loop inside the abdomen.

RICHTER'S HERNIA

- A portion of the circumference of the intestine becomes the content of the sac **(Fig. 4)**.
- Strangulation occurs when associated with femoral or obturator hernia.
- Diarrhea is seen in cases of strangulation.
- Unless more than half of the circumference is involved, there is no constipation.

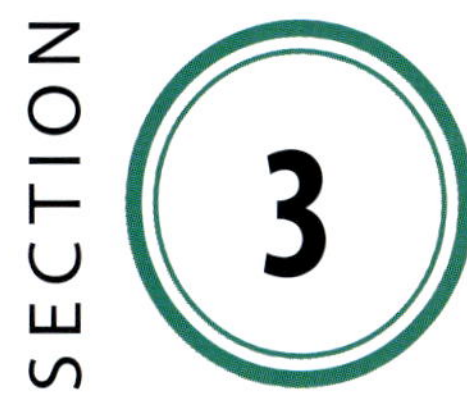

Hepatobiliary Pancreatic Emergencies

CHAPTER 14

Gallbladder

R Rajamahendran

INTRODUCTION

- One of the most common diseases of gallbladder in surgical practice is gallstones.
- More than 90% of gallstones remain silent without any symptoms.
- Symptomatic gallstones are the ones that result in various complications and have to be operated by laparoscopic cholecystectomy.

Various emergencies can result from the complications of gallstones, which are given as follows:

- Acute cholecystitis—most common complication
- Chronic cholecystitis
- Mucocele
- Empyema
- Gangrene
- Gallstone ileus
- Mirizzi syndrome
- Cholangitis due to common bile duct (CBD) obstruction
- Pancreatitis

ACUTE CHOLECYSTITIS

- Acute cholecystitis is the most common complication of gallstones, where the biliary colicky pain persists for >24 hours.
- This is because of the obstruction of the cystic duct by a small stone or due to edema causing bile infection inside the gallbladder.

Clinical Features

- Patient complaints of persistent pain in the right hypochondrium for >24 hours.
- On examination:
    - Murphy's sign is positive.

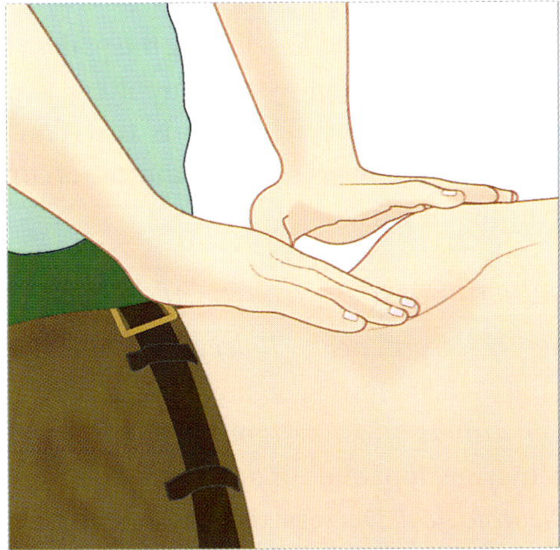

Fig. 1: Moynihan's method of examination.

    - In Moynihan's method of examination, patient is examined in lying down position showing tenderness in the right subcostal region **(Fig. 1)**.
    - Boas' sign is hyperesthesia in the right subcostal region.
- If the infection becomes severe, the patient develops fever and sepsis features.
- A grading system is used to classify and manage acute cholecystitis called as Tokyo guidelines.
- Ultrasonography (USG) is enough to confirm the diagnosis. Findings seen are:
    - Thickened gallbladder wall >3 mm
    - Pericholecystic fluid or edema
    - Sludge or stone in the gallbladder (GB)

Management

- 90% of acute cholecystitis subsides with conservative measures.
- Nonoperative treatment is based on 4 principles:
    1. Nil oral and intravenous (IV) fluids until pain resolves.
    2. Analgesics

3. Antibiotics (as the cystic duct is blocked, we have to give antibiotics that will concentrate in serum rather than in bile, e.g., cefazolin, cefuroxime, and ciplox)
4. Once the temperature and physical signs subside, oral fluids are started and investigations are done such USG; magnetic resonance cholangiopancreatography (MRCP), if jaundice is there; and computed tomography (CT) scan, if perforation is suspected.

- Recently, acute cholecystitis is taken for early cholecystectomy (within 7 days).
- Many criteria are used in selecting the patient for early surgery or interval cholecystectomy after 6 weeks.
- Laparoscopic cholecystectomy is the treatment of choice for acute cholecystitis, but the rate of conversion to open cholecystectomy is high.

Management Based on "Tokyo Guidelines"

- *Grade III (severe) acute cholecystitis:* Associated with any one of the following organ dysfunction:
  - *Cardiovascular system (CVS):* Hypotension requiring dopamine or noradrenaline
  - *Neurological:* Decreased consciousness level
  - *Respiratory:* PaO_2/FiO_2 ratio <300
  - *Renal dysfunction:* Oliguria: creatinine > 2 mg/dL
  - *Liver dysfunction:* Prothrombin time (PT)-International Normalized Ratio (INR) elevated
  - *Hematological dysfunction*: Platelet count <1 lakh/mm^3
- *Grade II (moderate cholecystitis)*
  - Elevated white blood cell (WBC) count >18,000/mm^3
  - Palpable tender mass in right upper quadrant
  - Duration of complaints >72 hours
  - Marked local inflammation (gangrene, abscess, biliary peritonitis, and emphysematous cholecystitis)
- *Grade I (mild acute cholecystitis)*
  - Grade 1 has none of the earlier-mentioned features.
  - Healthy person with mild inflammations only
  - Cholecystectomy is a safe and low risk procedure.
  - Most grade I and II cases are taken up for early laparoscopic cholecystectomy if patient is fit for surgery.
  - In grade III high-risk cases, sometimes if patient is unfit for a cholecystectomy, a percutaneous cholecystostomy can be performed by Radiologist **(Fig. 2)**.

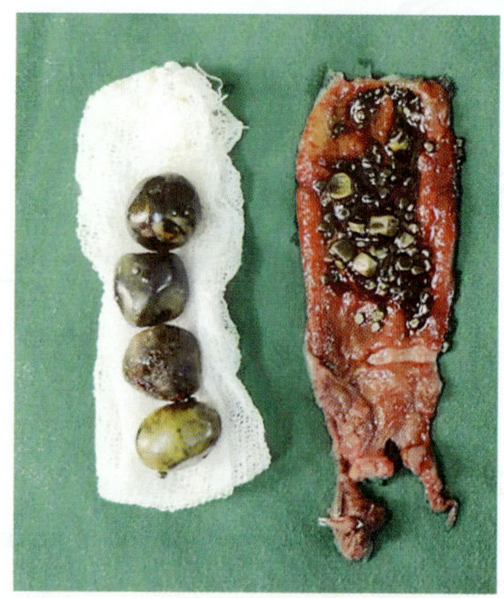

Fig. 2: Laparoscopic cholecystectomy—early surgery done for acute cholecystitis.

MUCOCELE

- Obstruction of stone at *neck* of GB results in collection of mucus inside the GB. The mucocele can get infected forming empyema or gangrene of GB.
- *Treatment:* Early cholecystectomy **(Figs. 3A to C)**

MIRIZZI SYNDROME

- Mirizzi syndrome refers to the obstruction or stricture of the common hepatic duct as result of extrinsic compression by a gallstone in the cystic duct or Hartmann's pouch in GB.
- As per *Csendes classification*, 5 types are there **(Fig. 4)**.
  1. *Type 1 (11%):* Extrinsic compression of common hepatic duct (CHD) by a large stone in neck of GB
  2. *Type 2 (41%):* Stone has now eroded into the hepatic duct to form a fistula involving less than one-third of circumference.
  3. *Type 3 (44%):* Lesions involve two-third of circumference.
  4. *Type 4 (<4%):* Completely destroyed hepatic duct **(Figs. 5A and B)**.
  5. *Type 5:* Associated with cholecystoenteric fistula.

FISTULAS FROM GALLBLADDER

- Most common site is duodenum (cholecystoenteric fistula)
- Diagnosis suspicious by presence of air in bile duct.
- *Complication:* Gallstone ileus
- *Other sites of fistula:* Colon

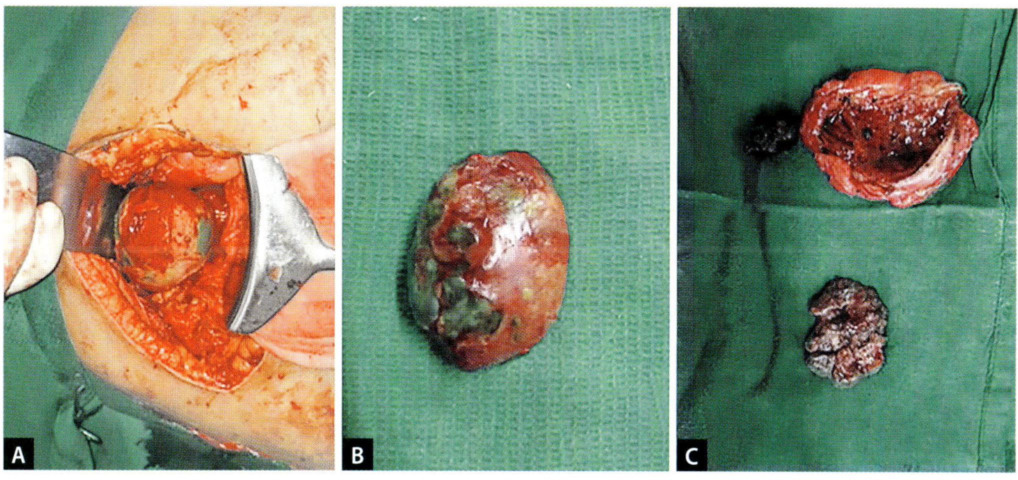

Figs. 3A to C: Infected gangrenous gallbladder.

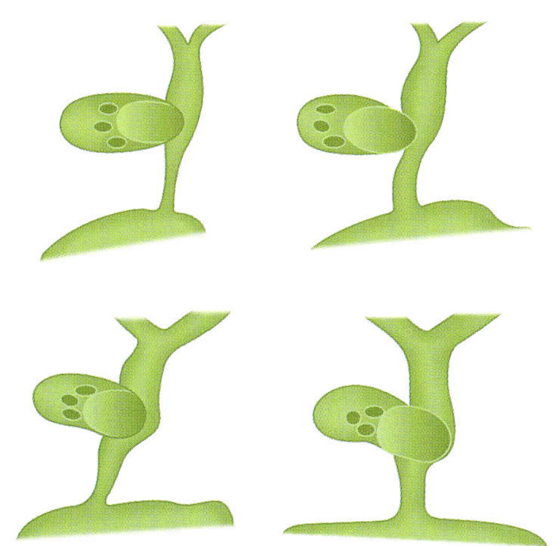

Fig. 4: Mirizzi syndrome—Csendes classification.

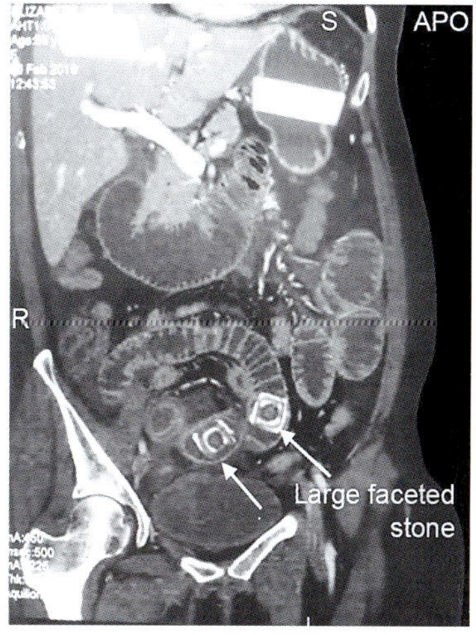

Fig. 6: Gallstone obstructing in the bowel.

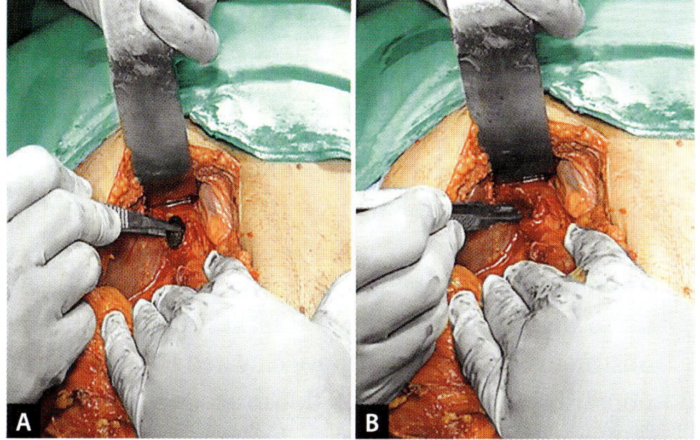

Figs. 5A and B: Gallstone eroding into bile duct.

Gallstone Ileus

- Gallstone ileus is characterized by tumbling intermittent small intestine obstruction by the gallstone, which has passed via the choledochoduodenal fistula.
- *Rigler's triad:* Pneumobilia, intestinal obstruction, and cholecystoenteric fistula **(Fig. 6)**
- Duodenal obstruction due to gallstones usually in the bulb is known as Bouveret's syndrome **(Figs. 7A and B)**
- Most common in old age > 70 years
- Most common site of obstruction is terminal ileum.
- *Management:*
  - *Stable cases:* Enterotomy and stone removal + closure of fistula + cholecystectomy **(Fig. 8)**

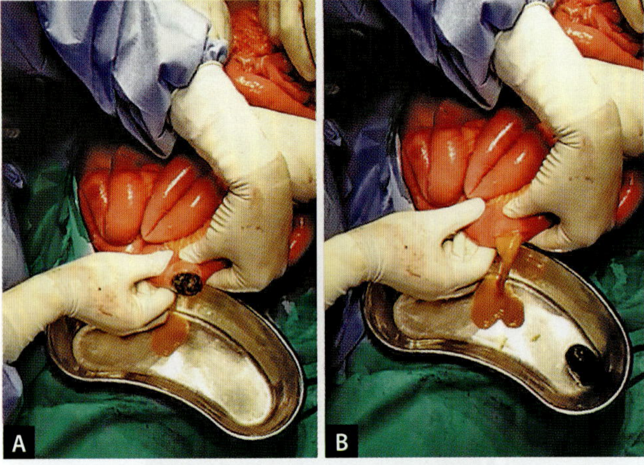

Figs. 7A and B: Gallstone obstructing the bowel removed.

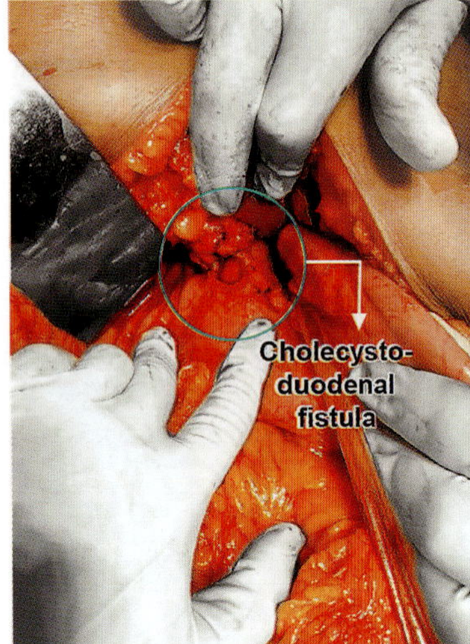

Fig. 8: Fistula between gallbladder (GB) and duodenum.

- *Unstable cases:* Only stone removal and obstruction relief

ACALCULOUS CHOLECYSTITIS

- Acute inflammation of GB without gallstones.
- Incidence is 5–10%.
- Highest mortality
- Most common in patients recovering from major surgery (such as abdominal aneurysm repair/ cardiopulmonary bypass), burns, trauma, and in patients on long-term total parenteral nutrition (TPN)
- *Uncommon causes:* GB torsion and adenocancers, *Leptospira*, *Streptococcus*, *Salmonella*, *Vibrio*, and parasitic infections.
- Most commonly missed diagnosis and most commonly progresses to empyema, gangrene, and perforation.
- Ultrasonographyis the investigation of choice (IOC)
- Hepatobiliary iminodiacetic acid scan (HIDA) scan demonstrates absent gallbladder filling. It is done only in doubtful cases.
- Most important causative factors are GB stasis and ischemia.
- *Best treatment is emergency open cholecystectomy.*
- *If unfit for surgery, percutaneous cholecystotomy (USG drainage of gallbladder)*

CHOLANGITIS

Inflammation of biliary duct due to obstruction of the bile duct.

Etiological factors:

- Common bile duct (CBD) stone (Most common cause)
- Endoscopic retrograde cholangiopancreatography (ERCP)
- Benign and malignant strictures
- Parasites

Most common organisms: Escherichia coli, Klebsiella, Streptococcus faecalis, and Bacteroides.

Clinical Features

- *Most common presentation:* Fever with chills and rigors
- *Charcot's triad:* CBD stone causing cholangitis:
  1. Pain
  2. Jaundice
  3. Rigors
- *Reynold's pentad:* Includes Charcot's triad + septic shock + mental status changes

Treatment of Cholangitis

- Immediately start intravenous (IV) fluids and broad-spectrum antibiotics.
- Urgent biliary decompression is the priority in management of cholangitis if they do not respond to antibiotics.
- Prothrombin time/INR must be done before proceeding to any surgical intervention as these patients having obstructive jaundice may have elevated PT/INR due to nonabsorption of vitamin K due to absence of bile salts (vitamin K is essential for production of the factors 2, 7, 9, and 10).

Flowchart 1: Management of common bile duct (CBD) stones.

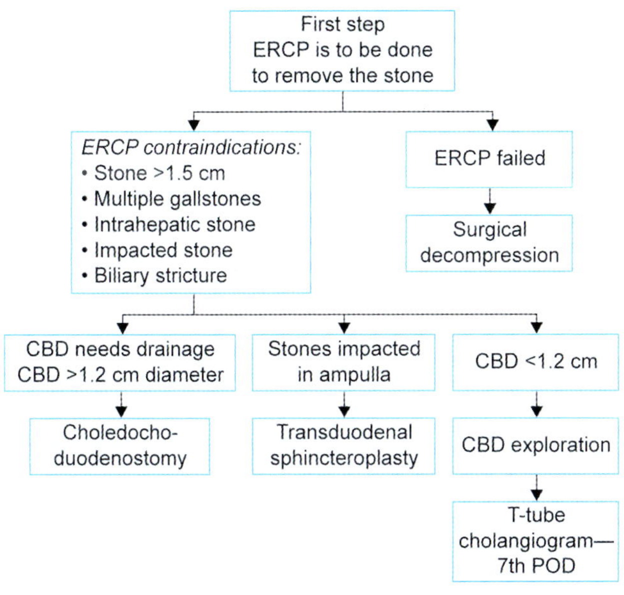

(ERCP: Endoscopic retrograde cholangiopancreatography; POD: postoperative day)

- *Correction of PT/INR:* Injection vitamin K is given or in cases of emergency, fresh frozen plasma is given to prevent severe bleeding during any intervention.

Protocol for management of CBD stones is given in **Flowchart 1**.

Management of common bile duct (CBD) stone:
- *In presence of cholangitis:*
  - ERCP with sphincterotomy and stone extraction (Treatment of choice)
  - *Percutaneous biliary drainage:* ERCP failed cases
  - *Surgery:* Only when above two procedures not possible, decompression of CBD with T-tube is done.
- *CBD exploration and T-tube removal:* A T-tube cholangiogram is taken about 5–7 days after the operation. If it appears normal, the tube is removed *on day 7 or 8 by gentle traction.*
- *Author's preference: The author and most gastrosurgeons prefer to remove the T-tube after 14 days.*

Figures 9A to C show ERCP and stone removal and **Figures 9D to F** show CBD exploration and T-tube placement.

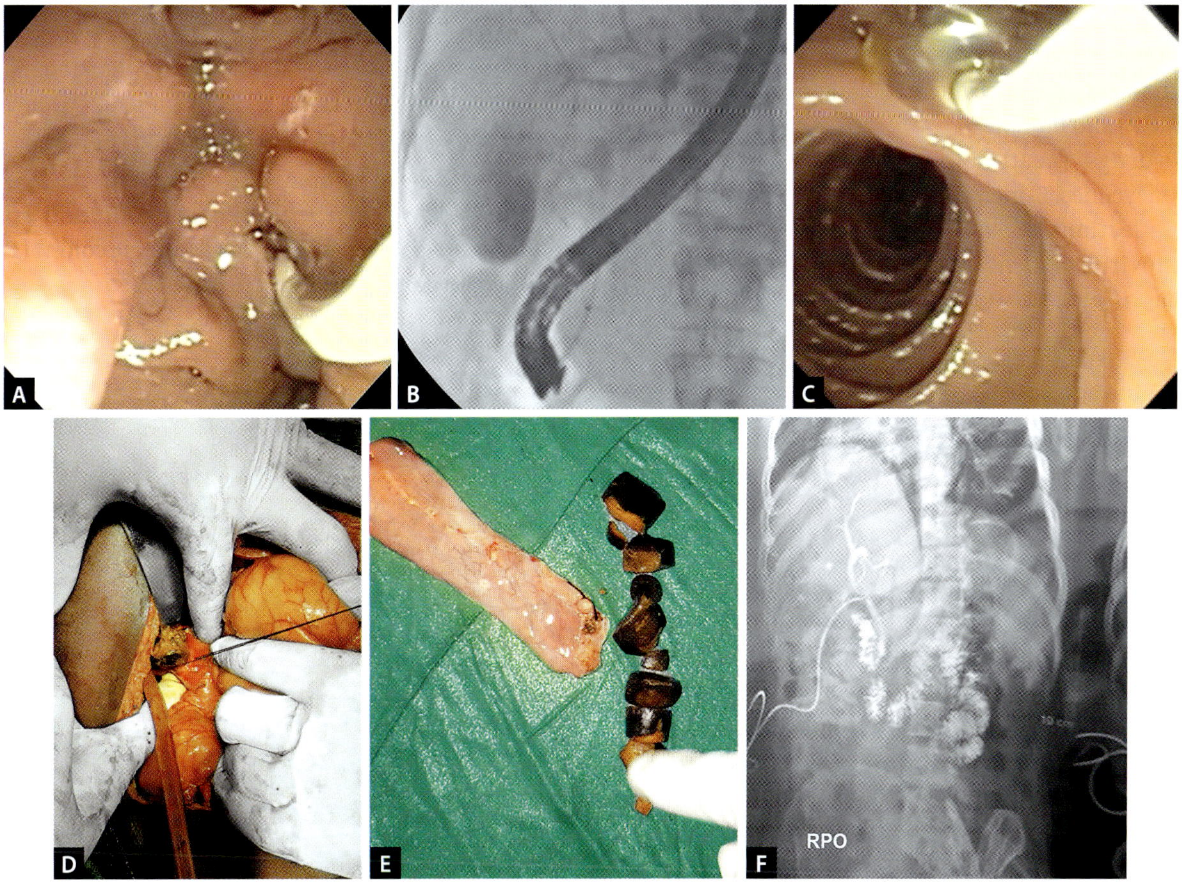

Figs. 9A to F: (A to C) Endoscopic retrograde cholangiopancreatography (ERCP) and stone removal; (D and E) Common bile duct (CBD) stone removal; (F) T-tube cholangiogram.

CHAPTER 15

Pancreatic Emergencies

R Rajamahendran

ACUTE PANCREATITIS

Etiology of Pancreatitis (GET-SMASHED-I)

- *G*—gallstones (most common cause in adults)
- *E*—ethanol
- *T*—trauma (most common cause in children)
- *S*—steroids
- *M*—mumps
- *A*—autoimmune [polyarteritis nodosa (PAN), systemic lupus erythematosus (SLE), etc.]
- *S*—scorpion venom
- *H*—hyperlipidemia, hypercalcemia, and hypothermia
- *E*—endoscopic retrograde cholangiopancreatography (ERCP) and emboli
- *D*—drugs (azathioprine, thiazides, furosemide, tetracyclines, 6-mercaptopurine, etc.)
- *I*—infections [Coxsackie, *Cytomegalovirus* (CMV), echovirus, *Ascaris lumbricoides*, and *clonorchis sinensis*, etc.]

Drugs that cause acute pancreatitis are:
- Corticosteroids
- Azathioprine
- Asparaginase
- Valproic acid
- Thiazide diuretics
- Estrogens

Pathophysiology

- As a result of pancreatic injury, inflammatory mediators such as tumor necrosis factor alpha (TNF- α) and interleukin 1 (IL-1) are mainly released.
- This stimulates more and more mediators of inflammation such as IL-2, 6, 8, 10, bradykinin, and platelet-activating factors, which results in systemic inflammatory response syndrome (SIRS) and multiple organ dysfunction syndrome (MODS).

Symptoms	*Signs*
• Pain • Nausea • Vomiting • Retching • Hiccough • Sudden abdominal pain with partial relief on leaning forward *(Mohammed prayer sign)* **(Fig. 1)**	• Tachypnea • Tachycardia • Hypotension • Icterus • Facial flushing • *Grey Turner's sign:* Hemorrhagic pigmentation around the flanks • *Cullen's sign:* Pigmentation around umbilicus **(Fig. 2)** • *Fox sign:* Inguinal ecchymosis • Abdominal distension—ileus • Ascites

Radiology Findings

- *Sentinel loop* of jejunum
- *Colon cut-off sign* (gas-filled hepatic and splenic flexures separated by gasless transverse colon) **(Fig. 3)**
- Calcified gallstones

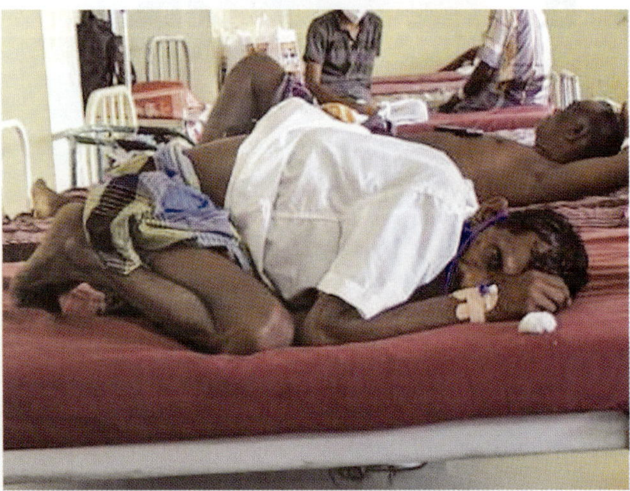

Fig. 1: Mohammed prayer sign.

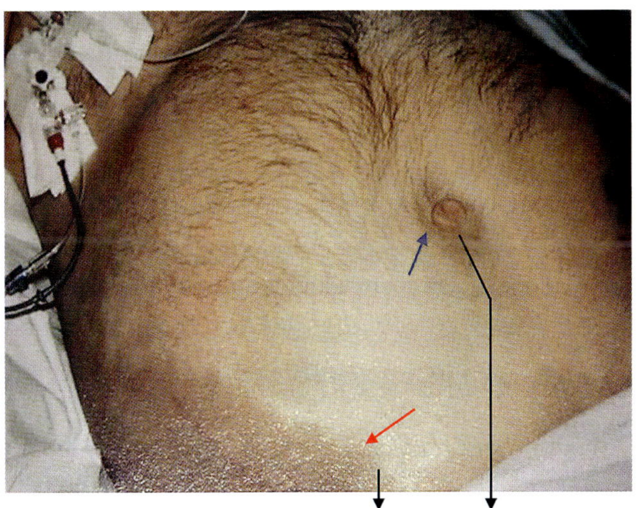

Fig. 2: Cullen's sign (blue arrow) and Grey Turner (red arrow) sign.

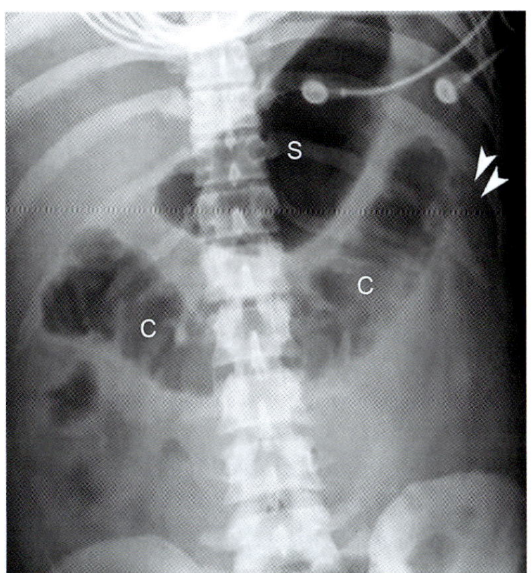

Fig. 3: Colon cut-off sign.

Investigations

- Serum amylase (three-fold elevation seen) in the initial 24–48 hours
- *Serum lipase: Most specific*
- Serum lipase will be more sensitive after 24–48 hours.
- Elevation of alanine transaminase (ALT) implies *acute gallstone pancreatitis* (95% sensitive)
- Urinary amylase may be more accurate than serum amylase and may be elevated for several days.
- Serum trypsin
- *Hyperglycemia*
- *Hypocalcemia*

Latest Updates

Imaging investigations:

- *Computed tomography (CT) scan:* Multidetector CT scan is the imaging investigation of choice (IOC)
- *Ideal phase:* Portal venous phase (60–70 seconds after contrast injection)
- *To look for necrosis:* CT scan must be taken after 72 hours of onset of symptoms
- Magnetic resonance cholangiopancreatography (MRCP) is used in suspected cases of gallstone pancreatitis

Normal serum amylase is seen in following cases:

- Greater than 3 days after attack
- Massive gland destruction
- Completely destroyed gland by previous attacks
- In hyperlipidemia-induced acute pancreatitis, the amylase level may be normal.

Prediction of Severity of Acute Pancreatitis

Prognostic indicators:

- *Ranson's scoring:* Most widely used—*>3 is severe.*
- *Acute Physiology and Chronic Health Evaluation 2 (APACHE 2):* >8 is severe.
- Modified Glasgow scoring
- Computed tomography severity index (CTSI) **(Table 1)**/ Balthazar et al. scoring are based on contrast-enhanced

TABLE 1: Computed tomography (CT) severity index for acute pancreatitis.

Feature	*Points*
Pancreatic inflammation	
Normal pancreas	0
Focal or diffuse pancreatic enlargement	1
Intrinsic pancreatic alterations with peripancreatic fat inflammatory changes	2
Single fluid collection or phlegmon	3
Two or more fluid collections or gas, in or adjacent to the pancreas	4
Pancreatic necrosis	
None	0
≤30%	2
30–50%	4
>50%	6

computed tomography scan (CECT) scan and necrosis in pancreas.

- *C-reactive protein:* >150 mg/dL is severe.
- Bedside index for severity in acute pancreatitis (BISAP) score
- Revised Atlanta scoring (RAS) system

Bedside index for severity of acute pancreatitis (BISAP) scoring:

The more recently proposed (BISAP) is calculated from:

- *B*—blood urea nitrogen (>25 mg/dL)
- *I*—impaired mental status [Glasgow Coma Scale (GCS) <15]
- *S*—systemic inflammatory response syndrome (SIRS)
- *A*—age >60 years
- *P*—pleural effusion

It can be performed in first 24 hours

Ranson's Scoring

Mnemonic to remember Ranson's score is "LAGAW-BUCHOW".

On admission	Within 48 hours
• L—lactate dehydrogenase (LDH) >700 u/L • A—aspartate aminotransferase (AST) >250 sigma Frankel units % • G—Glucose >10 mmol/L • A—Age >55 years • W—white blood cell (WBC) count >16,000/mm^3	• B—base deficit > 4 mmol/L • U—blood urea nitrogen >5 mg% • C—calcium < 2.0 mmol/L • H—hematocrit fall > 10% • O—arterial O_2 saturation (PaO_2) <60 mm Hg • W—water sequestration >6 litres

APACHE-II Scoring

There are 12 factors.

General examination:

- Pulse rate
- Blood pressure (BP)
- Respiratory rate
- Temperature

Blood values:

- Creatinine
- White blood cell count
- Sodium
- Potassium
- Hematocrit

Arterial blood gas analysis:

- Oxygenation
- Arterial pH
- Glassgow Coma Scale

TABLE 2: Correlation of computed tomography severity index (CTSI) score with morbidity and mortality in acute pancreatitis.

CTSI score	Morbidity	Mortality
0–3	8%	3%
4–6	35%	6%
7–10	92%	17%

Correlation of CTSI score with morbidity and mortality in acute pancreatitis is given in **Table 2**.

Atlanta Criteria for Acute Pancreatitis

Organ failure, as defined by:

- Shock [systolic blood pressure (BP) <90 mm Hg]
- Pulmonary insufficiency [partial pressure of arterial oxygen (PaO_2) <60 mm Hg]
- Renal failure (creatinine level >2 mg/dL after fluid resuscitation)
- Gastrointestinal bleeding (>500 mL/24 hour)

Systemic complications:

- Disseminated intravascular coagulation (platelet count ≤100,000)
- Fibrinogen <1 g/L
- Fibrin split products >80 µg/dL
- Metabolic disturbance (calcium level ≤7.5 mg/dL)

Local complications:

- Necrosis
- Abscess
- Pseudocyst
- *As per Atlanta criteria, acute severe pancreatitis is presence of one organ failure or a local complication.*
- *Example: If a patient has low BP or a pseudocyst, it is a case of severe pancreatitis.*

Recent updates:

- Ranson's scoring includes all except serum amylase and serum lipase.
- Ranson's scoring is not used nowadays because the important factors to predict severity range between 0–48 hours.
- APACHE-II scoring advantage is that it can be scored at any time and can be repeated easily (but it is a more complex scoring).
- Revised Atlanta classification is used to classify acute pancreatitis complications.

Management of Acute Pancreatitis

- *Key for survival is intravenous (IV) fluids. Fluids are infused adequately to have a urine output >0.5 mL/kg/hour*

- Nonsteroidal anti-inflammatory drugs (NSAIDs) of choice is *metamizole* for mild pain and buprenorphine for severe pain.
- Best fluid of choice to resuscitate is Ringer lactate.
- Investigation imaging of choice is *CECT abdomen after 72 hours.*
- *Enteral nutrition must be started in 24 hours via a nasogastric (NG) tube* in mild cases of acute pancreatitis.
- Supplement oxygen
- Invasive monitoring of central venous pressure (CVP), urine output, and blood gas analysis
- Monitor liver function test (LFT), renal function test (RFT), coagulation profiles, serum calcium, and blood glucose.
- *Total parenteral nutrition (TPN) may be given if patient is in shock and having severe pancreatitis.*
- For gallstone pancreatitis without cholangitis, there is no need of ERCP (ERCP is indicated only if there is pancreatitis + cholangitis).
- No prophylactic antibiotics must be used. Antibiotics are used if there is confirmed infective necrosis.
- For gall stone pancreatitis, *index cholecystectomy* (performed during the same admission) for mild-to-moderate cases is recommended. For severe cases, cholecystectomy is done after 6 weeks.

Local Complications of Acute Pancreatitis

Usually develop after the 1st week.

- *Sterile and infected fluid collections:* Without epithelium
- *Pancreatic necrosis:* The nonviable pancreatic parenchyma is diagnosed by low attenuation value on CECT scan. The major complication of this is infection.
- *Infected pancreatic necrosis:*
    - 20% cases of acute pancreatitis develop pancreatic necrosis.
        - Organisms isolated are *Klebsiella*, *Escherichia coli*, *Pseudomonas* spp., etc.
        - Characterized by fever, unwellness, and increased white blood count (WBC) count.
        - Presence of air confirms the diagnosis.
        - CECT is the investigation of choice (IOC) for pancreatic necrosis.
        - Fine-needle aspiration cytology (FNAC) is advocated to confirm the infection in the necrosis.
        - Carbapenems are the drug of choice (DOC).
        - Surgical debridement is advocated in STEP-UP approach starting from percutaneous drainage to open drainage.
        - Patients who develop MODS will usually have pancreatic necrosis.
- *Pseudocysts:* Capsule formed by granulation tissue with no epithelium. It takes 4–8 weeks to form.
- *Pancreatic ascites:*
    - Pancreatic ascites is a high protein ascites [low serum ascites albumin gradient (SAAG) ascites/exudate].
    - Communication with pancreatic duct is seen in 80% cases.
    - 50–60% resolve with conservative management [nil oral, renal tubular acidosis (RTA), and somatostatin]
    - Repeated paracentesis was found helpful.
    - ERCP with pancreatic stenting is the initial treatment of choice for nonresolving cases.
- *Vascular complications:*
    - Most common vessel affected = Splenic artery
    - Pseudoaneurysms (due to elastase enzyme from pancreas) due to acute pancreatitis is most commonly seen in splenic artery
    - Most common vessel affected in vascular thrombosis is splenic vein thrombosis.

Systemic Complications of Acute Pancreatitis

Usually develops in 1st week.

- *Cardiovascular system (CVS):* Arrythmias and shock
- *Pulmonary:* Acute respiratory distress syndrome (ARDS)
- Renal failure
- Hematological: Disseminated intravascular coagulation (DIC)
- *Metabolic:* Hypocalcemia, hyperglycemia, and hyperlipidemia
- *Gastrointestinal:* Ileus
- *Neurological:* Visual problems and confused states
- *Miscellaneous:* Fat necrosis and arthralgia

Extra Edge

- Most common cause of death in these cases in multiple organ dysfunction syndrome (MODS)
- Mortality in first 2 weeks—MODS
- Mortality after 2 weeks—septic complications

PSEUDOCYSTS

- Pseudocysts *are the most common cause of cystic lesion in pancreas.*
- These are most common complication of chronic pancreatitis **(Fig. 4)**.
- It arises from acute pancreatic fluid collection (APFC) that has not resolved >4 weeks.
- Follows 10% of acute and 20–30% of chronic pancreatitis.
- Acute (3–4 weeks) and chronic (>6 weeks)
- Acute pseudocyst resolves spontaneously in 50% cases.
- *Complications:* Splenic vein thrombosis, splenic artery aneurysm, infection, duodenal obstruction, and hemorrhage.
- Infection is the most common complication.
- Usually, solitary. It is multiple in 17% cases.
- Elevated serum amylase level after an episode of acute pancreatitis gives the suspicion of pseudocyst.
- 80% of pseudocysts have communication to the duct, so internal drainage by endoscopic or surgical method is the best treatment.
- *Surgical options:* Cystogastrostomy, cystoduodenostomy, or cystojejunostomy (best method) based on the site.
- *Old concept:* Rule of 6: >6 cm and >6 weeks cyst must be operated *(New concept—pseudocyst of any size can be observed is they are asymptomatic).*

Factors that may cause delayed healing:

- Thick-walled pseudocysts
- Large >6 cm size

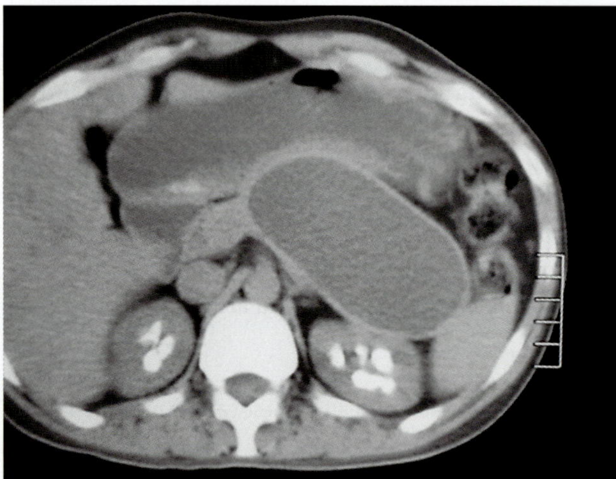

Fig. 4: Pseudocyst pancreas.

- Long time >12 weeks
- Cysts occurred from chronic pancreatitis

Above are the indications of intervention. Intervention is needed only if there is symptoms.

Intervention Methods of Pseudocyst

- Percutaneous drainage
- Endoscopic ultrasound (EUS)-guided puncture and drainage into stomach (cystogastrostomy)
- ERCP can be done and stent placed against the communication of the duct can resolve the pseudocyst with communication.
- Surgical cystogastrostomy or cystojejunostomy.

PANCREATIC NECROSIS

- Diffuse or focal area of nonviable parenchyma.
- Computed tomography (CT) scan used to diagnose this—absence of parenchymal; enhancement of contrast
- Pancreatic necrosis is associated with lysis of peripancreatic fat.
- This lysis leads to acute necrotic collection, with no definite wall in initial period.
- Over a period of 4 weeks, this may develop a pancreatic inflammatory capsule and known as walled off pancreatic necrosis (WOPN).
- Initially, necrosis is sterile, but as days prolong, the intestinal bacteria translocate and result in infection.
- Risk of mortality in infected necrosis = 50%

Management

- If there is no infection and if it is a sterile necrotic material, there is *no need to drain.*
- If there is sepsis and infection is collected, then it must be aspirated by *CT guidance* and if the aspirate if purulent, percutaneous drainage is done. Pus is sent for culture and appropriate antibiotics are used.
- If in spite of percutaneous aspiration, sepsis worsens then one must take the decision of *pancreatic necrosectomy* **(Figs. 5 and 6)**.
- *Necrosectomy can be done by following ways:*
  - Laparoscopic method
  - Midline abdominal incision
  - Retroperitoneal incision
  - In all above methods, blunt dissection is done and never use sharp instruments.

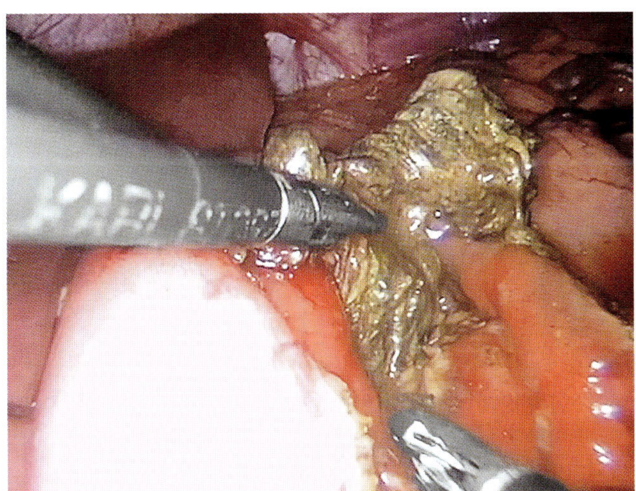

Fig. 5: Laparoscopic necrosectomy.

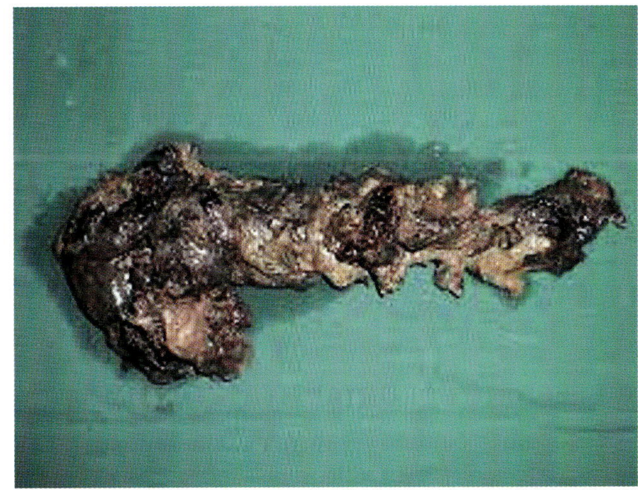

Fig. 6: Pancreatic necrotic tissue.

- After draining the necrotic materials, the following methods are used to drain the cavity:
  - Closed continuous lavage
  - Closed drainage
  - Open packing (reoperating at regular intervals)
  - Closure and relaparotomy—every 48–72 hours

CHAPTER 16

Liver Emergencies

R Rajamahendran

BLEEDING IN PORTAL HYPERTENSION

- The most common cause of bleeding in portal hypertension (PHT) patients is esophagogastric varices (esophagus 80% and gastric 20%).
- The only nonvariceal cause of portal hypertensive bleeding is PHT gastropathy.
- Esophagogastric varices will not bleed until the pressure exceeds 12 mm Hg.

Clinical Features

- Esophageal varices bleeding most commonly presents with massive hematemesis. hematochezia may be seen sometimes.
- Patient presents with hemorrhagic shock features.
- If Ryle's tube has been inserted elsewhere, there will be blood in the Ryle's tube.

Resuscitation

Step 1: Resuscitation

- Intravenous (IV) fluids are started.
- If this is a known case of esophageal variceal bleeding, Ryle's tube is avoided as it may injure the esophageal varices causing more bleeding when inserted blindly **(Fig. 1)**.
- *Injection octreotide (somatostatin analogue)* has been used more commonly now-a-days, it decreases the portal blood flow and reduces the pressure in portal vein.
- *Injection terlipressin* is very commonly used, but has the risk of coronary spasm and hence, must be given along with glyceryl trinitrate.

Step 2: Endoscopic Management

- Upper gastrointestinal (GI) endoscopy must be done at the earliest and is the investigation of choice **(Figs. 2A and B)**. It identifies the active bleeding from the esophageal varices and also the clotted blood in the stomach **(Figs. 1 and 3)**.
- Endoscopy can grade the varices:
  - *Grade 1:* Varices just above mucosal level
  - *Grade 2:* Enlarged varices occupies <one-third esophagus
  - *Grade 3:* Enlarged varices occupies >one-third esophagus
  - *Grade 4:* Cherry red spots and red wale marks are signs suggestive of varices about to rupture.
- Endoscopic banding is advantageous over sclerotherapy because it does not lead to necrosis or ulceration of esophagus but both are equally effective in controlling bleeding **(Fig. 4)**.
- Sclerosants used are ethanolamine oleate, cyanoacrylate, sodium morrhuate, or sodium tetradecyl sulphate.

Step 3: Sengstaken–Blakemore Tube (Figs. 5 and 6)

- When endoscopic procedure fails, we have to insert Sengstaken–Blakemore tube.

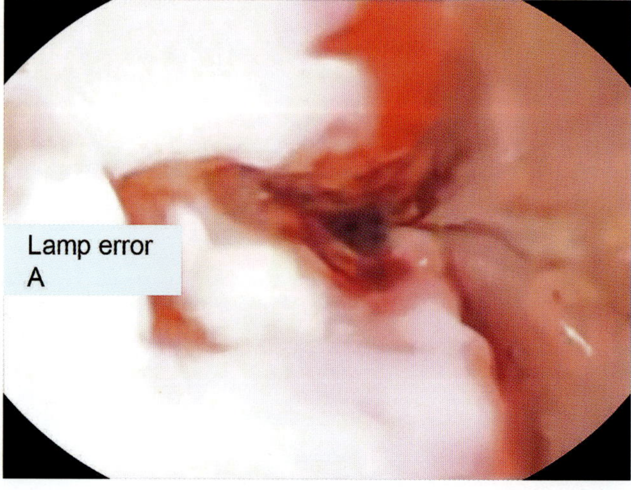

Fig. 1: Active bleeding varices.

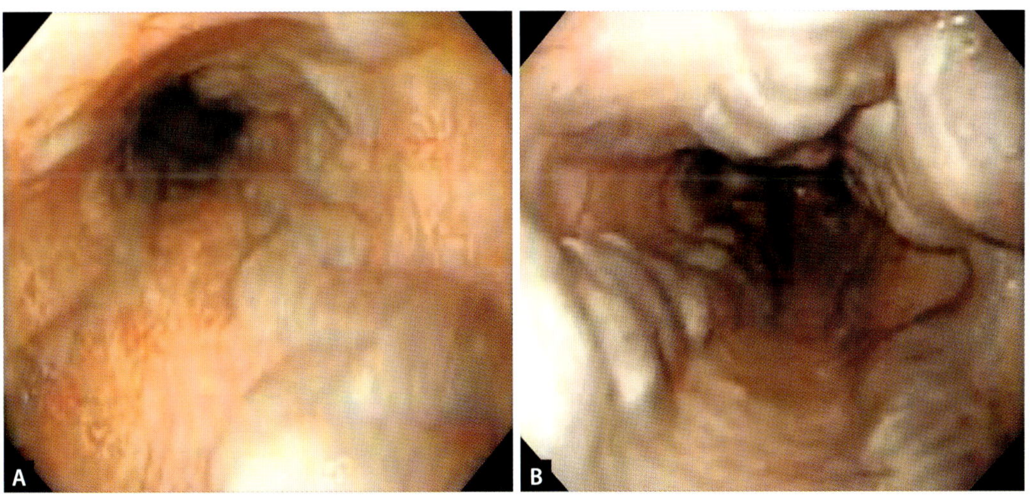

Figs. 2A and B: Esophageal varices grade 3.

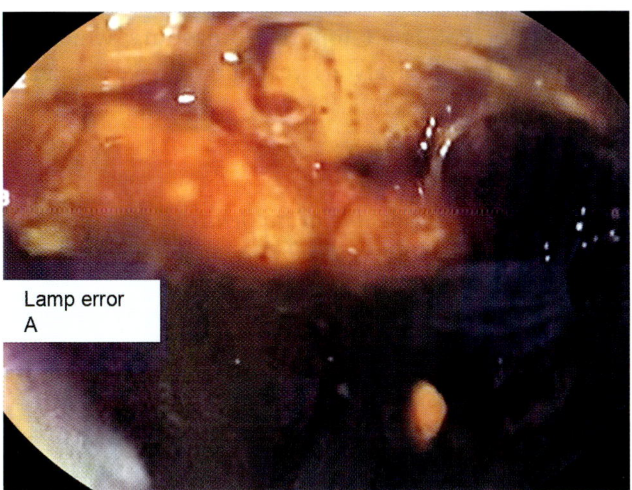

Fig. 3: Stomach full of bleeding.

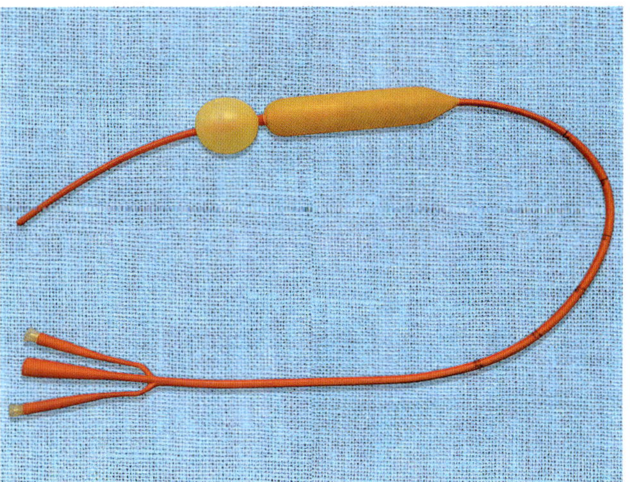

Fig. 5: Sengstaken–Blakemore tube.

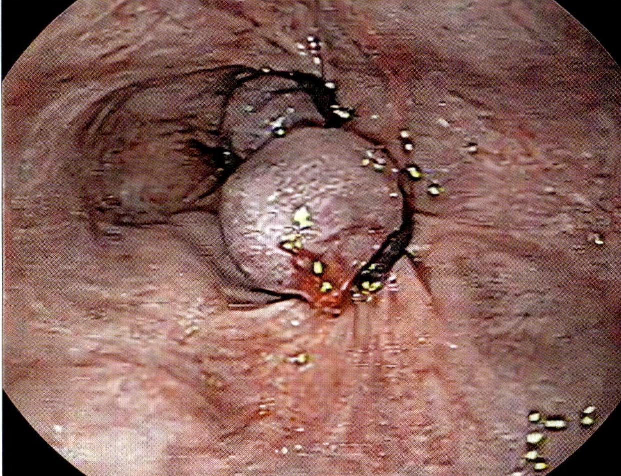

Fig. 4: Endoscopic banding done.

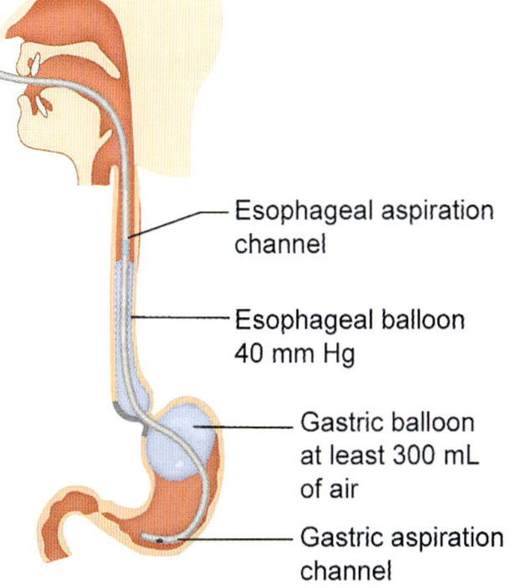

Fig. 6: Pressures in Sengstaken–Blakemore.

- Modified Sengstaken tube (known as Minnesota tube) contains *4 lumens.*

(old Sengstaken-Blakemore tube contains 3 tubes)—one for aspiration from stomach, one from esophagus, one for esophageal balloon dilatation, and last one for gastric balloon dilatation.

- The tube is inserted via the mouth and gastric balloon inflated first.
- The gastric balloon inflated first through 250 mL of air and esophageal balloon to a pressure of *40 mm Hg using air.*
- The potentially lethal complication is accidentally inflating gastric balloon inside the esophagus resulting in *perforation of esophagus.*
- Balloons should be temporarily deflated after 12 hours to prevent esophageal necrosis.
- This is a temporary procedure, and we must plan redo endoscopy at the earliest.

Step 4: Redo Endoscopy

- Endoscopic sclero or banding can be retried.
- Gastric varices are usually treated by cyanoacrylate glue as banding is not possible.

Step 5: Transhepatic Porto Systemic Shunt

- Transhepatic porto systemic shunt (TIPSS) is a short-term bridge to liver transplant.
- It is inserted via internal jugular vein by interventional radiologist.
- Access the portal vein inside the liver via a branch of hepatic vein and dilate the tract to 10 mm through which expandable metallic stent is inserted **(Fig. 7)**.
- It is not used as initial therapy but can be used if endoscopy and pharmacotherapy fails.
- It is a type of *nonselective shunt* between portal vein (PV) and hepatic vein (HV).
- It is an IH shunt.

Complications:

- Main early complication is *perforation of liver capsule* and fatal intraperitoneal hemorrhage.
- Post shunt encephalopathy, the confusional state due to the toxic metabolites bypassing the metabolism in liver, is the most common complication and happens in 30 days.
- Another short-term complication is shunt thrombosis.
- Long-term complication is *shunt stenosis* which may occur in <1 year.

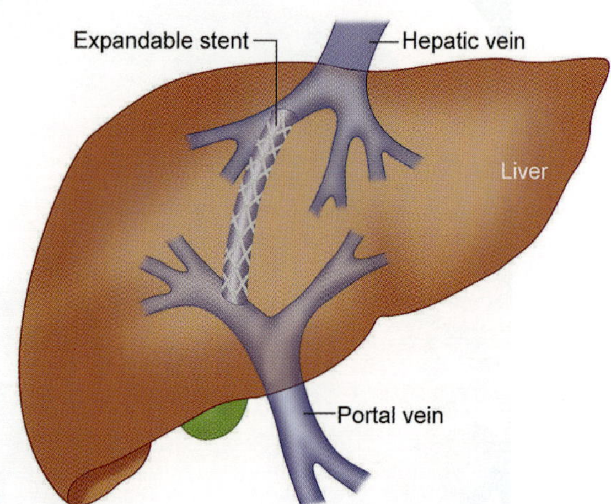

Fig. 7: Transhepatic porto systemic shunt (TIPSS)

- Hence, TIPSS is a temporary procedure, which can prolong the survival for 1 year and we have to plan for transplant at the earliest.

Step 6: Shunt Operations

- *If TIPSS is not possible or not feasible, surgical shunt operations are undertaken by hepatic surgeons.*

Nonselective shunts ***(Fig. 8)***
- End-to-side portocaval shunt (Eck's fistula)
- Side-to-side portocaval shunt
- Large diameter interposition shunts (>16 mm)
- Conventional splenorenal shunts

Selective shunts:
- Warren's shunt
- Inokuchi shunt

Conventional splenorenal shunt: (Linton shunt/proximal splenorenal shunt)

- Involves removal of spleen and insertion of proximal splenic vein into renal vein.
- *Complication: Portal shunt encephalopathy is more common in this procedure.*
- *Advantages:* This type of shunt also decompresses the splanchnic venous system and intrahepatic sinusoidal network; hence, side-to-side shunts are effective in controlling ascites and preventing rebleed.

Selective shunts:

- *Splenorenal shunt:* Distal (Warren's)
- *Inokuchi:* Left gastric vena caval shunt—vein graft interposed between the left gastric vein and inferior vena cava.

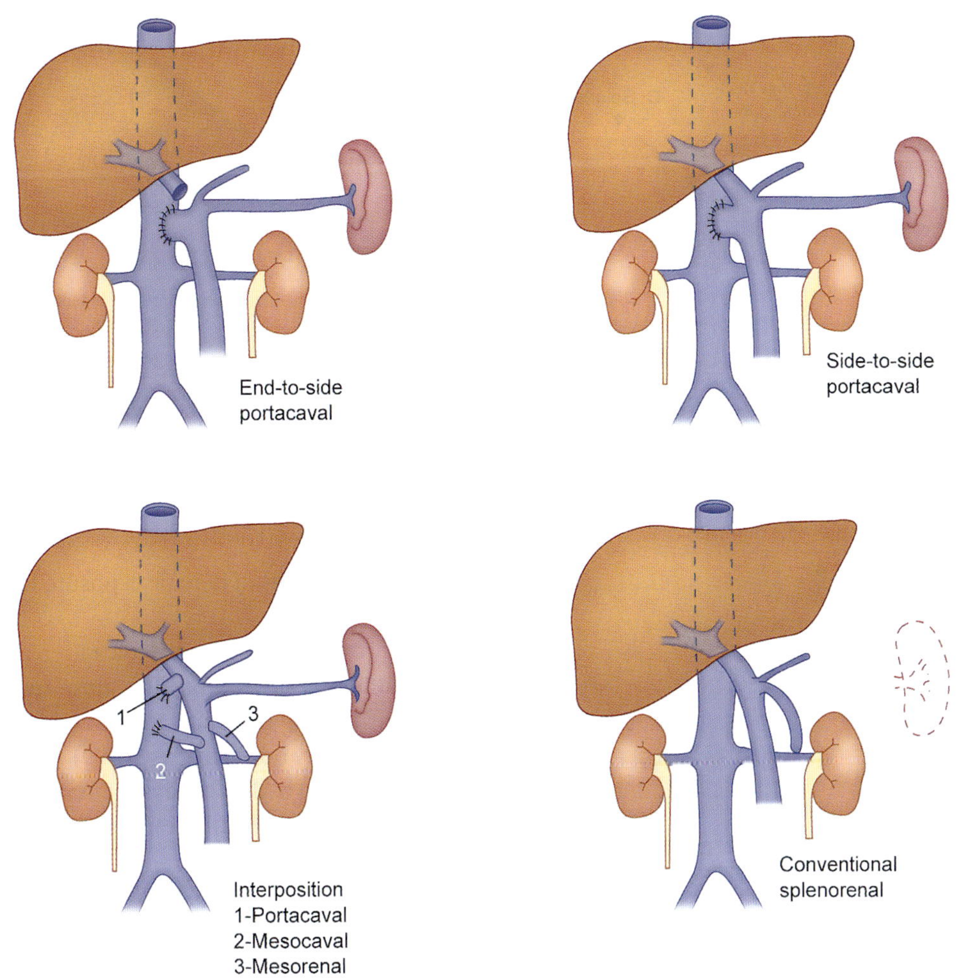

Fig. 8: Nonselective shunt operations.

Distal splenorenal shunt (Warren's shunt):

- Anastomosis of distal end of splenic vein to the left renal vein along with interruption of all collaterals **(Fig. 9)**
- *This shunt aggravates the ascites* because sinusoidal and mesenteric hypertension is maintained and important lymphatic pathways are transected during dissection.

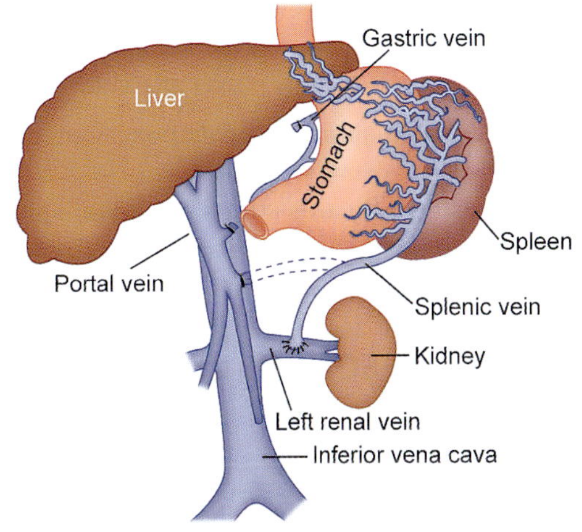

Fig. 9: Distal splenorenal shunt.

Step 7

- If shunt operations are not possible, a procedure to devascularize all the collaterals entering the esophagus and stomach called as Sugiura operation is done.
- Extensive esophagogastric devascularization combined with splenectomy and esophageal transection (Sugiura operation) is shown in **Figure 10**.

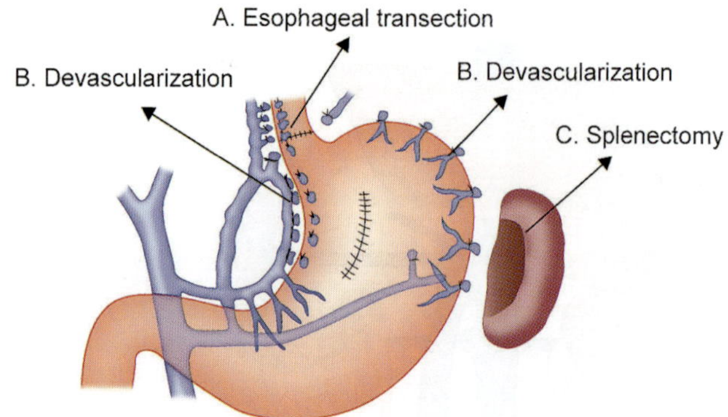

Fig. 10: Sugiura operation.

Flowchart 1: Protocol for bleeding esophageal varices

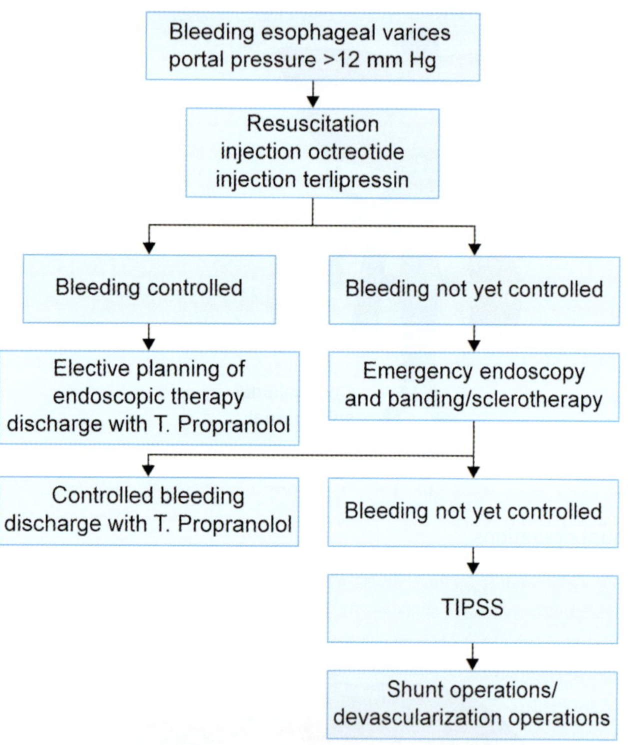

(TIPSS: transjugular intrahepatic portal shunt)

- Main indication for this surgery is distal splanchnic venous thrombosis and patients with distal splenorenal shunt thrombosis **(Flowchart 1)**.

SURGICAL INFECTIONS IN LIVER

Pyogenic Abscess

Children:
- MC organism is *Staphylococcus* in Children
- MC organism is *Escherichia coli* in adults in West and *Klebsiella* in Eastern countries

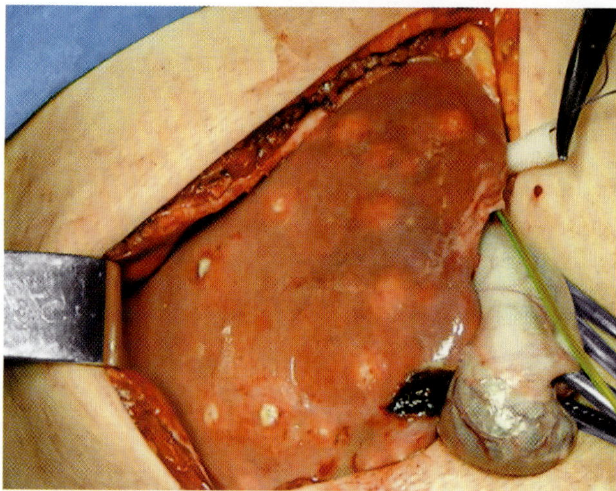

Fig. 11: Multiple macroabscess liver.

The potential routes of hepatic exposure to bacteria are as follows:

- Biliary tree (most common route)
- Portal vein (Pylephlebitis due to diverticulitis, appendicitis, primary immunodeficiency (PID), inflammatory bowel disease (IBD), perforation, etc.)
- *Hepatic artery:* This type of hematogenous spread is usually monomicrobial especially with *Staphylococci* or *Streptococci*.
- Direct extension
- Trauma

Must Know Table:
- Solitary abscess is more common than multiple abscess.
- Multiple abscess is seen in patients of biliary origin.
- Multiple macroabscess are seen in Biliary origin **(Fig. 11)**.
- Multiple microabscess are seen in hematogenous origin.
- Solitary abscess is usually polymicrobial.
- Hematogenous route is mostly monomicrobial.

Clinical Features

- Most common in right lobe.
- *Most common presenting symptom:* Fever, chills, and abdominal pain
- A rare complication of *Klebsiella* abscess is endogenous endophthalmitis (3%), common in diabetics.

Management

- *Treatment* involves *percutaneous catheter drainage along with broad-spectrum antibiotics.*

- Surgery is reserved for those who fail percutaneous technique and for those in whom surgery is required for some other pathology such as appendicectomy.

Amoebic Abscess

Pathogenesis

- The major mechanism of abscess formation is enzymatic cellular hydrolysis. The abscess contains acellular proteinaceous debris *surrounded by a rim of invasive amoebic trophozoites.*
- Due to liquefaction necrosis of liver, the abscess results—*anchovy sauce colored and odorless.*
- Characteristic feature of amoebic abscess is Glisson's capsule, it is resistant to amoebic invasion; hence, abscess is limited to Glisson's capsule.

Features of pyogenic and Amoebic liver abscess are given in **Table 1**.

Clinical Features

- Most common LFT abnormality is elevated prothrombin time.
- Enzyme immunoassays (EIA) have sensitivity of 99% and specificity of >90% in patients with amebic abscess.
- *Ultrasonography (USG) characters: Hypoechoic and nonhomogeneous rounded lesion abutting liver capsule without significant rim echoes.*

Investigation

- *Computed tomography (CT) scan:* More sensitive in differentiating pyogenic from amoebic.
- *Contrast-enhanced computed tomography (CECT) scan shows well-defined hypodense abscess.*

Treatment

- *Oral metronidazole:* 750 mg three times/10 days is the drug of choice.
- Emetine intramuscular (IM) injections are very effective for invasive amoebiasis.
- After treatment of liver abscess, luminal agents like iodoquinol, paromomycin, and diloxanide furoate are administered to treat carrier state.

Percutaneous Aspiration

- Therapeutic aspiration is usually avoided.
- Metrogyl is the treatment of choice and about 90% cases respond well.
- *Indications for aspiration:*
- Abscess wall diameter larger than 5 cm (abscess with high risk of rupture)
- Abscess in the left lobe of liver
- For diagnostic uncertainty
- Failure to respond in 3–5 days

Extra Edge

- In menstruating women, low incidence is seen.
- The most frequent complication of liver abscess is rupture.
- *Active amoebic colitis:* One third have synchronous liver abscess.
- Recent history of diarrhea is very uncommon.
- Most common site of rupture is peritoneum.
- *Treatment of rupture into bronchus:* Self-limiting (bronchodilators + postural drainage)

TABLE 1: Features of pyogenic and amoebic liver abscess.

Features	*Pyogenic liver abscess*	*Amoebic liver abscess*
Most common symptom	Fever (classical presentation—fever + jaundice + RUQ pain)	Pain abdomen
Most common sign	RUQ tenderness	Hepatomegaly
Lesion	Usually single (50%)	Single in 80%
Age group	>50 years	20–40 years
M:F ratio	1.5:1	10:1
Diabetes	More common	Very rare
LFT (most common abnormality)	Elevated ALP	Raised PT
Jaundice	+++ (25% cases)	–
Blood culture	+	–
Amoebic serology	–	+
CT scan	• Hypodense • Gas produced inside • Irregular margins • Peripheral rim enhancement+	• Hypodense • Rounded margins • Rim enhancement not seen

(ALP: alkaline phosphatase; CT: computed tomography; PT: prothrombin time; RUQ: right upper quadrant)

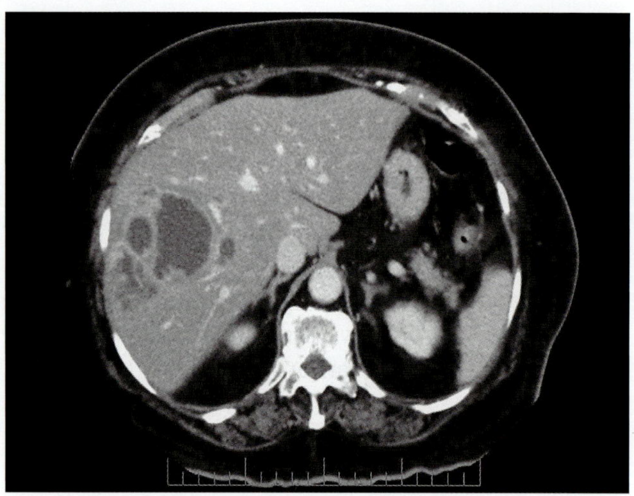
Fig. 12: Pyogenic abscess liver.

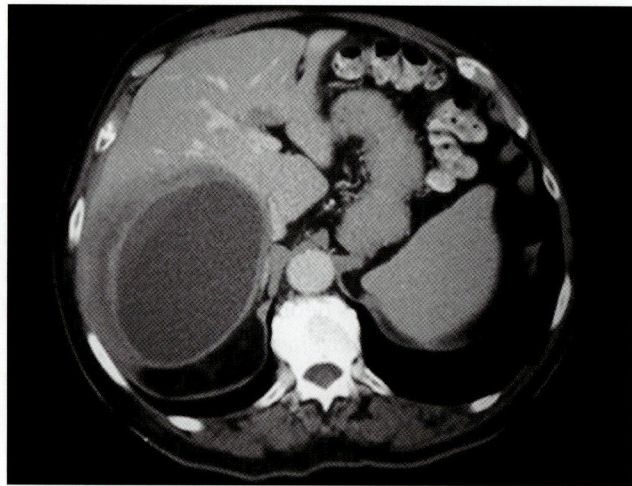
Fig. 13: Amoebic liver abscess.

Computed tomography scan findings in Pyogenic abscess ***(Fig. 12)***:

- Clustering of abscess
- No well-defined border.
- Peripheral rim enhancement seen (double target sign seen)

Computed tomography scan findings of amoebic liver abscess ***(Fig. 13)***:

- Well-defined border
- Peripheral rim enhancement is absent as per Sabiston.
- Peripheral edema is seen.

HYDATID CYST

- *Echinococcus granulosus* is most common.
- Others are *Echinococcus multilocularis* are *Echinococcus oligartus.*
- *Dogs are definitive hosts* in which adult tapeworm is attached in villi of small intestine.
- *Sheep are intermediate hosts* that consume the ova passed by the feces of dog over grasses.
- *Humans are accidental hosts* consuming these eggs that coverts to embryo in duodenum and releases oncosphere-containing hooklets that penetrate the mucosa and reach the blood stream.
- The oncosphere reaches the liver (most common) or lungs where the parasite develops into larval stage called as hydatid cyst.
- Remember, humans are end-stage host.

Extra Edge

Layers of hydatid cyst ***(Fig. 14)***:

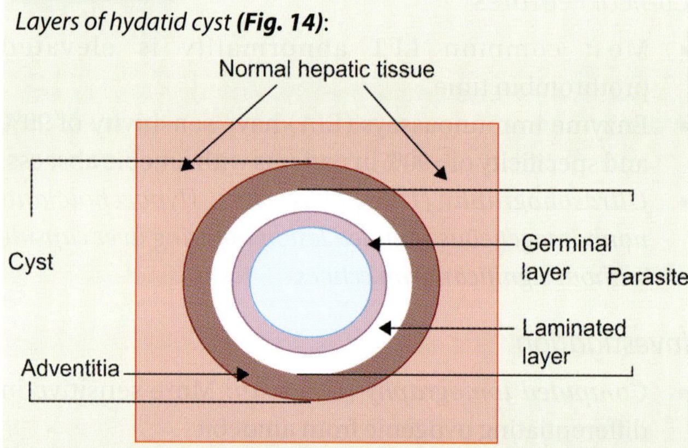

Fig. 14: Hydatid cyst.

- Made up of 3 layers
  - Germinal layer
  - Laminated layer
  - Ectocyst (pericyst)
- Endocyst is formed by inner germinal layer and laminated layer.

Innermost germinal layer:

- *Thin layer*
- *Living component*
- Produces invaginations into cavity forming brood capsules that contain protoscolices
- It is the *source of daughter cyst.*
- *Daughter cyst contains* germinal layer, laminated membrane, cyst fluid, brood capsules and protoscolices. *The only difference is it does not have adventitial layer.*

Contd...

Contd...

Middle laminated layer:
- 1–2 mm thick
- Acellular layer separable easily from pericyst (3rd layer)
- Permeable to potassium, water, and chloride
- *Not permeable to Bile, bacteria*, and enzymes.

Satellite hydatid cysts:
- Formed when there is a small leak or defect in laminated membrane and germinal layer passes out (ectogenic vesiculation)

Pericyst/ectocyst/adventitial layer:
- Derived from the host tissue
- Thick layer.
- *This layer is present in liver and spleen.*
- *Absent in lungs and brain hydatids*
- Blood supply is abundant in this layer—appear as hypervascular rim in CT scan.
- No clear plane is seen between adventitial layer and surrounding host tissue.

Hydatid fluid nature
- Clear
- Colorless
- Odorless
- Compared to plasma, sodium, chloride and bicarbonate are same. Calcium and potassium are decreased.

Clinical Features

- Most common in right lobe of liver (most common lobe affected is segment 7 and 8).
- Equal in males and females.
- Most are asymptomatic.
- Most frequent sign is hepatomegaly.
- Most common symptoms are abdominal pain, dyspepsia, and vomiting.
- *Complications:* Rupture into biliary tree, bronchial tree, pleural, peritoneal, and pericardial cavity.'

Biliary communication: Most common complication of hydatid cyst:
- Incidence of cystobiliary communication = 37%
- Clinically apparent biliary leakage = 26%
- *Major biliary communication (>5 mm diameter) = 5–10%*

Risk of biliary-cyst communication:
- *Male patients*
- Abnormal preoperative serum alkaline phosphatase and γ-glutamyl transferase (GGT);
- Multiple cysts, multilocular and degenerated cysts
- Cysts near the *biliary bifurcation*
- Presence of bile-stained or purulent cyst
- Cyst diameter *greater than 10 cm* was an independent clinical predictor for the presence of intrabiliary rupture

Investigations

- *Ultrasound:* Rosette-like appearance or water-lily appearance **(Figs. 15A and B)**.
- *Calcifications* in the wall are highly diagnostic.
- *Serological tests:* Enzyme-linked immunosorbent assay (ELISA), arc 5 test, indirect hemagglutination (IHA)

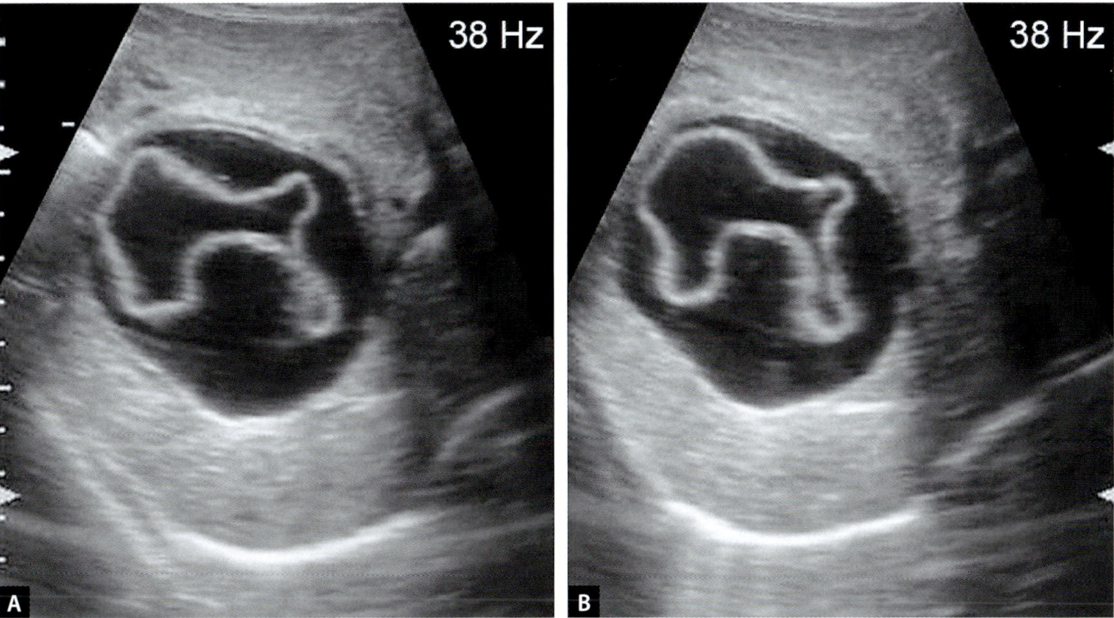

Figs. 15A and B: Ultrasonography (USG) showing water–lily sign.

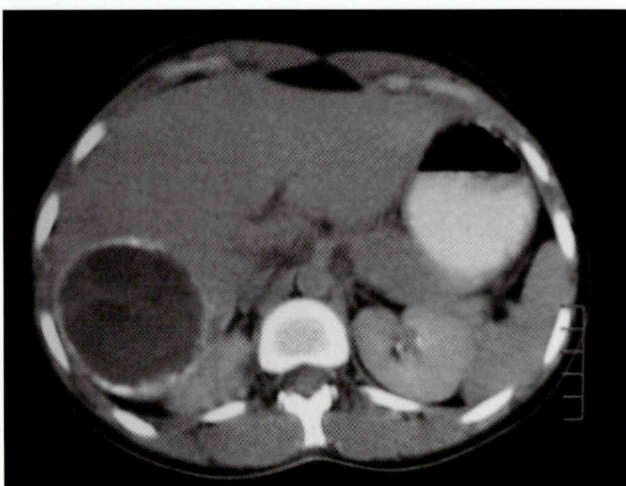

Fig. 16: Calcifications in hydatid cyst in computed tomography (CT) scan.

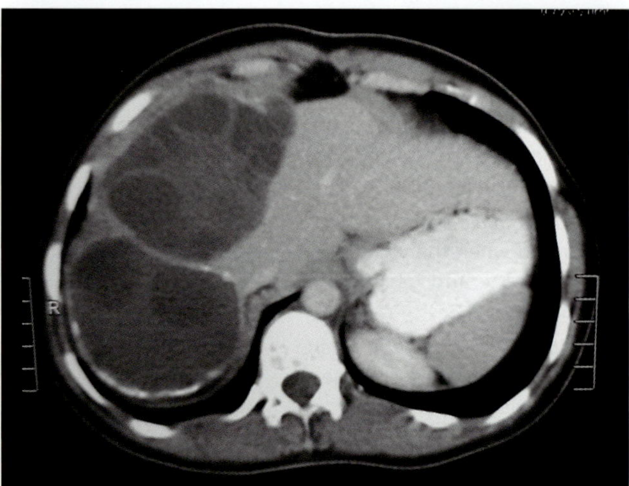

Fig. 17: Daughter cyst in computed tomography (CT) scan.

test, and *immunoblast test where available is the test of choice.*

- *Casoni's test:* Intradermal injection of sterile hydatid fluid. It is not done nowadays.
- *CT scan will show calcifications and daughter cysts* **(Figs. 16 and 17)**.

Extra Edge

- Enzyme-linked immunosorbent assay (ELISA) can also be automatized for large-scale epidemiologic studies.
- Selected test antibodies affect its value on post-treatment follow-up.
- *Immunoglobulin (Ig) G assay may remain positive for 4 years* after successful treatment, so it is not a suitable test for post-treatment follow-up.
- *IgM assay has been reported to be negative after 6 months* of successful treatment.
- Circulating *Echinococcus granulosus* antigens are small, and most are in the form of immune complexes.
- *Detection of these antigens is less sensitive than antibody detection.*

Extra Mile

- Gharbi et al. classification of hydatid cysts is old classification.

Latest classification is World Health Organization (WHO) classification

- *CE 1:* Unilocular cyst
- *CE 2:* Multiseptated (honey comb/rosette like)
- *CE 3:* Floating membrane (water lily sign)
- *CE 4:* Heterogenous cysts with partial calcification
- *CE 5:* Calcified wall

Type 1, 2, 3 are active cysts.

Type 4 and 5 are inactive and dead cysts.

Treatment

Medical management:

- Albendazole or mebendazole alone can shrink <50% of cysts.
- Preoperative treatment also helps in decreasing the spillage of the cyst.
- Chemotherapy without resection is indicated only for widely disseminated disease or poor surgical risks.

Interventions:

- Primarily surgical but introduction of percutaneous aspiration, infusion of scolicidal agents and reaspiration (PAIR) has totally replaced it.
    - Remember, surgery is now preferred where PAIR is not possible or when it does not respond to PAIR or when there is any communication to biliary tree.

Surgical approaches:

- Cystectomy
- Pericystectomy/radical cystectomy/capsulectomy/Cystopericystectomy
- Liver resection

Partial Pericystectomy (Figs. 18A to E)

- *Simplest and safest approach:* Removal of germinal layer and laminated layer leaving the ectocyst there itself.
- Scolicidal agents are used to wash the cavity.
- 20% hypertonic saline is the best, which has 100% scolicidal property (6 minutes).

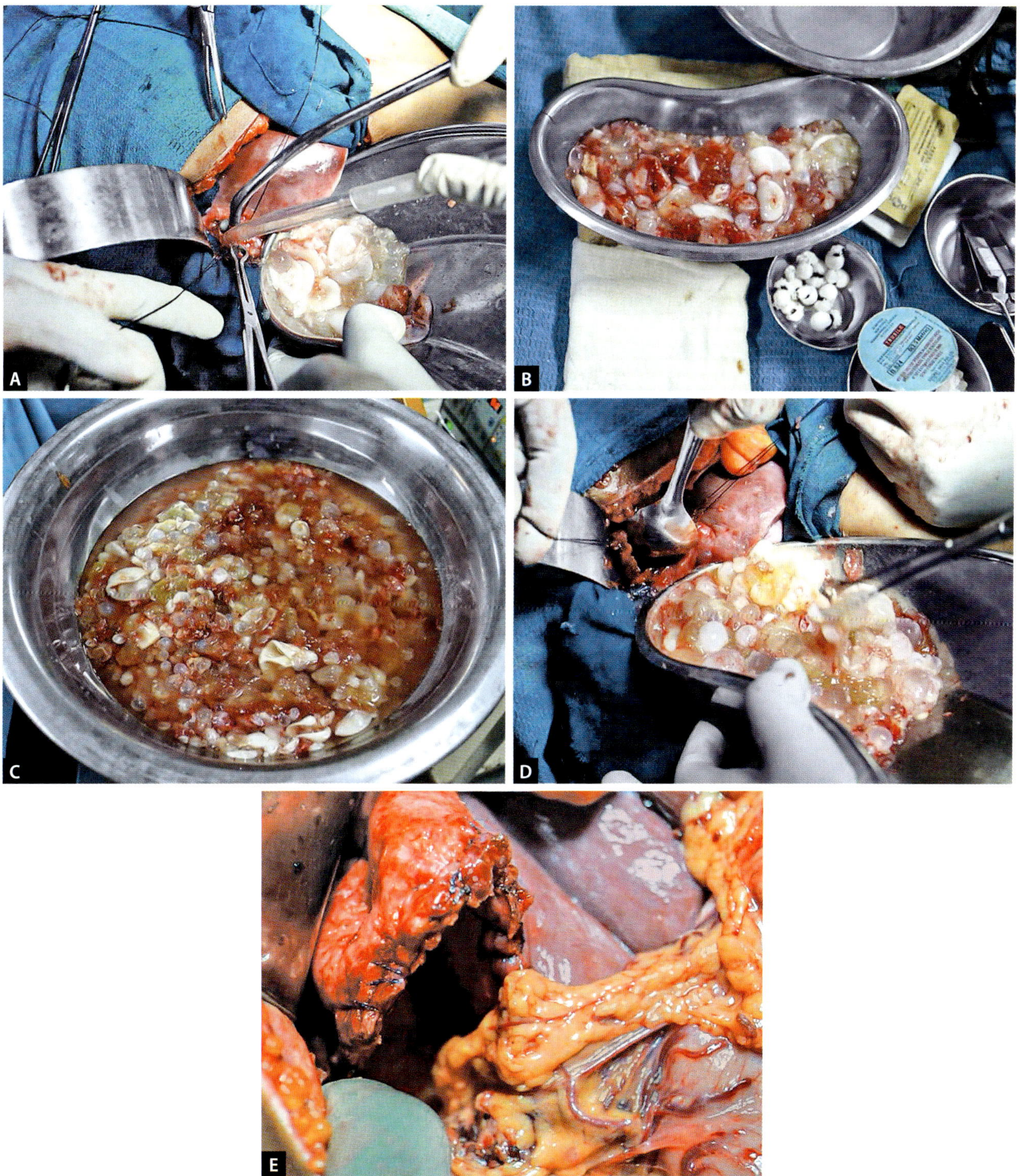

Figs. 18A to E: Partial pericystectomy and removal of hydatid cyst.

- 0.5% cetrimide + chlorhexidine 0.05% is also used.
- Povidone iodine 10% was once an effective agent. It no more used due to caustic cholangitis and difficulty in identification of biliary communication.
- Formalin is no longer used.

Indications for Liver Resection

- *Echinococcus multilocularis: The only option is resection of liver.*
- Atrophic liver parenchyma due to obstruction
    - Large bile leak that cannot be safely closed.

Percutaneous aspiration, infusion of scolicidal agents, and reaspiration (PAIR):
- Given with prophylactic cover of albendazole.
- *Scolicidal agents:* 20% hypertonic saline, 0.5% silver nitrate, 95% ethanol, absolute alcohol, mebendazole 2.4 μg/mL, and 10% povidone iodine

Contraindications for PAIR:
- Superficially located cyst (chance of rupture)
- Honey combing of cysts (multiple thick internal septae)
- Communication with biliary tree
- Dead or inactive cysts
- Lung/brain cysts
- Peritoneal rupture or pleural rupture

Also know:
- *PAIR: <6 cm cyst (<100 mL)*
- *PAIR catheter: >6 cm cyst (>100 mL)*
- *Percutaneous evacuation of cyst content (PEVAC)*

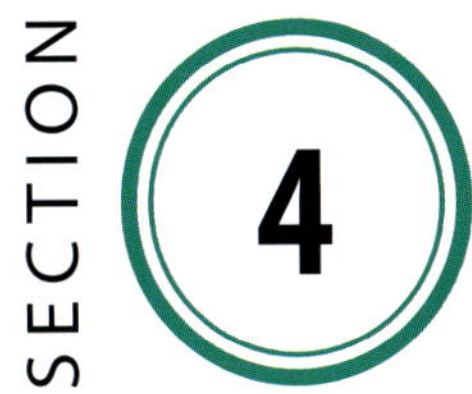

Neurosurgical Emergencies

Head Injury

Premnath Susendran

INTRODUCTION

Commonest cause of death in Trauma is a type of head injury and hence as surgeons we must know the basics behind the various pathophysiology of head injury.

CLASSIFICATION

Based on Glasgow Coma Scale (GCS) and in particular, Motor Score, best predictor of neurological outcome is given in **Table 1**.

TABLE 1: Head injury severity: Clinical classification

Head injury severity	*Glasgow Coma Scale (GCS) and LOC*
Minor head injury	GCS 15 with no LOC
Mild head injury	GCS 14 or 15 with LOC
Moderate head injury	GCS 9–13
Severe head injury	GCS 3–8

(LOC: loss of consciousness)

MINOR AND MILD HEAD INJURY

- Decisions on imaging and discharge are best made guided by published criteria.
- In preverbal children and other vulnerable groups, nonaccidental injury must be considered.
- Amnesia, confusion, headaches, and somnolence are typical features of concussion.

MODERATE AND SEVERE TRAUMATIC BRAIN INJURY

- Resuscitation and evaluation
- Advanced trauma life support (ATLS) guideline
- Airway with cervical spine control
- Breathing
- Circulation

HISTORY

Bystanders and paramedics may give vital information on the:

- Preinjury state (fits, alcohol, and chest pain)
- Mechanism and energy involved in the injury (speed of vehicles and height fallen)
- Conscious state and hemodynamic stability of the patient after the accident
- Length of time taken for extrication
- Check the medication history, especially anticoagulants and antiplatelet agents.

PRIMARY SURVEY

- Ensure adequate oxygenation and circulation
- Exclude hypoglycemia.

Pupils

- The pupil size should be recorded in millimeters and the reactivity is documented as present, sluggish, or absent.
- Uncal herniation can compress the third nerve, compromising the parasympathetic supply to the pupil. Unopposed sympathetic activity produces a sluggish enlarged pupil, progressing to fixed and dilated under continued compression.
- Established pupil changes may reflect pathology anywhere in the eye or the reflex loop made up by the optic nerve, the oculomotor nerve, and the brainstem.
- Direct ocular trauma or nerve injury in association with a skull base fracture can cause mydriasis (dilated pupil) to be present from the time of injury.
- Pre-existing discrepancy in the pupil size (anisocoria), as a result of Holmes-Adie pupil or cataracts, for example, may also complicate assessment.

TABLE 2: Glasgow Coma Scale (GCS) scoring.

Component	*Response*	*Score*
Eyes open	Spontaneously	4
	To verbal command	3
	To painful stimulus	2
	Do not open	1
Verbal	Normal	5
	Confused	4
	Inappropriate/words only	3
	Sounds only	2
	No sounds	1
	Intubated patient	T
Motor	Obeys commands	6
	Localizes to pain	5
	Withdrawal/flexion	4
	Abnormal flexion	3
	Extension	2
	No motor response	1

Glasgow Coma Scale score (Table 2)

- Score represents the best performance elicited, so a patient flexing in response to a painful stimulus on the left and localizing on the right scores "M5".
- Sternal *or*
- Supraorbital rub *or*
- Trapezius squeeze represents an appropriate painful stimulus

Neurological Deficit

- Gross focal neurological deficits, such as paraplegia, may be evident in the primary survey.
- Assessment to exclude such a deficit should be carried out, especially if the patient is to be intubated so that subsequent examination will be impossible.
- Detailed neurological examination is included in the secondary survey.

EXAMINATION: SECONDARY SURVEY

A full secondary survey will be required. Particular attention must be paid to the head, neck, and spine.

Head

- *Scalp:* Subgaleal hematoma and lacerations, which may bleed profusely and potentially overlie fractures

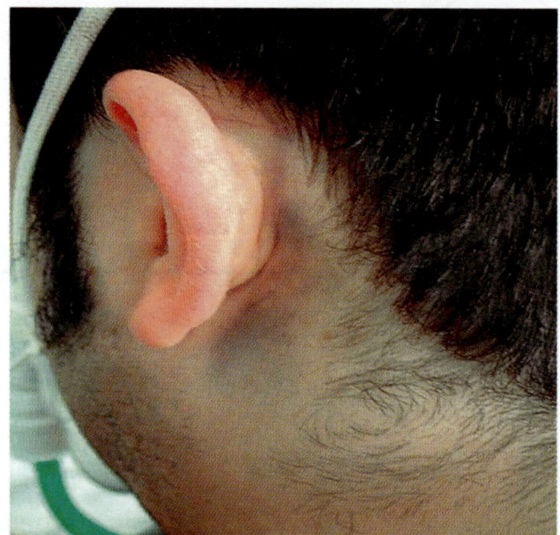

Fig. 1: Battle sign.

- *Face:* For evidence of fractures, especially to the orbital rim, zygoma and maxilla.
- Skull base fracture.

Battle's Sign

- "Racoon" or "panda" eyes (bilateral periorbital bruising)
- Hemotympanum or overt bleeding from the ear if the tympanic membrane has ruptured.
- Cerebrospinal fluid (CSF) rhinorrhea or otorrhea are highly suggestive **(Fig. 1)**.
- Cranial nerves damage associated with skull base fracture.
- Midbrain or brainstem dysfunction:
    - Gaze paresis (inability of the eye to look across beyond the midline)
    - Dysconjugate gaze (inability of eyes to work together)
    - Roving eye movements

Eye Examination

Conjunctiva and cornea, retina using an ophthalmoscope, looking for hyphema (blood in the anterior chamber of the eye), papilledema or retinal detachment

- Blood in the mouth may be due to tongue-biting at seizure
- The GCS score and pupil status.

Neck and Spine

- Cervical fracture of up to 10% in association with moderate and severe traumatic brain injury (TBI).
- Managed in a hard collar until the neck can be cleared clinically.

- Log-rolled to palpate for thoracic or lumbar deformity, and any cervical collar should be removed at this stage to allow palpation of the cervical spine before it is then replaced again.
- *Per rectum examination:* Assessing for anal tone, sensation in the awake patient and anal wink (sphincter seen to contract in response to a pinprick stimulus).
- Priapism is a strong predictor of severe cord injury even in intubated patients.

SURGICAL PATHOLOGY

Fractures: Skull Vault

- Closed linear—conservatively
- Open or comminuted—debridement and prophylactic antibiotic therapy
- Depressed skull fractures with at least thickness of skull wall, Dural breech-exploration, and elevation.
- Fractures that involve the air sinuses—manage like open fractures using broad-spectrum antibiotics with or without exploration **(Figs. 2 and 3)**.

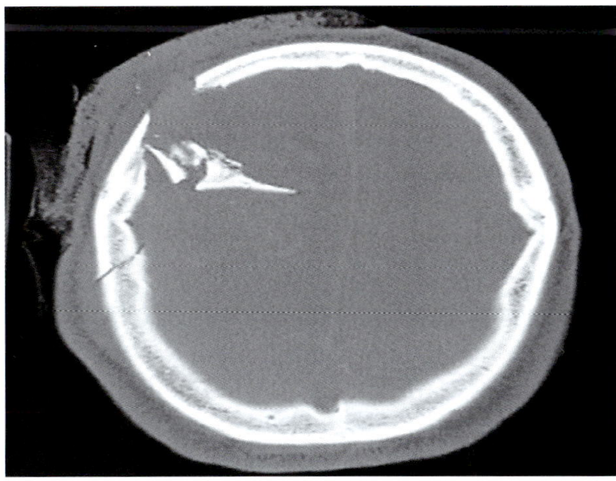

Fig. 2: Frontal comminuted depressed skull fracture.

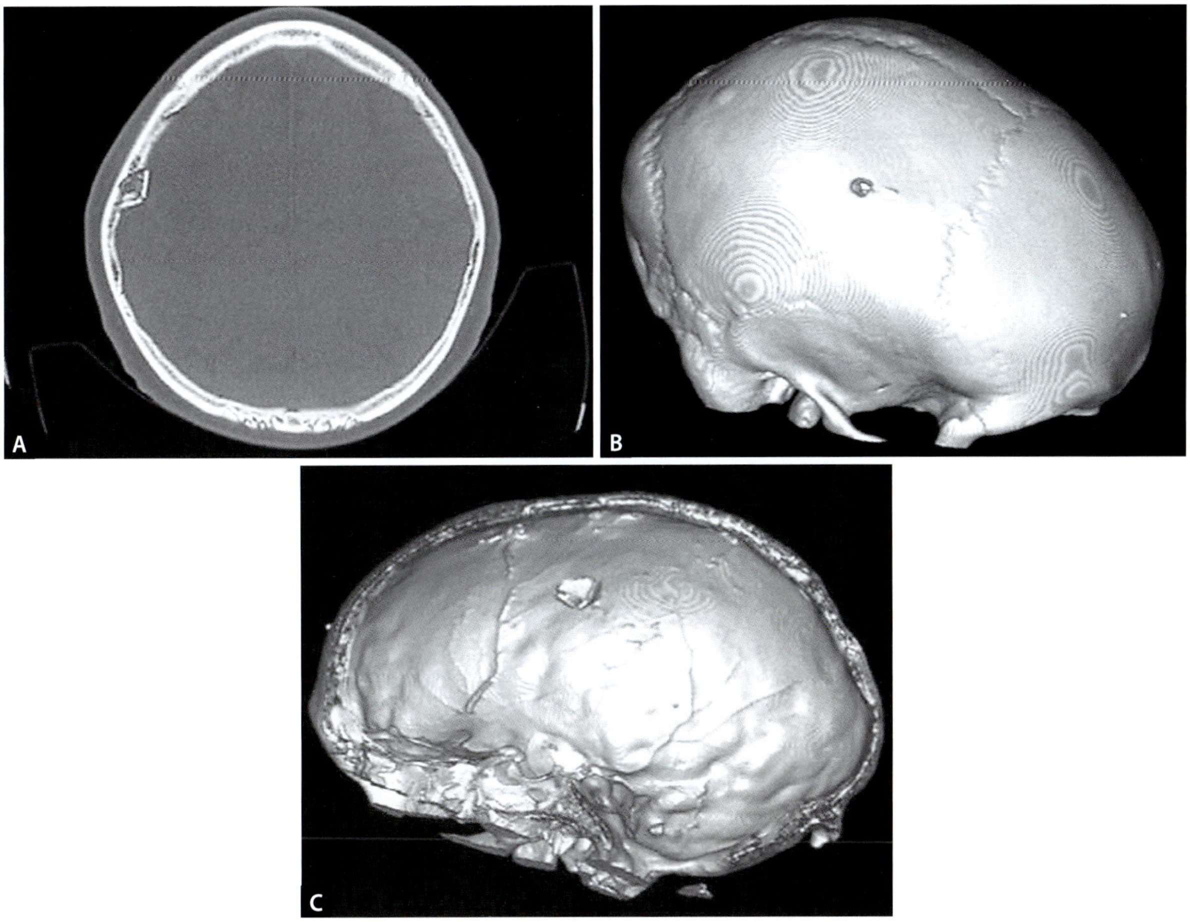

Figs. 3A to C: (A) A small depressed skull fracture of the parietal bone visible on an axial bone window; (B) Visualized on bone vault reconstructions; and (C) with an underlying breach of the dura.

Fractures: Skull Base

- Skull base fractures may be complicated by pituitary dysfunction, arterial dissection or cranial nerve deficits, with anosmia, facial palsy, or hearing loss typical.
- CSF leak will generally resolve spontaneously but persistent leak can result in meningitis so repair may be required.
- Blind nasogastric tube placement is contraindicated in these patients.

EXTRADURAL HEMORRHAGE

- Rupture of an artery, vein, or venous sinus, in association with a skull fracture
- Classical injury to the thin squamous temporal bone, with associated damage to the middle meningeal artery
- Transient loss of consciousness is typical, then present in lucid interval with headache but without any neurological deficit.
- As the hematoma expands, compensation is exhausted with rapid deterioration.
- Contralateral hemiparesis, a reduced conscious level and ipsilateral pupillary dilatation, the cardinal signs of brain compression and herniation
- Although this "talk and die" pattern of deterioration occurs in only one-third of cases.

Computed Tomography Brain (Figs. 4A to C)

- Lentiform (lens-shaped or biconvex) hyperdense lesion
- A mass effect may be evident, with compression of the surrounding brain and midline shift
- Areas of mixed density suggest active bleeding.
- A skull fracture will usually be evident.

Treatment

- Immediate evacuation
- In deteriorating *or*

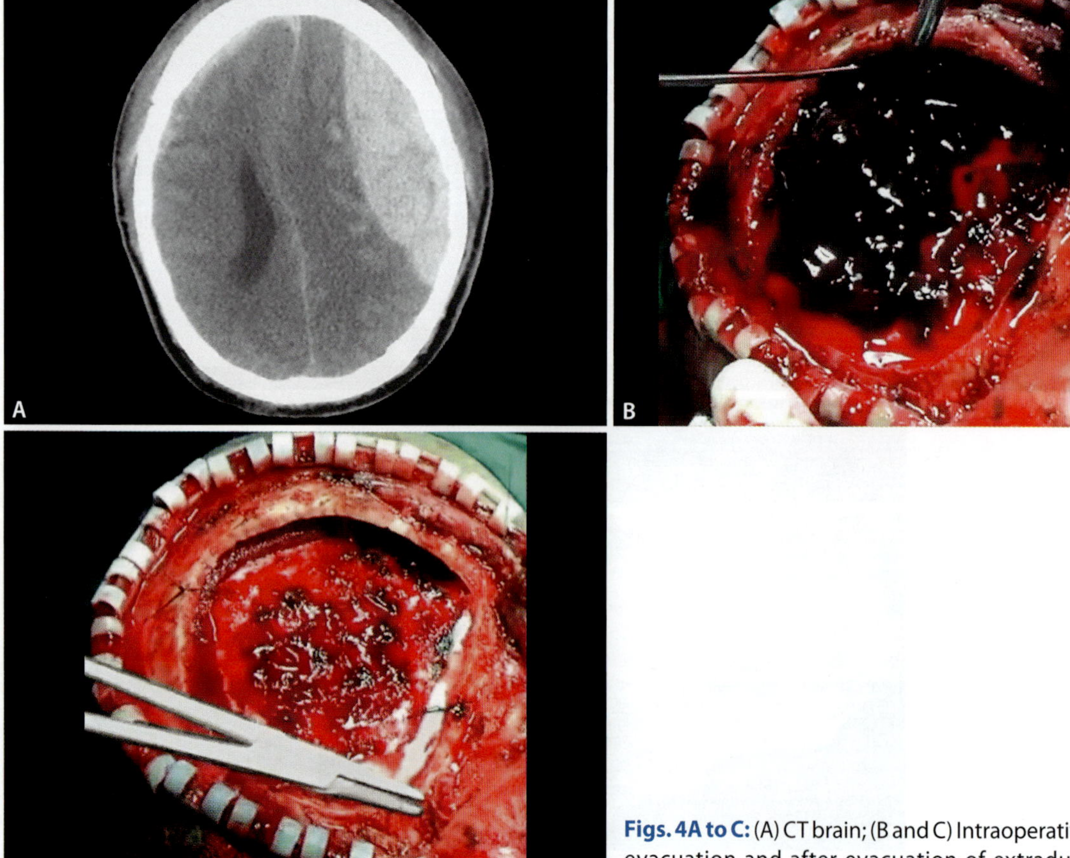

Figs. 4A to C: (A) CT brain; (B and C) Intraoperative images before evacuation and after evacuation of extradural hemorrhage (EDH) with intact dura.

- Comatose patients *or*
- Those with large bleeds
- Close observation is required in other stable cases.

Prognosis is excellent in evacuated hematoma, without associated primary brain injury.

ACUTE SUBDURAL HEMATOMA

Etiology

- *High-energy* injury mechanisms: Rupture of cortical surface vessels with significant associated primary brain injury
- Results in an expanding hematoma with rapid deterioration
- Development of signs of raised intracranial pressure (ICP) without lucid interval
- *In a second group:* Older and often anticoagulated, a lower energy injury leads to venous bleeding around the brain.
- Depending on time, develops into acute, chronic subdural hematoma (SDH) or may even remain clinically silent.

Treatment

- Urgent evacuation
  - Bleeds of significant size
  - With significant associated midline shift *or*
  - With deteriorating neurology
- *Conservative:* Smaller bleeds in neurologically stable patients.
- *Liquefaction of the clot over 7–10 days:* Burr holes

  Acute SDH is shown in **Figure 5.**

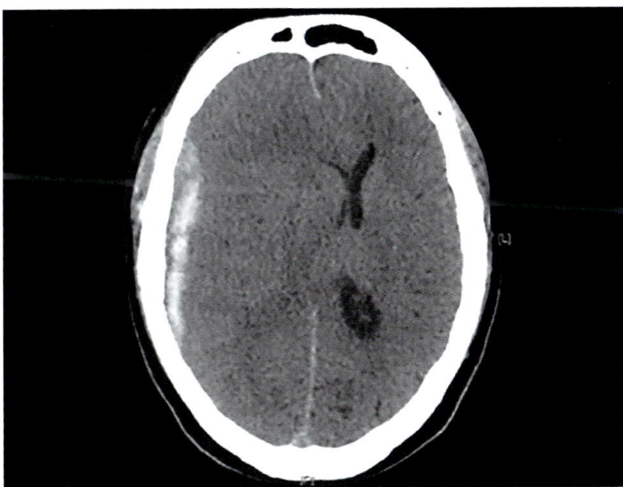

Fig. 5: Acute subdural hematoma (SDH). Right-sided acute SDH (hyperdense); the substantial midline shift reflects brain swelling as well as bleeding—this is a high-energy injury.

Bilateral Subdural Hematomas

The left is mixed density, the hypodense material represents old blood and the higher density indicates more recent bleeding, probably loculated so requiring a craniotomy to evacuate. The bleed on the right is isodense, indicating intermediate age **(Fig. 6)**.

Steps of surgery for SDH is shown in **Figures 7A to 7D**.

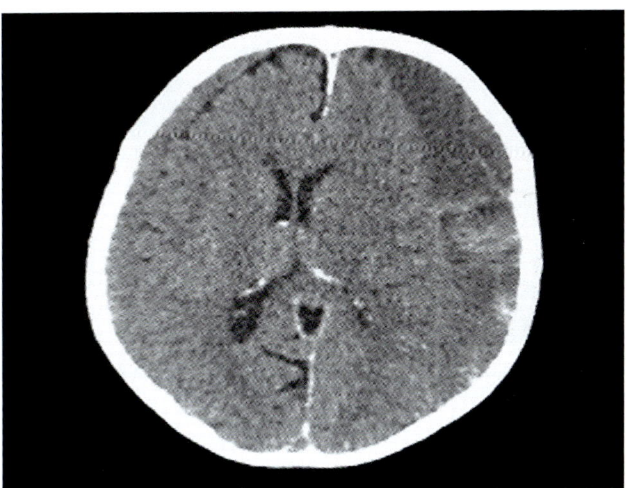

Fig. 6: Bilateral subdural hematomas. The left is mixed density, the hypodense material representing old blood and the higher density indicating more recent bleeding, probably loculated so requiring a craniotomy to evacuate. The bleed on the right is isodense, indicating intermediate age.

CHRONIC SUBDURAL HEMATOMA

Pathophysiology

- Acute neurological deterioration in older adults
- Cerebral atrophy results in stretching of the cortical-dural bridging veins, then vulnerable to rupture.
- Hematoma can expand over days or weeks by osmosis, producing symptoms of raised ICP or focal deficits.

Risk Factor

- History of recent injury
- In context of antiplatelet or anticoagulant medication, it may trigger.

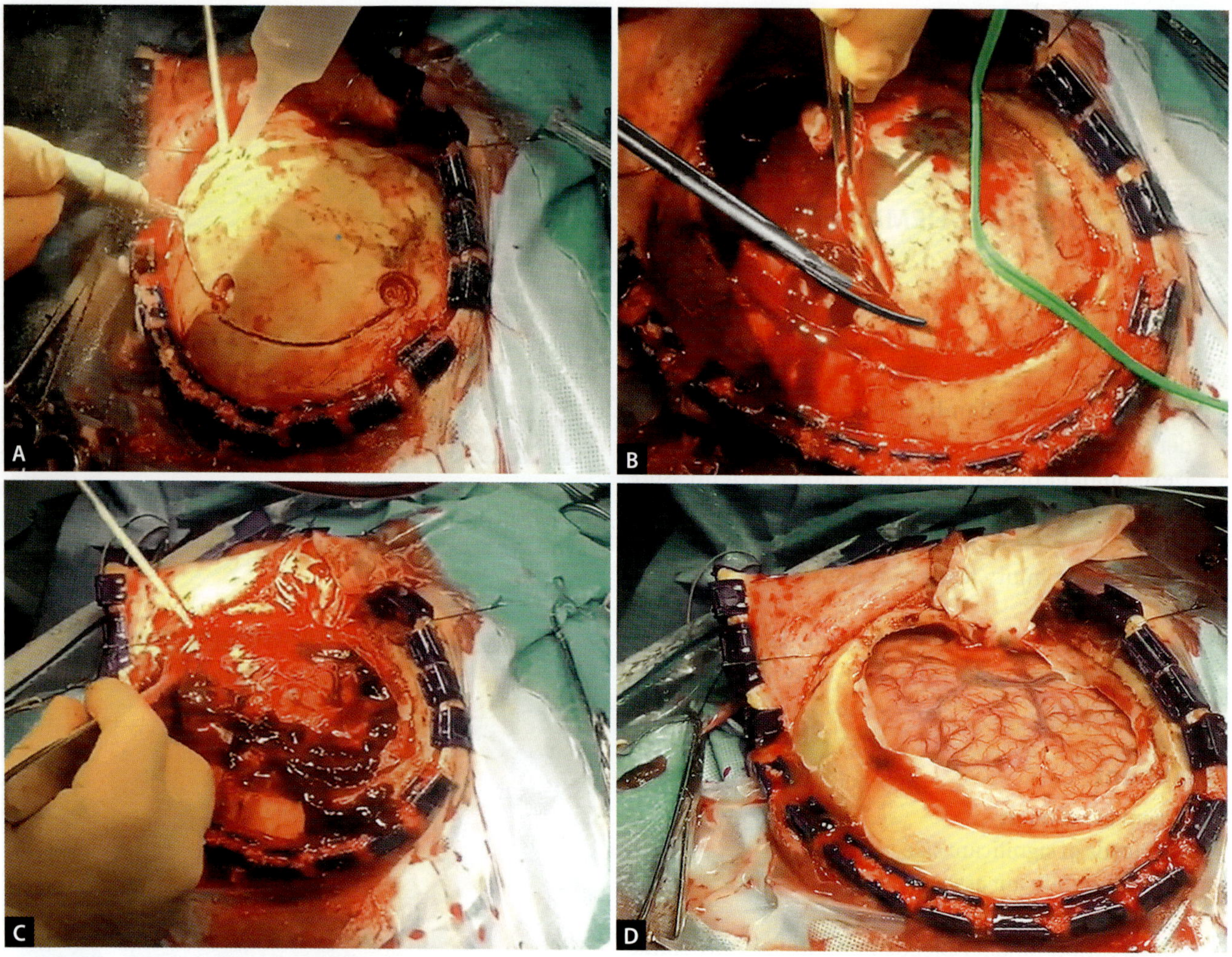

Figs. 7A to D: (A) Craniotomy; (B) Opening of dura with underlying hematoma; (C) Hematoma evacuation; and (D) After evacuation.

Diagnosis

Computed tomography brain:

- Diffuse hypodensity overlying the brain surface
- Recent bleeding may be isodense or hyperdense, and mixed density acute-on chronic SDH **(Fig. 8)**

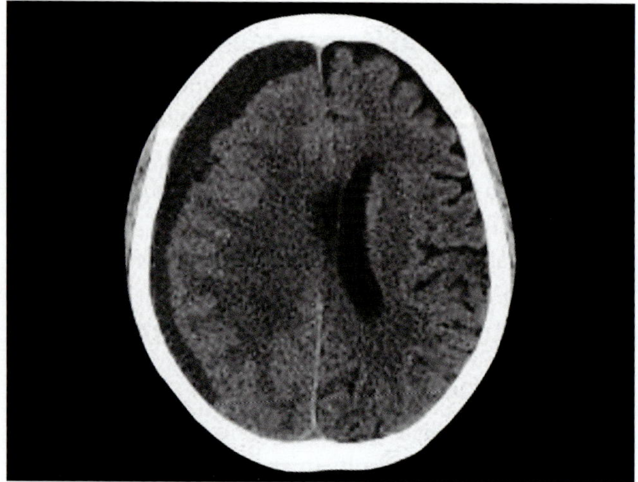

Fig. 8: Chronic subdural hematoma.

Treatment

- Anticoagulation should be reversed, either by administration of vitamin K or urgently by transfusion of recombinant clotting factors in patients who have deteriorated acutely.
- Conservative management include corticosteroids.
    - Small bleeds without symptoms *or*
    - With headache alone

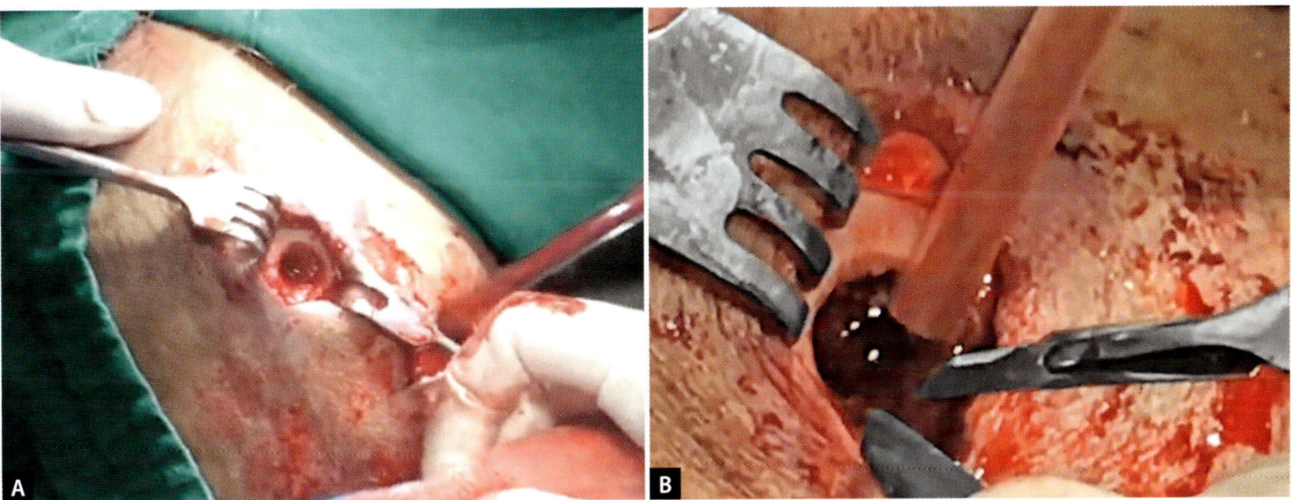

Figs. 9A and B: (A) Burr hole made; (B) Cruciate-shaped incision made over dura with drainage of chronic SDH.

Majority—burr holes drainage (Figs. 9A and B)

- If not drained or thick membrane present, craniotomy and evacuation
  - *Urgency:* Based on clinical condition
- Imaging evidence of mass effect
  - *Delayed:* Clinically stable, a delay of 7–10 days to allow platelet function to normalize after withdrawal of aspirin/clopidogrel may be considered **(Figs. 10A to D)**.

TRAUMATIC BRAIN INJURY IN CHILD

- Child heads are large compared with rest of their body, predisposing to both head and neck injury.
- Nonaccidental injury should always be considered.
- The pediatric Glasgow Coma Scale is applied in the under 2-year-olds.

Management

Minor head injury requires identifying risk factors, requiring further admission for observation or CT scan.

Moderate and severe head injury:

- Trauma team in a resuscitation room
- Using pediatric ATLS protocols to prevent secondary brain injury.
- Intensive care unit (ICU) involvement for airway management.
- Open sutures can lose substantial blood volumes into the head.
- Palpating the fontanelle allows direct assessment of ICP.
- All cases—head and neck CT imaging.

Specific Injury

- Traumatic versus primary subarachnoid hemorrhage is an important distinction.
- Cerebral contusions arise adjacent to rough bone surfaces.
- Diffuse axonal injury results from extreme accelerations of the skull contents.
- Arterial dissection is associated with fractures of the skull base (**Box 1** and **Table 3**).

NEUROSURGICAL MANAGEMENT OF INTRACEREBRAL HEMORRHAGE

Clinical Presentation

- Sudden focal deficit
- Reduced conscious level **(Box 2)**

Etiology

- Spontaneous ICH = 10–15% of strokes
  - The majority—hypertension or amyloid angiopathy, *or*
  - Complication of ischemic stroke
- Coagulation disorders, especially on warfarin treatment, are a major risk factor.

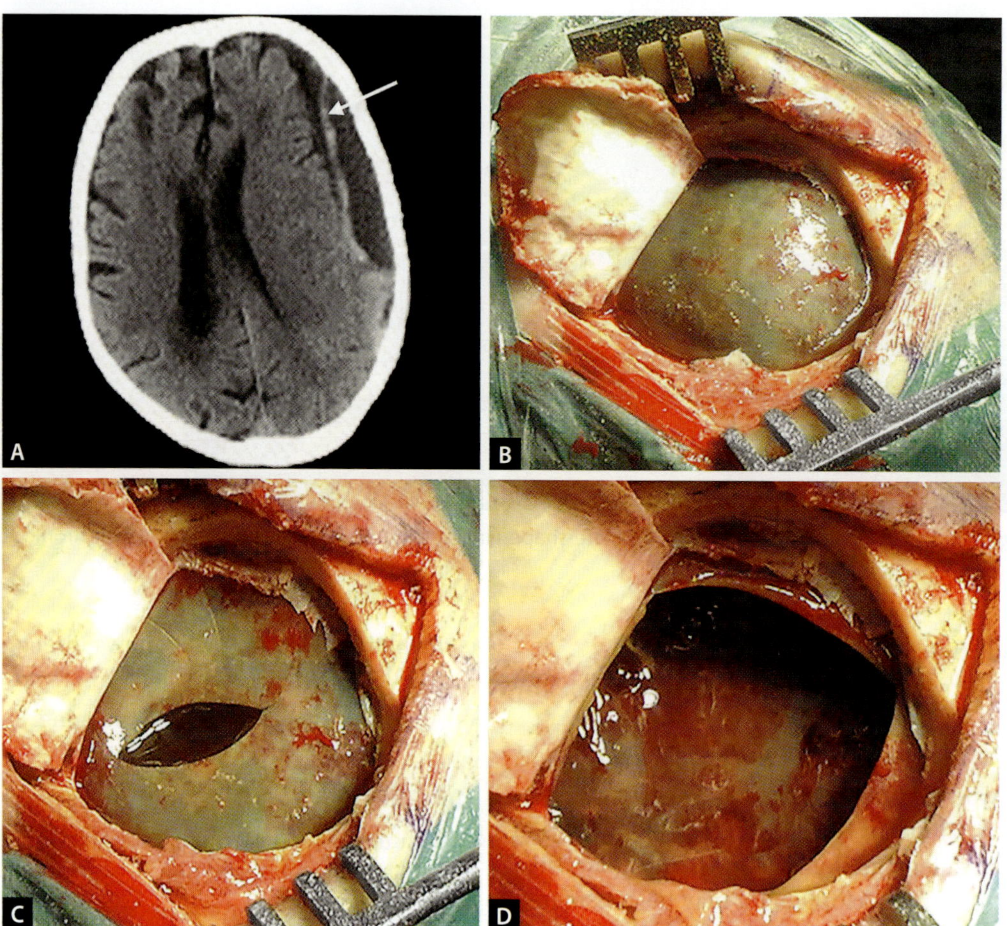

Figs. 10A to D: Minicraniotomy for laminar type chronic subdural hematoma (CSDH). (A) Computed tomography scan demonstrating a laminar-type CSDH. The hyperdense inner septum of the parietal membrane is marked with an arrow; (B) Dural flap was raised, demonstrating the parietal membrane; (C) The parietal membrane was incised, showing yellow–green subdural fluid; (D) The parietal membrane was widely excised, and the subdural fluid from the outer compartment was washed out, revealing the hemorrhagic inner septum of the membrane. The septum was subsequently disrupted and the fluid from the inner compartment was washed out (not shown). The patient made a good recovery.

BOX 1: UK National Institute for Health and Care Excellence (NICE) criteria for computed tomography (CT) scan in children following head injury

- Suspicion of nonaccidental injury (NAI)
- First seizure
- GCS <14 or <15 in under 1-year-old
- GCS <15 two hours postinjury
- Signs of fracture of the base of skull
- Focal neurological deficit
- Bruise/swelling/laceration >5 cm in under-ones
- More than one of the following:
  - Loss of consciousness >5 minutes
  - Abnormal drowsiness
  - Four or more episodes of vomiting
  - Dangerous mechanism
  - Amnesia >5 minutes

(GCS: Glasgow Coma Scale score)

TABLE 3: Pediatric Glasgow Coma Scale score.

Eye opening	Spontaneously	4
	To verbal stimulus	3
	To pain	2
	No response	1
Verbal response	Coos/babbles	5
	Irritable cries	4
	Cries in response to pain	3
	Moans in response to pain	2
	No response	1
Motor response	Purposeful/spontaneous movements	6
	Withdraws to touch	5
	Withdraws to pain	4
	Flexes to pain	3
	Extends to pain	2
	No response	1

BOX 2: Causes of spontaneous intracerebral hemorrhage.

- Hypertension
- Vascular anomaly
- Cerebral aneurysm
- Arteriovenous malformation
- Cavernous malformation
- Cerebral infarction (stroke) transformation
- Cerebral amyloid angiopathy
- Coagulopathy
- Tumors
- Drug abuse
- Other

- In younger patients—to rule out an underlying vascular anomaly or tumor.

Diagnosis (Figs. 11A and B)

Initial resuscitation followed by CT brain.

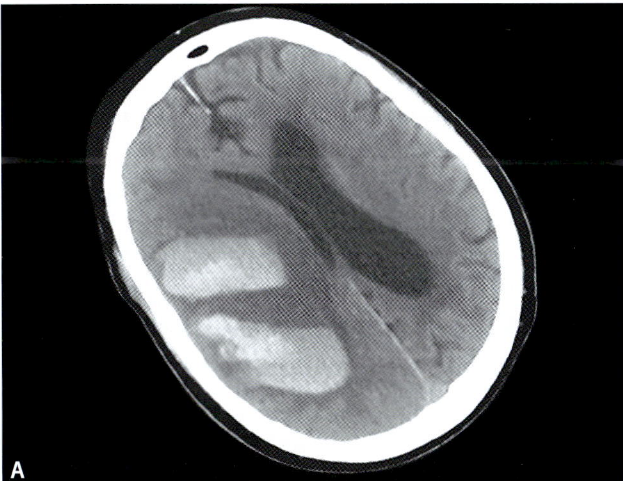

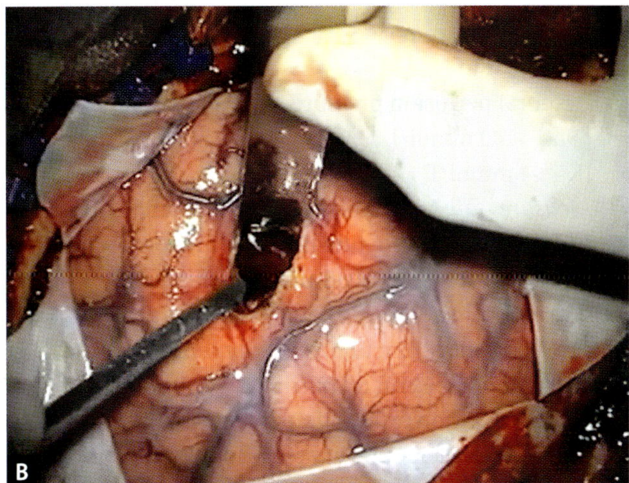

Figs. 11A and B: Computed tomography (CT) brain; (B) Evacuation of intracerebral hemorrhage (ICH).

Management

- Reversal of anticoagulation
- Ongoing hourly neuro-observations
- Blood pressure monitoring.
  - High blood pressure (BP) may be longstanding and associated with adaptations to autoregulation.
  - So, attempts at lowering it acutely with intravenous (IV) antihypertensives should be made only if values are very high [e.g. mean arterial pressure (MAP) >130 mm Hg].
- Due to aneurysm rupture or arteriovenous malformation (AVM) before considering surgical intervention.
- Craniotomy and evacuation—in raised ICP cases.
- May be life-saving by relieving raised ICP but cannot reverse resulting deficits.
- Good option for:
  - Younger, fitter patients with signs of raised ICP
  - Hematomas close to cortical surface or in posterior fossa

Medical Management

- Minimize secondary brain injury through avoidance of hypoxia and hypotension and control of ICP.
- Unchecked, secondary injury leads to a further cycle of deterioration **(Fig. 12)**

Control of Intracranial Pressure

- First-line ICP control involves optimizing sedation, ventilation, and serum sodium levels

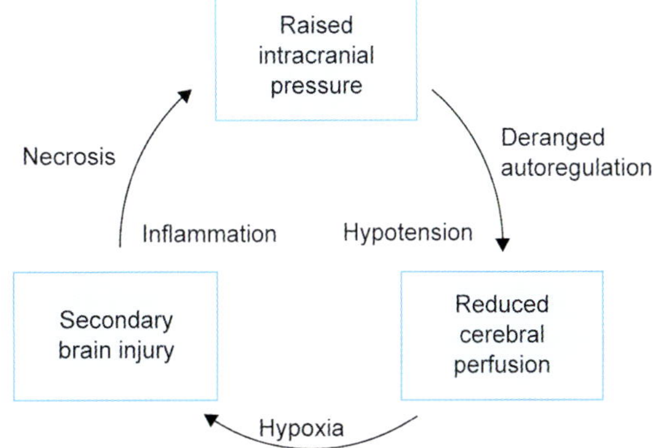

Fig. 12: Cycle of deterioration.

- Bolus of mannitol or hypertonic saline
- ICP monitoring using a bolt ICP monitor or external ventricular drain
- Raising the head of the bed
- Loosening the collar to improve venous drainage
- Seizures and pyrexia should be actively controlled
- Escalating doses of sedatives, analgesics, and muscle relaxants.

Key Parameters to Maintain in Head-Injured Patients in Neuro Intensive Care Unit

- Partial pressure of arterial carbon dioxide ($PaCO_2$) = 4.5–5.0 kPa
- Partial pressure of arterial oxygen (PaO_2) >11 kPa
- MAP = 80–90 mm Hg
- ICP <20 mm Hg
- Cerebral perfusion pressure (CPP) > 60 mm Hg
- [Na^+] >140 mmol/L
- [K^+] >4 mmol/L
- *Measures fail:* Mannitol or hypertonic saline infusions
- Induction of therapeutic hypothermia or thiopentone coma and surgical decompressive craniectomy—long-term outcome benefit is limited or absent.
- Check pituitary function, consider seizure prophylaxis, and commence enteral nutrition within 72 hours.
- Administration of corticosteroids in severe head injury is associated with increased mortality and is not recommended.

Outcomes and Sequelae (Table 4)

TABLE 4: Glasgow outcome scale.

Outcome	*Score*
Good recovery	5
Moderate disability	4
Severe disability	3
Persistent vegetative state	2
Dead	1

SPINAL CORD INJURY

Classification

- Complete
- *Incomplete:*
  - Central cord syndrome
  - Brown-Séquard syndrome (hemisection)
  - Anterior spinal syndrome
  - Posterior cord syndrome
  - Cauda equina syndrome

Pathophysiology

- *Primary injury:*
  - Direct insult to the neural elements
  - Occurs at the time of the initial injury
- *Secondary injury:*
  - Hemorrhage, edema, and ischemia.
  - Accentuated by hypotension, hypoxia, spinal instability, and/or persistent compression of the neural elements.
- Management focuses on minimizing secondary injury.

Identification of Shock

- Hypovolemic shock
- Hypotension with tachycardia and cold, clammy peripheries
- Due to hemorrhage
- Treated with appropriate resuscitation

Neurogenic Shock

- Hypotension, a normal heart rate or bradycardia, and warm peripheries
- Due to unopposed vagal tone resulting from cervical spinal cord injury at or above the level of sympathetic outflow (t5).
- Treated with inotropic support, and care should be taken to avoid fluid overload.

Spinal Shock

- Temporary physiological disorganization of spinal cord function that starts within minutes following the injury
- Length of effect is variable, but it can last 6 weeks or longer.
- Paralysis, decreased tone, and hyporeflexia
- Once it has resolved, the bulbocavernosus reflex returns **(Fig. 13)**.

Assessment

- Use ATLS principles in all cases of spinal injury.
- In polytrauma, cases suspect a spinal injury.
- A second spinal injury at a remote level may be present in 10% of cases.

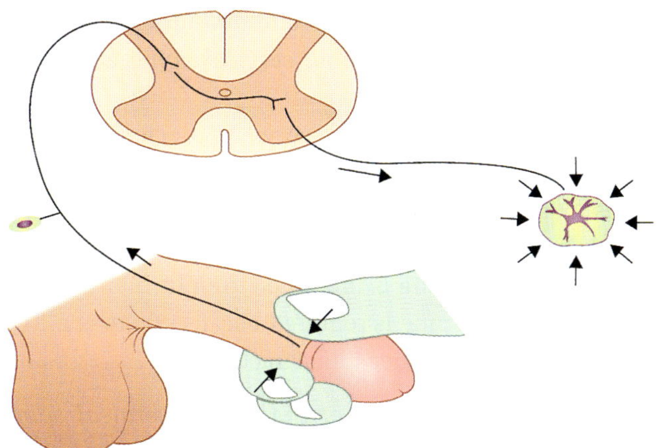
Fig. 13: Bulbocavernosus reflex.

- Spinal boards cause pressure sores **(Figs. 14A and B)**
- The unconscious patient-immobilization should be maintained until magnetic resonance imaging (MRI) or equivalent can be used to rule out an unstable spinal injury.

Pertinent History

- The mechanism and velocity of injury should be determined at an early stage.
- A check for the presence of spinal pain should be made.
- The onset and duration of neurological symptoms should also be recorded.

Physical Examination

Initial assessment:

- The primary survey always takes precedence, followed by careful systems' examination paying particular attention to the abdomen and chest.
- Spinal cord injury may mask signs of intra-abdominal injury.

Spinal Examination

Overlying skin inspection (e.g., for possible penetrating wounds) and the entire spine must be palpated.

A formal spinal log roll must be performed to achieve this.

Significant swelling, tenderness, palpable steps, or gaps suggest a spinal injury. Seatbelt marks on the abdomen and chest must be noted, as these suggest a high-energy accident **(Fig. 15)**.

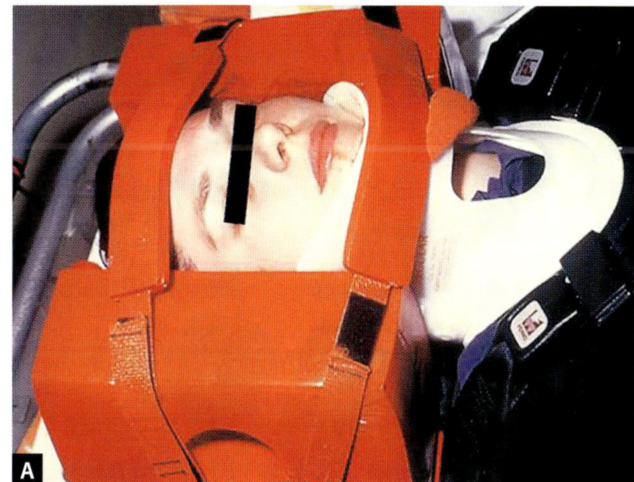

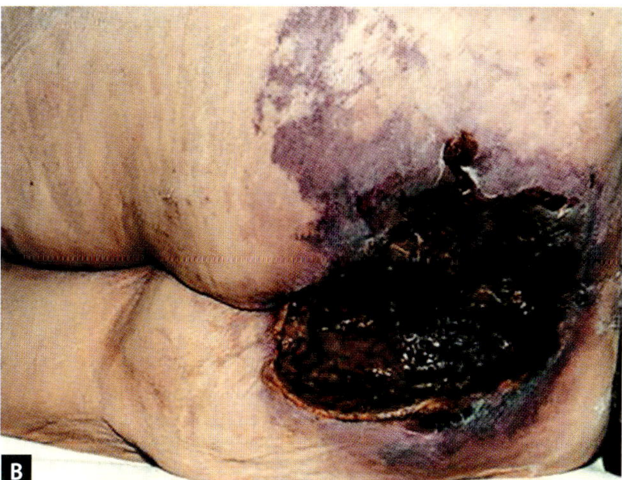

Figs. 14A and B: Pressure sores may develop rapidly in insensate patients.

Neurological Examination

- The American Spinal Injury Association (ASIA) neurological evaluation system is an internationally accepted method of neurological evaluation **(Fig.16)**.
- Motor function is assessed using the Medical Research Council (MRC) grading system (0–5) in key muscle groups. A motor score can then be calculated (maximum 100).
- Sensory function (light touch and pin prick) is assessed using the dermatomal map.
- A total sensory score is then calculated.
- Rectal examination is performed to assess anal tone, voluntary anal contraction, and perianal sensation.

Diagnostic Imaging

- Plain radiograph

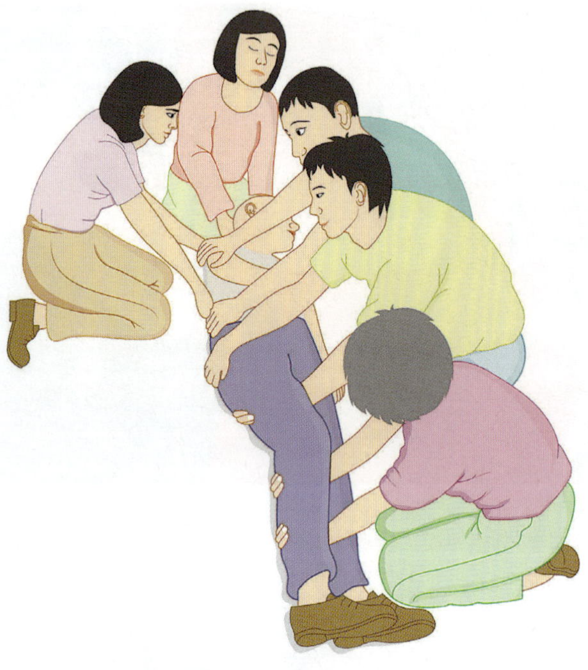

Fig. 15: Spinal log roll.

- *A full cervical spine series:* Anteroposterior and lateral radiographs of the whole cervical spine and open mouth views.
- Clear visualization of the cervicothoracic junction is essential in all cases of suspected spinal injury, as this is a common site for injury and often not seen on a plain radiograph.
- If a spinal fracture is identified then further imaging of the whole spine is required because there is a 15% incidence of a further spinal fracture.

A system for evaluation of the lateral cervical spine radiograph:

- Assess prevertebral soft-tissue swelling **(Figs. 17 and 18)**.
- Assess sagittal alignment using three imaginary lines.
- Assess for instability:
  - 3.5 mm of sagittal translation **(Fig. 19)**
  - Sagittal angulation of >11° (compared with the adjacent level).

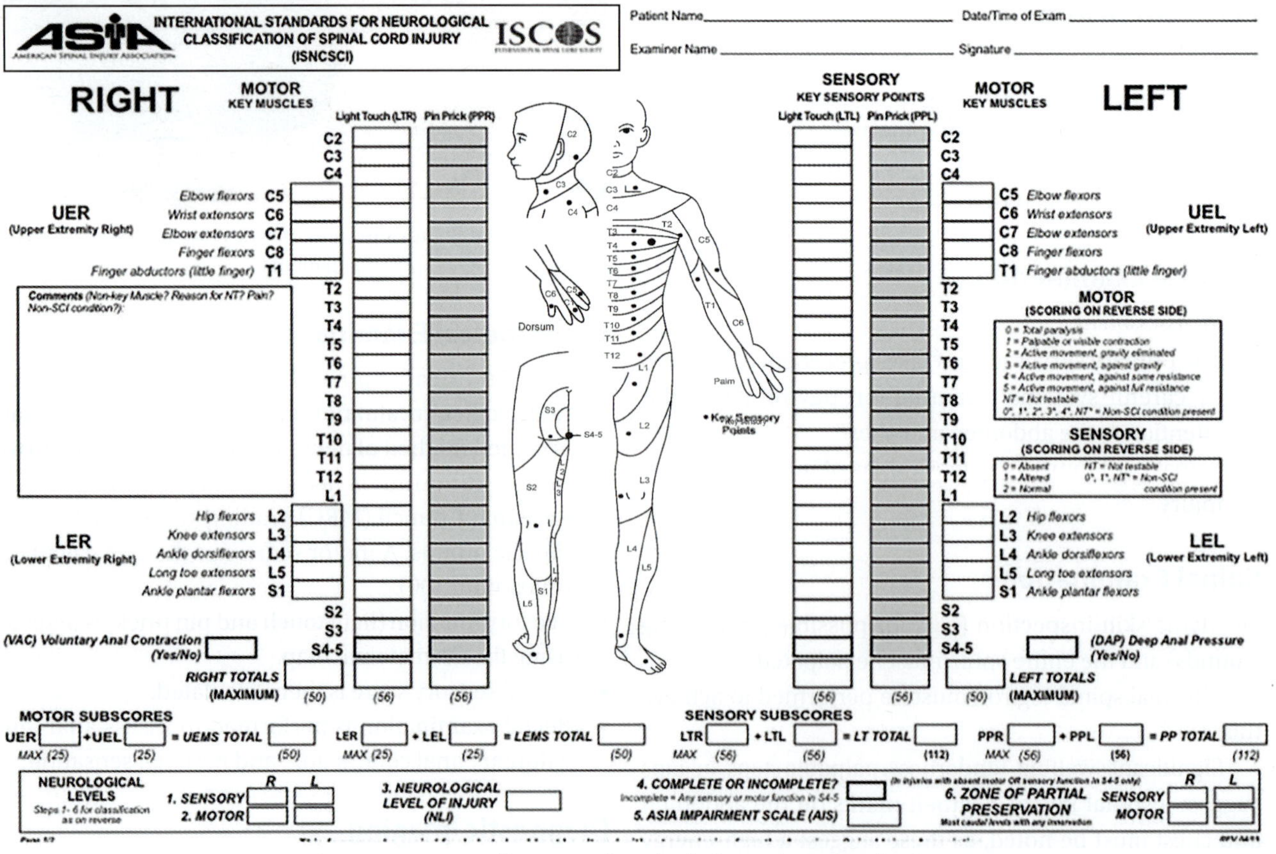

ASIA — AMERICAN SPINAL INJURY ASSOCIATION

INTERNATIONAL STANDARDS FOR NEUROLOGICAL CLASSIFICATION OF SPINAL CORD INJURY (ISNCSCI)

ISCOS

Patient Name ______ Date/Time of Exam ______

Examiner Name ______ Signature ______

RIGHT — MOTOR KEY MUSCLES — SENSORY KEY SENSORY POINTS: Light Touch (LTR), Pin Prick (PPR)

C2, C3, C4

UER (Upper Extremity Right): Elbow flexors C5; Wrist extensors C6; Elbow extensors C7; Finger flexors C8; Finger abductors (little finger) T1

Comments (Non-key Muscle? Reason for NT? Pain? Non-SCI condition?):

T2, T3, T4, T5, T6, T7, T8, T9, T10, T11, T12, L1

LER (Lower Extremity Right): Hip flexors L2; Knee extensors L3; Ankle dorsiflexors L4; Long toe extensors L5; Ankle plantar flexors S1

S2, S3, S4-5

(VAC) Voluntary Anal Contraction (Yes/No)

RIGHT TOTALS (MAXIMUM) (50) (56) (56)

LEFT — MOTOR KEY MUSCLES — SENSORY KEY SENSORY POINTS: Light Touch (LTL), Pin Prick (PPL)

C2, C3, C4

UEL (Upper Extremity Left): C5 Elbow flexors; C6 Wrist extensors; C7 Elbow extensors; C8 Finger flexors; T1 Finger abductors (little finger)

T2, T3, T4, T5, T6, T7, T8, T9, T10, T11, T12, L1

MOTOR (SCORING ON REVERSE SIDE)
0 = Total paralysis
1 = Palpable or visible contraction
2 = Active movement, gravity eliminated
3 = Active movement, against gravity
4 = Active movement, against some resistance
5 = Active movement, against full resistance
NT = Not testable
0*, 1*, 2*, 3*, 4*, NT* = Non-SCI condition present

SENSORY (SCORING ON REVERSE SIDE)
0 = Absent; 1 = Altered; 2 = Normal
NT = Not testable
0*, 1*, NT* = Non-SCI condition present

LEL (Lower Extremity Left): L2 Hip flexors; L3 Knee extensors; L4 Ankle dorsiflexors; L5 Long toe extensors; S1 Ankle plantar flexors

S2, S3, S4-5

(DAP) Deep Anal Pressure (Yes/No)

LEFT TOTALS (MAXIMUM) (56) (56) (50)

Body diagram labels: C2, C3, C4, T2, T3, T4, T5, T6, T7, T8, T9, T10, T11, T12, C5, C6, C8, T1, L1, L2, L3, L4, L5, S1, S2, S3, S4-5, Dorsum, Palm, • Key Sensory Points

MOTOR SUBSCORES

UER ☐ + UEL ☐ = UEMS TOTAL ☐ — MAX (25) (25) (50)

LER ☐ + LEL ☐ = LEMS TOTAL ☐ — MAX (25) (25) (50)

SENSORY SUBSCORES

LTR ☐ + LTL ☐ = LT TOTAL ☐ — MAX (56) (56) (112)

PPR ☐ + PPL ☐ = PP TOTAL ☐ — MAX (56) (56) (112)

NEUROLOGICAL LEVELS (Steps 1-6 for classification as on reverse): 1. SENSORY R ☐ L ☐; 2. MOTOR R ☐ L ☐

3. NEUROLOGICAL LEVEL OF INJURY (NLI) ☐

4. COMPLETE OR INCOMPLETE? ☐ (Incomplete = Any sensory or motor function in S4-5)

5. ASIA IMPAIRMENT SCALE (AIS) ☐

6. ZONE OF PARTIAL PRESERVATION (In injuries with absent motor OR sensory function in S4-5 only; Most caudal levels with any innervation): SENSORY R ☐ L ☐; MOTOR R ☐ L ☐

Fig. 16: Internationally accepted method of neurological evaluation.

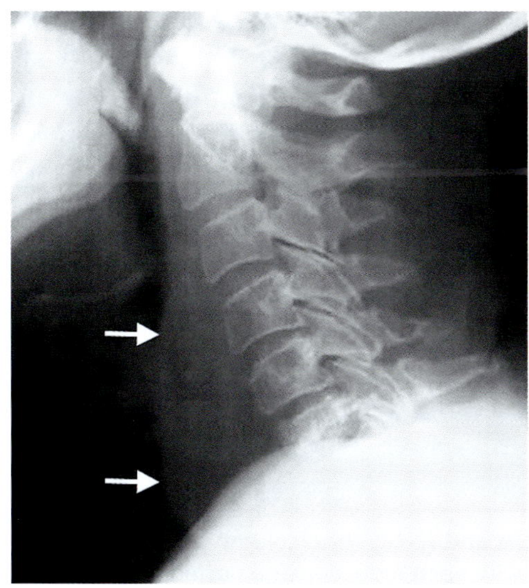

Fig. 17: Prevertebral soft tissue swelling

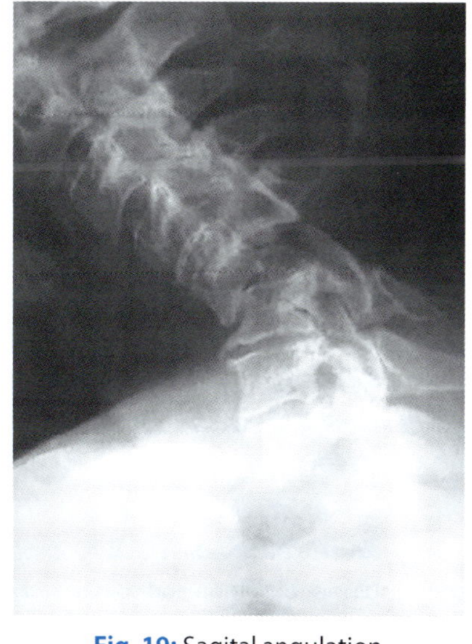

Fig. 19: Sagital angulation

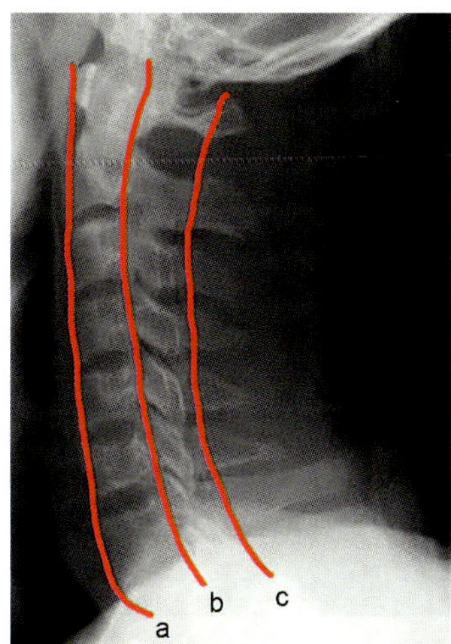

Fig. 18: (a) Anterior, (b) posterior, and (c) spinolaminar lines are useful in identifying anterior translation on lateral radiographs of the neck.

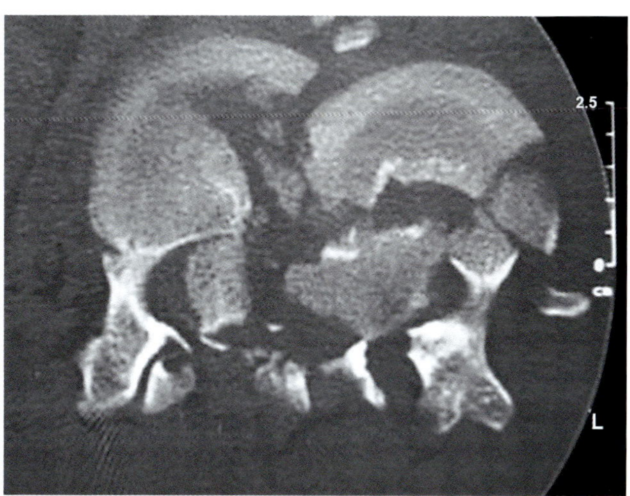

Fig. 20: Axial computed tomography demonstrating a thoracolumbar facture dislocation.

Computed Tomography

- Two-dimensional CT reconstruction is the gold standard in spinal trauma.
- *Indication:* Suspected or visible injuries on plain radiographs
- Patients undergoing a head CT scan for closed head injury should also have a cervical screening CT.
- Often, CT scans of the chest and abdomen are performed as part of the assessment of polytrauma patients and will usually include the spine **(Fig. 20)**.

Magnetic Resonance Imaging

Indication:

- All patients with neurological deficit and where assessment of ligamentous structures is important **(Figs. 21 and 24)**

Dynamic Imaging

- Lateral flexion-extension radiographs of the cervical spine should not be undertaken acutely
- Role in assessing spinal stability in the longer term

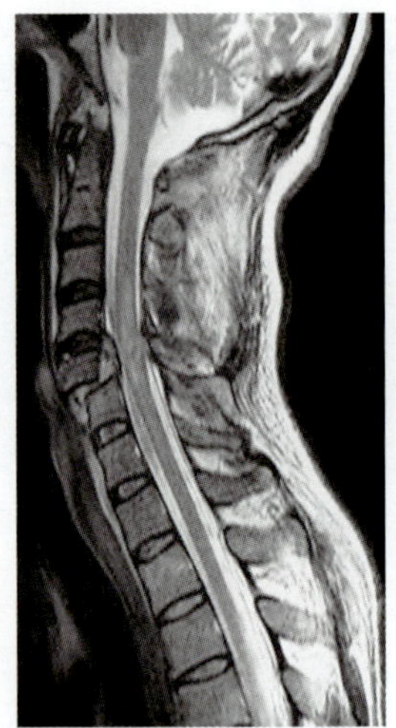

Fig. 21: Cervical spine subluxation and spinal cord contusion.

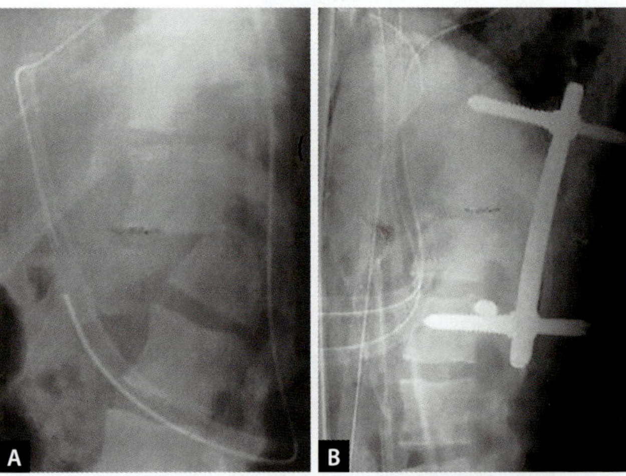

Figs. 23A and B: (A) Thoracolumbar fracture dislocation (B) treated with open reduction and posterior fixation as shown in **Figures 23A and B**.

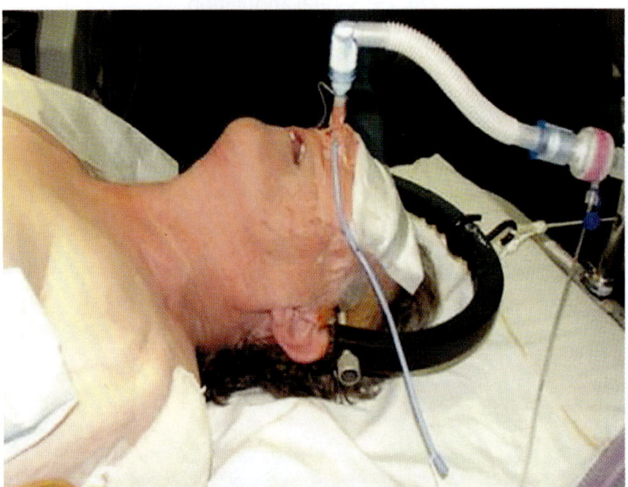

Fig. 22: Skeletal traction using skull tongs.

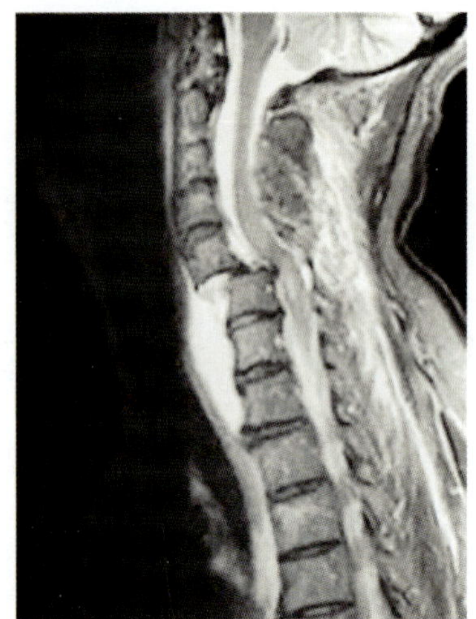

Fig. 24: Bifacetal cervical spine dislocation.

Basic Management Principles

Spinal Realignment

- Skeletal traction is necessary to achieve anatomical realignment—skull tongs **(Fig. 22)**
- Reduction and stabilization with internal fixation **(Figs. 23A and B)**
- Halo brace **(Fig. 26)**

Performed a closed realignment and immobilization of cervical fractures.

Stabilization Surgery

Absolute indication for surgery in spinal trauma is deteriorating neurological function **(Fig. 25)**

Decompression of Neural Elements

- Realignment of the spine and correction of the spinal deformity may achieve an indirect decompression.
- Direct decompression of the neural elements may also be indicated if there are bone fragments causing residual compression or a significant hematoma.

The timing of surgery in spinal cord trauma remains controversial **(Figs. 27 and 28)**.

Corticosteroids

- No longer indicated in acute spinal cord injury because of a lack of evidence to support efficacy

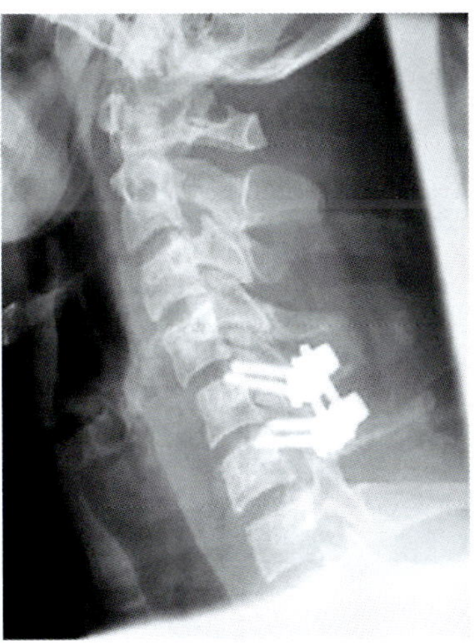

Fig. 25: Posterior stabilization following closed reduction.

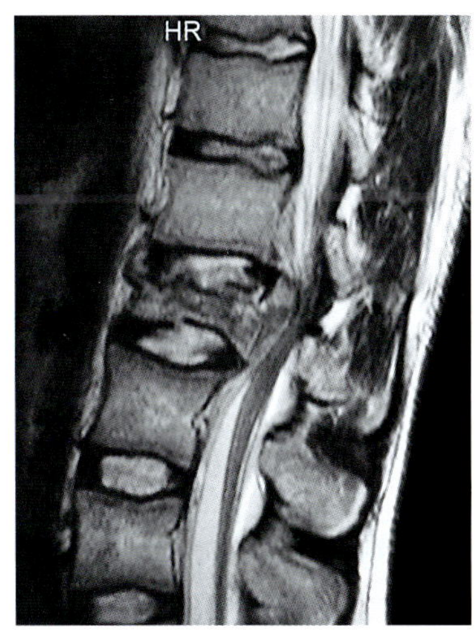

Fig. 27: Combined anterior and posterior surgery.

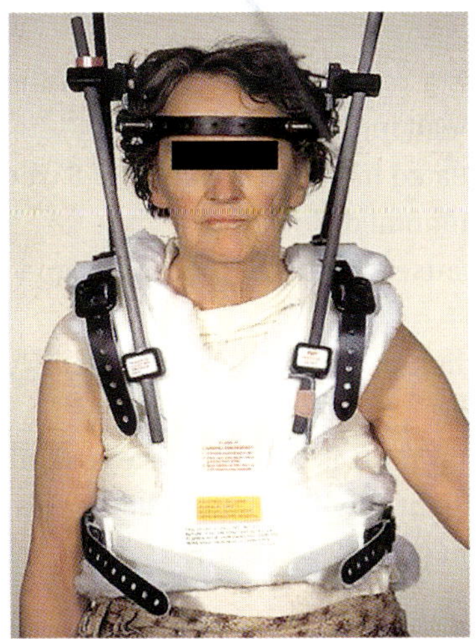

Fig. 26: External immobilization using a halo jacket.

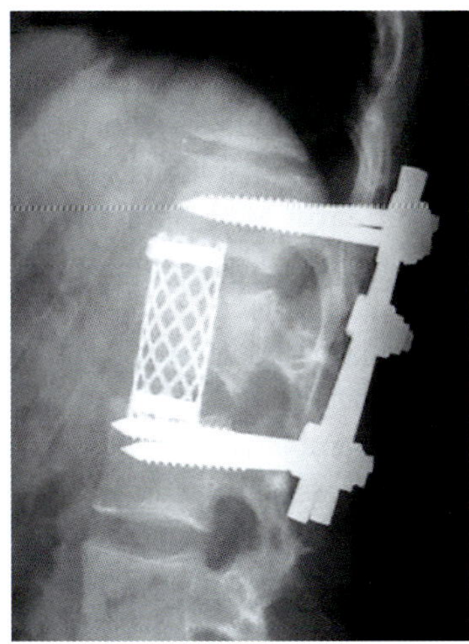

Fig. 28: L1 burst fracture with neural compression.

- Role in nontraumatic spinal cord compression, for example, malignant spinal cord compression

Complications Associated with Spinal Cord Injury

- *Pressure ulcers*: Many of these are preventable. Patients should be turned regularly on an appropriate mattress to minimize the risk of skin breakdown.
- *Pain and spasticity* Neurogenic pain is common. Once reflex activity returns following cord injury, spasticity may occur and can be problematic. Intrathecal infusion of baclofen may be required in resistant cases.
- Autonomic dysreflexia
    - This is a paroxysmal syndrome of hypertension, hyperhidrosis (above the level of injury), bradycardia, flushing, and headache in response to noxious visceral and other stimuli.
    - It is most commonly triggered by bladder distension or rectal loading from fecal impaction.

Neurological Deterioration

- Post-traumatic syringomyelia may occur in around 28% of patients with spinal cord injury up to 30 years following injury. Approximately, 30% of cases are symptomatic.

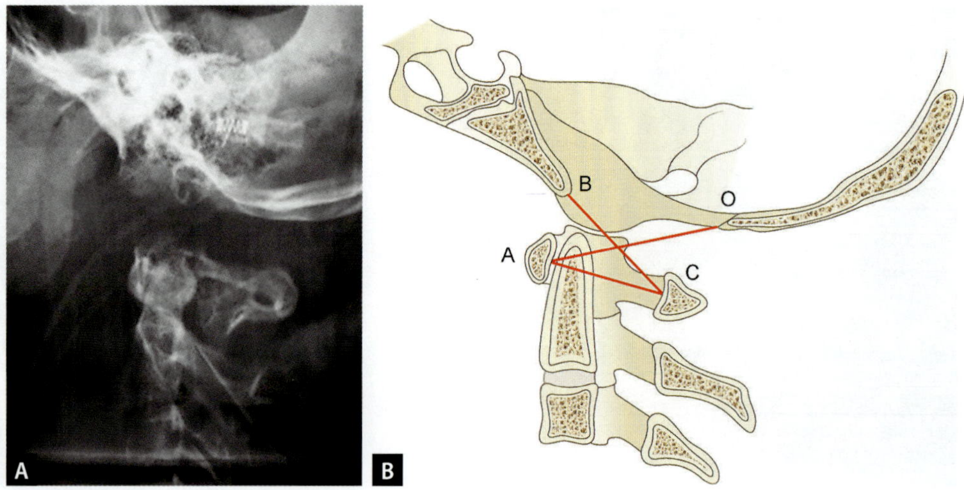

Figs. 29A and B: (A)Vertical occipitocervical dislocation; (B) Powers' ratio = BC/OA ≥1 indicates anterior translation; ≤0.75 indicates posterior translation.

- Clinically, patients present with segmental pain at or above the level of injury, sensory loss, progressive asymmetrical weakness, or increased spasticity.
- This warrants early MRI assessment. Expanding cavities require neurosurgical intervention.
- Thromboembolic events
- Deep vein thrombosis occurs in 30% of patients with spinal cord injury.
- Fatal pulmonary embolus is reported in 1–2% of cases. Thromboprophylaxis with compression stockings and low-molecular- weight heparin is indicated, provided there are no contraindications.

Osteoporosis, Heterotopic Ossification, and Contractures

- Disuse osteoporosis is an inevitable consequence of spinal cord injury and fragility fractures may occur.
- Heterotopic ossification may affect the hips, knees, shoulders and elbows.
- It occurs in 25% of patients with spinal cord injury. Surgery is appropriate in selected cases.
- Soft-tissue contractures around joints may occur as a result of spasticity but can be avoided by appropriate physical therapy, positioning, and splinting.

Cervical Spine Injury

Upper Cervical Spine (Skull–C2)

- Occipital condyle fracture
    - This is a relatively stable injury often associated with head injuries.
    - It is treated in a hard collar for 6–8 weeks.
- Occipitoatlantal dislocation
    - It is caused by high-energy trauma and is often fatal.
    - The dislocation may be anterior, posterior, or vertical.
    - Powers' ratio is used to assess skull translation. Treatment is with a halo brace or occipitocervical fixation **(Figs. 29A and B)**.

Atlas Fracture (Jefferson Fracture)

- Fracture of the C1 ring is associated with axial loading of the cervical spine and may be stable or unstable
- Associated transverse ligament rupture may occur

Most are treated nonoperatively in a cervical collar or halo brace **(Figs. 30A to C)**.

Open mouth view of C1/2:

- C1 lateral mass deviation (arrows in **Figure 30C**).
- Rupture of the transverse ligament is present when the combined

Atlantoaxial Instability

- This is defined as nonphysiological movement between C1 and C2.
- It can be translational or rotatory.

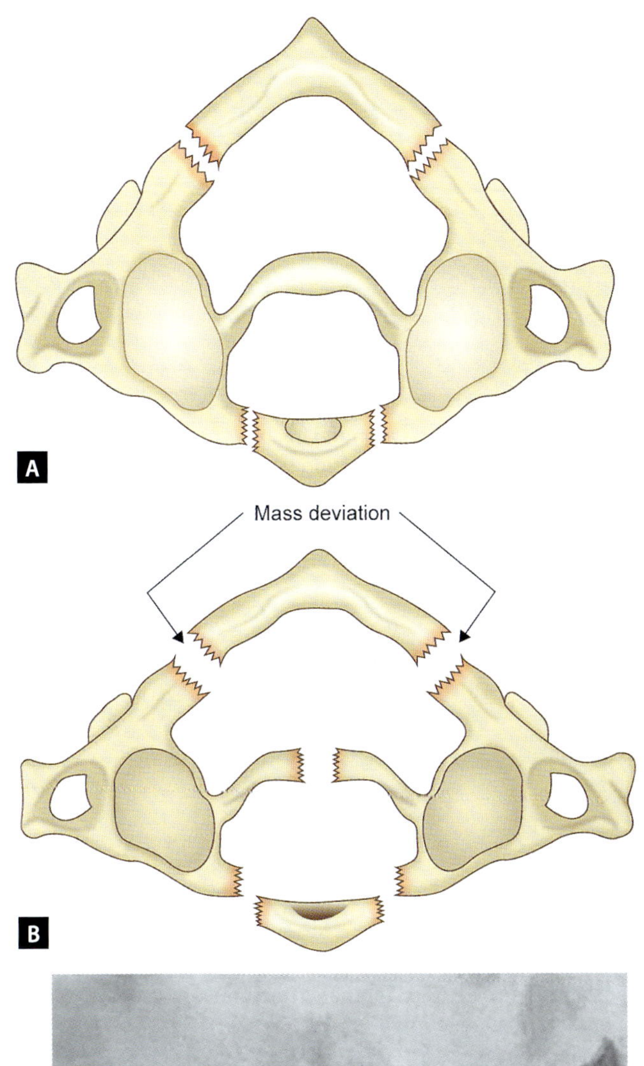

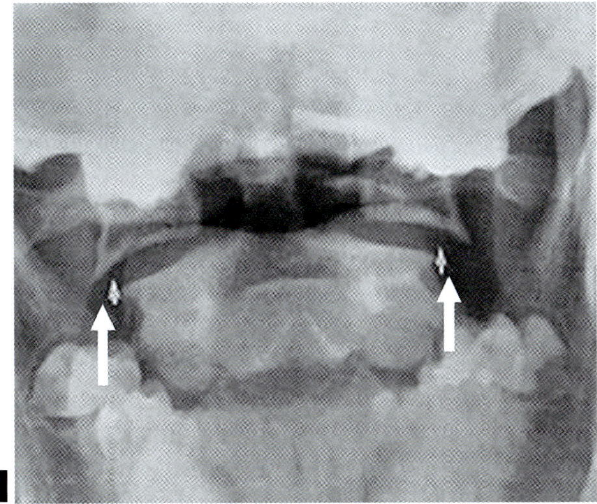

Figs. 30A to C: Atlas fracture (Jefferson fracture). (A) Stable; (B) unstable; and (C) Open mouth view of C1/2.

- It resolves either spontaneously or with traction followed by a cervical collar.

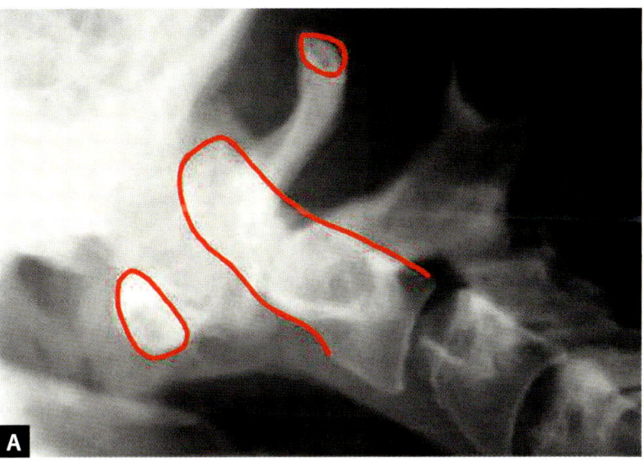

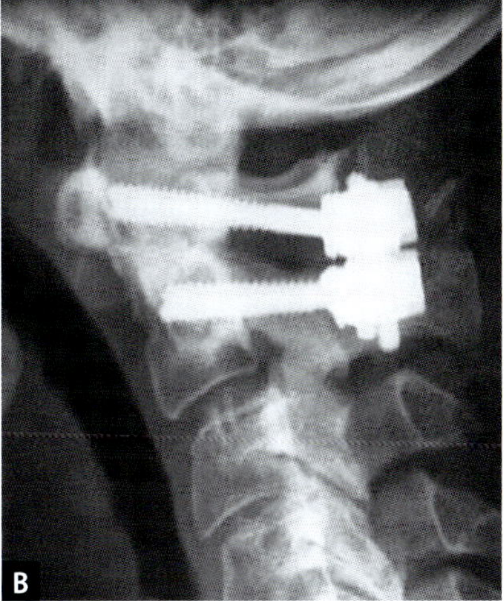

Figs. 31A and B: (A) Atlantoaxial instability. (A) C1/2 posterior fusion using C1 lateral mass and C2 pedicle screws. (B) Atlantoaxial subluxation.

- Isolated, traumatic transverse ligament rupture leading to C1/2 instability is uncommon and is treated with posterior C1/2 fusion **(Figs. 31A and B)**.

Odontoid Fractures (Figs. 32 and 33)

- These are of 3 types.
- Neurological injury is rare.
- The majority of acute injuries are treated nonoperatively in a hard collar or halo jacket for 3 months.
- Internal fixation with an anterior compression screw is indicated for displaced fractures.
- Posterior C1/2 fusion is considered in cases of nonunion.
- In the elderly, treatment in a soft collar should be considered on the basis that a relatively stable pseudarthrosis will occur.

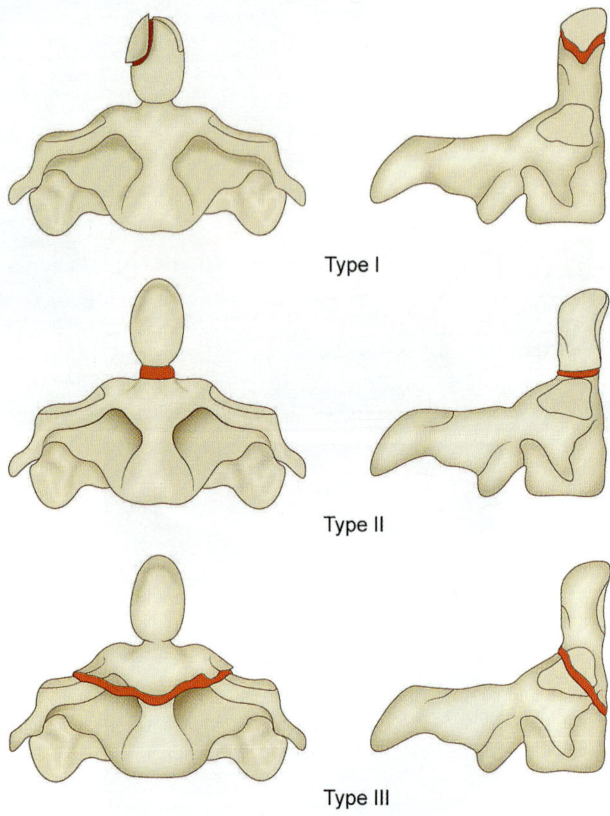

Fig. 32: Odontoid fractures.

Traumatic Spondylolisthesis of Axis (Hangman's Fracture)

- This is a traumatic spondylolisthesis of C2 on C3.
- There are four types with varying degrees of instability.
- Those with significant displacement or associated facet dislocation are treated operatively, usually with posterior stabilization **(Figs. 34A and B)**.

Subaxial Cervical Spine (C3–C7)

- Mechanism of trauma-compression fractures (hyperflexion), burst fractures (axial compression), facet subluxation/dislocation injuries (distraction-flexion), teardrop fractures (hyperextension), and fracture of posterior elements.
- The more severe injuries may have an associated spinal cord injury. Operative intervention may be required to decompress the spinal cord and to stabilize the spine with internal fixation.
- Facet subluxation/dislocation ranges in severity from minor instability to complete dislocation with spinal cord injury **(Figs. 35A to C)**.

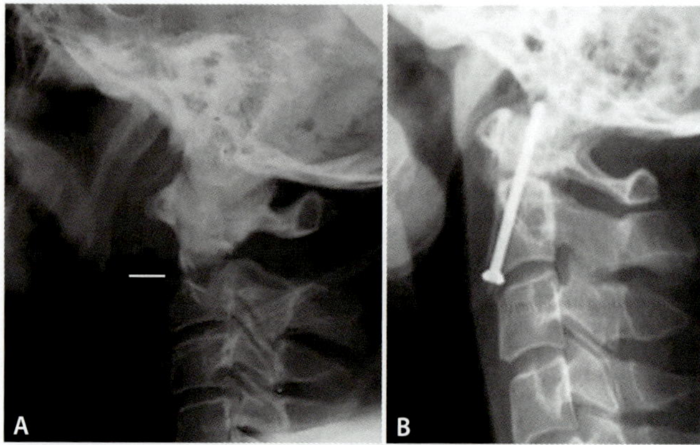

Figs. 33A and B: Odontoid fractures type II anterior compression screws.

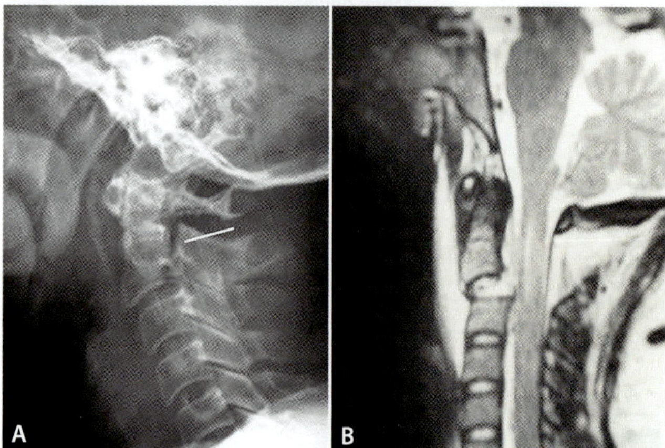

Figs. 34A and B: Hangman's fractures of C2 with minimal forward translation (arrow); (B) Hangman's fractures of C2 with minimal forward translation (arrow).

Fractures in Patients with Ankylosing Spondylitis

- Ankylosing spondylitis is a seronegative inflammatory disorder that causes autofusion of the spine.
- These patients have a higher risk of spinal fractures and spinal cord injury than the normal population.
- Senior advice should be obtained, because application of a cervical collar may be contraindicated, and patients should be managed instead in a position of comfort.
- Surgical stabilization is commonly indicated.

Thoracic and Thoracolumbar Fractures

- Arbeitsgemeinschaft für Osteosynthesefragen (AO) classifies these fractures.
- There are three main injury types, A, B, and C, with increasing instability and risk of neurological injury.
- *Type A:* Vertebral body compression fractures

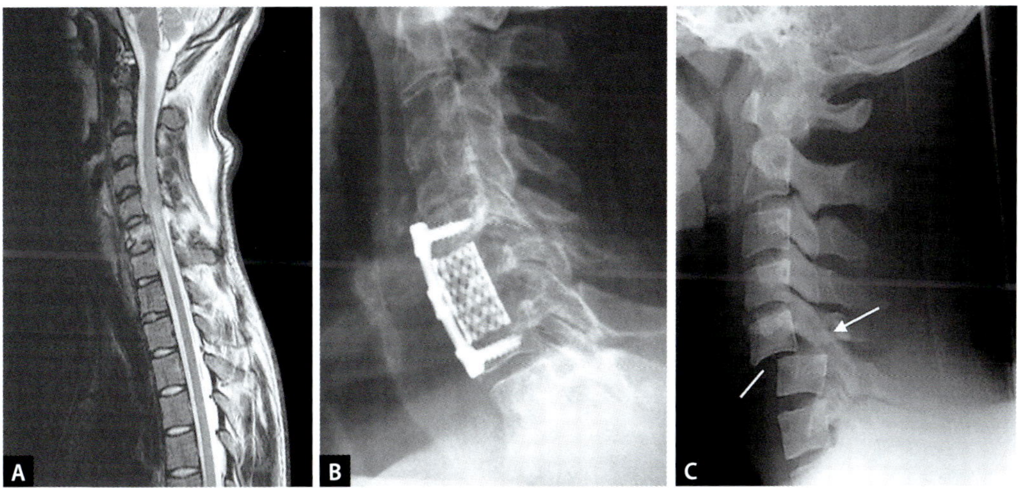

Figs. 35A to C: (A) Cervical burst fracture with spinal cord contusion; (B) treated with anterior decompression and reconstruction; (C) 5/6 bifacetal dislocation.

- *Type B:* Distraction of the anterior or posterior elements
- *Types C:* Rotational and often coexist with type A or B injuries.
- The majority of type B and type C injuries require surgical stabilization.

Thoracic Spine (T1–T10)

Osteoporotic wedge compression fractures.

- Most common injury in this group
- Mostly heal spontaneously
- *Symptomatic:* Percutaneous bone cement augmentation—vertebroplasty or kyphoplasty.
- Trauma cases
- Unstable fractures—significant energy transfer
- Associated with major internal injuries, such as pulmonary contusion and spinal cord injury

Note:

- Rib fractures (long arrow)
- Dislocation (short arrow)
- The presence of a chest tube **(Fig. 36)**.

Lateral radiograph showing multiple osteoporotic compression fractures.

Reduction in thoracic kyphotic deformity following four-level kyphoplasty

- The combination of thoracic spine disruption and a sternal fracture also carries a significant risk of aortic rupture
- Multiple posterior rib fractures and rib dislocations above and below a thoracic spinal injury signify a major rotational injury to the chest.

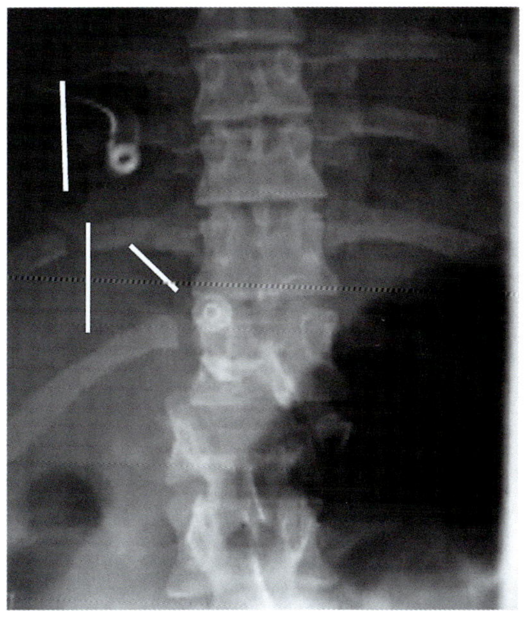

Fig. 36: Rotational (type C) injury at the thoracolumbar junction.

- It can be associated with vascular injury and significant pulmonary contusion.

Treatment

- Multimodality diagnostic imaging is recommended.
- Surgery is required, if unstable.

Thoracolumbar Spinal Fractures (T11–L2) (Fig. 37)

More prone to injury—minor wedge fracture to spinal dislocation.

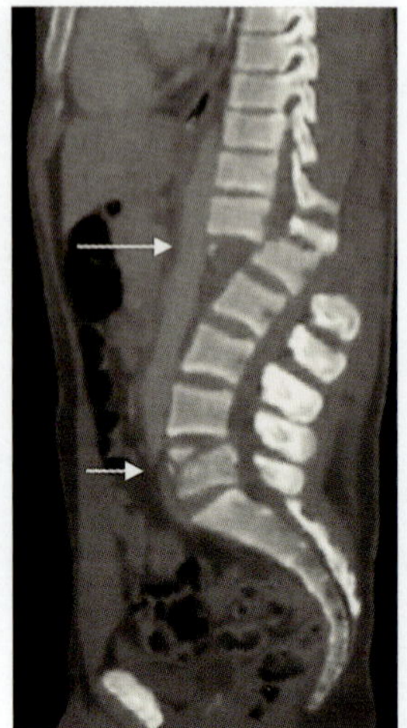

Fig. 37: Thoracolumbar junction injury. Thoracolumbar fractures dislocation (long arrow) fracture of L5 (short arrow).

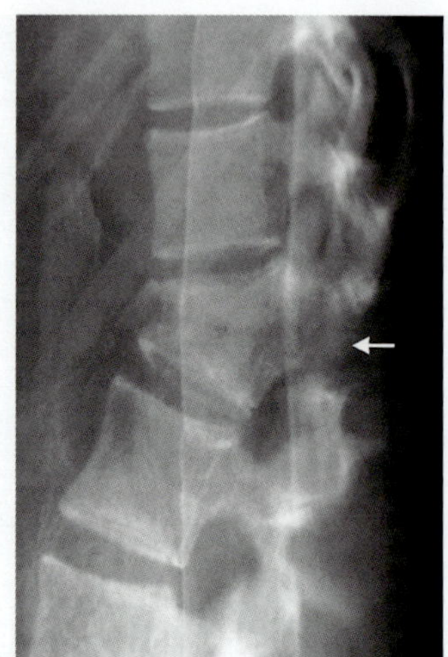

Fig. 39: Bony Chance fracture at the thoracolumbar junction (arrow) secondary to a lap-belt injury.

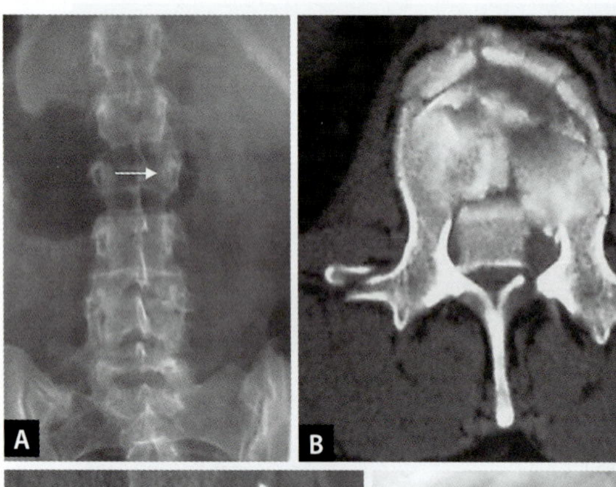

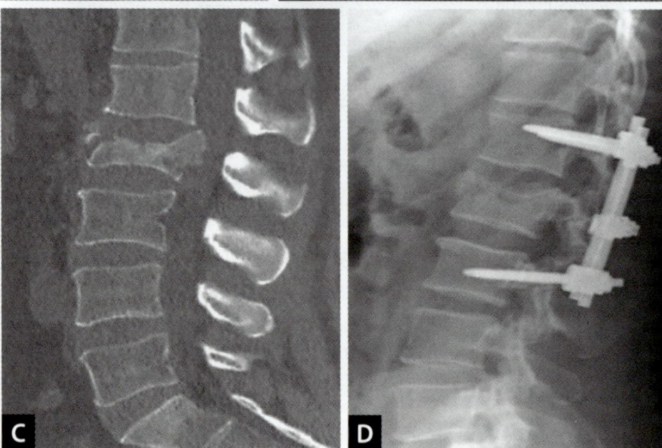

Figs. 38A to D: Lumbar burst fracture. (A) Increase in the interpedicular distance (arrow); (B) Spinal canal compromise; (C and D) Lumbar burst fracture at L2 posterior instrumentation with indirect reduction.

Burst Fracture (Figs. 38A to D)

- Comminuted fractures of the vertebral body
- Widening of the distance between the pedicles
- Associated with retropulsion of bone fragments into the spinal canal
- Current treatment principles—posterior fixation
- Anterior surgery is now rarely used.

Chance Fracture

- Flexion-distraction injuries of the thoracolumbar junction
- Associated with the use of lap belts
- Duodenal, pancreatic, and/or aortic ruptures are also associated with these injuries.

Lumbar Spinal Fractures (L3–S1)

- The incidence of neurological injury is lower.
- Neural canal is more capacious at this level (the spinal cord terminates at L1/L2).
- Most treated nonsurgically
- Owing to the, less likely for kyphotic deformity than injuries at the thoracolumbar junction **(Fig. 39)**

Urological Emergencies

Emergencies in Urology

U Venkatesh

INTRODUCTION

Emergencies in urology are relatively less when compared to other surgical specialties. However, they have to be attended at right time without much delay. Thorough clinical evaluation and supportive radiological imaging has to be done to arrive at the right diagnosis before any intervention.

Urological emergencies can basically be divided into traumatic and nontraumatic emergencies.

UROSEPSIS

Definition

Urosepsis refers to the complex immune response produced by the human body in response to the invasion of microorganisms into the urinary tract. These microbes release endogenous mediators, which lead to complex clinical phenomena. Urosepsis may progress to septic shock if left untreated and may increase the mortality.

Etiology of Urosepsis

Urosepsis is caused by:

- Gram-negative bacteria
  - *Escherichia coli*, 52%
  - *Enterobacteriaceae* spp., 22%,
  - *Pseudomonas aeruginosa*, 4%
- Gram-positive bacteria
  - *Enterococcus* spp., 5%,
  - *Staphylococcus aureus*, 10%

Pathophysiology

Sepsis is caused by the invasion of intact pathogenic bacteria or bacterial cell wall constituents, especially lipopolysaccharides (LPS) or toxins into systemic circulation. They bind to various cell surface receptors on white blood cell and endothelial cells and release various mediators that are responsible for a plethora of local and systemic effects in the host organism. This can lead on to a sequence of events starting from systemic inflammatory response syndrome (SIRS) to multiorgan dysfunction syndrome (MODS), which if not treated at the appropriate time, may lead to significant morbidity and mortality.

Risk Factors for Urosepsis

Risk factors for urosepsis:

- Advanced age
- Diabetes mellitus
- Malignancy
- Immunodeficiency
- Obstructive uropathy
- Nosocomial infections

Clinical Symptoms

Premonitory symptoms are:

- Tachypnea (>20 breaths/min)
- Tachycardia (>90 beats/min)
- Hyperthermia (>38°C)

Followed by intermittent bouts of fever with shaking chills during the invasion of bacteria.

Diagnostic Procedures

Diagnostic procedures are given in **Box 1**.

BOX 1: Laboratory findings in urosepsis.

- Erythrocyte sedimentation rate increased (normal range—females 1–25 mm/h; males 0–17 mm/h)
- C-reactive protein (CRP) increased (normal range: 0.1–≤8.2 mg/L, depends on the method used)
- Leukocyte counts (>12 × 10^9/L or <4 × 10^9/L) with toxic granulation and immature neutrophils (bands) >10%
- Thrombocytopenia (<80 × 10^9/L)
- Hyperbilirubinemia (normal range <1 mg/100 mL)
- Increased creatinine level (normal range <1.5 mg/100 mL)
- Proteinuria
- Initially, respiratory alkalosis then later on, metabolic acidosis
- Hypoxemia
- Biomarkers of sepsis (cytokines and procalcitonin) and of blood coagulation (D-dimer, protein C, protein S, and antithrombin) may be determined and provide further hints

Recommended Therapeutic Approach to Patients Suffering from Urosepsis

The general goals of therapy are:
- Stabilization of hemodynamics
- Improvement of oxygen saturation and sufficient organ perfusion
- Improved organ function (heart, lung, liver, and kidney)
- Antimicrobial treatment of sepsis
- Sanitization of the focal source of infection

Patients should immediately be transferred to the ICU and:
- The patient should be treated with intravenous (IV) bolus followed by IV fluids to maintain adequate intravascular volume.
- Patients may require inotropes and vasopressors, especially in those with septic shock.
- Start on appropriate broad-spectrum IV antibiotics.
- Take aggressive measures to eradicate the source of infection.
- Continuous vitals monitoring is recommended.
- Patient may require assisted ventilation, especially in those with severe sepsis and metabolic acidosis.

EMPHYSEMATOUS PYELONEPHRITIS

Emphysematous pyelonephritis (EPN) is a urological emergency. It has an overall mortality rate ranging between 19 and 43%. It refers to acute necrotizing infection of renal parenchyma caused by gas-forming organisms.

Etiopathogenesis

Emphysematous pyelonephritis is often associated with type-2 diabetes mellitus. Very high tissue glucose levels seen in these patients may form the substrate for these microorganisms, which ferment this glucose and produce carbon dioxide (CO_2). This CO_2 is responsible for the characteristic air pockets seen in radiological images in these patients. EPN is also seen in patients with urinary tract obstruction associated with calculi or papillary necrosis.

Clinical Presentation

Emphysematous pyelonephritis is more often seen in adults and female preponderance is seen. Patients often present with features of acute severe pyelonephritis. Patients present with high grade fever, vomiting, and loin pain. Passing air bubbles in urine often termed as pneumaturia may be present if collecting system is involved.

Radiologic Findings

Radiologic findings include:
- *X-ray kidneys, ureters, and bladder (KUB):* X-ray shows typical mottled gas appearance in the renal region. Crescent-shaped collection of gas over upper pole of kidney is more distinctive.
- *Ultrasonography (USG):* Presence of intraparenchymal gas appears as strong focal echoes in the renal fossa.
- *Computed tomography (CT)* ***(Fig. 1):*** It is the investigation of choice. It shows the severity and extent of infection and also guides in management of these patients. CT often reveals the presence of streaky or mottled gas, and it is associated with rapid destruction of renal parenchyma with 50–60% mortality rate.

Huang and Tseng (2000) developed a radiologic classification system for EPN. It is based on the extent of gas involvement in the renal tissue on CT scan and it helps to guide management **(Table 1)**.

Management

Many of these patients present with sepsis or septic shock. They must be adequately resuscitated with IV fluids, inotropes, and should be started on broad-spectrum antibiotics. Strict glycemic control and electrolyte imbalance if any had to be strictly addressed. If CT reveals any distal ureteric obstruction, it must be promptly

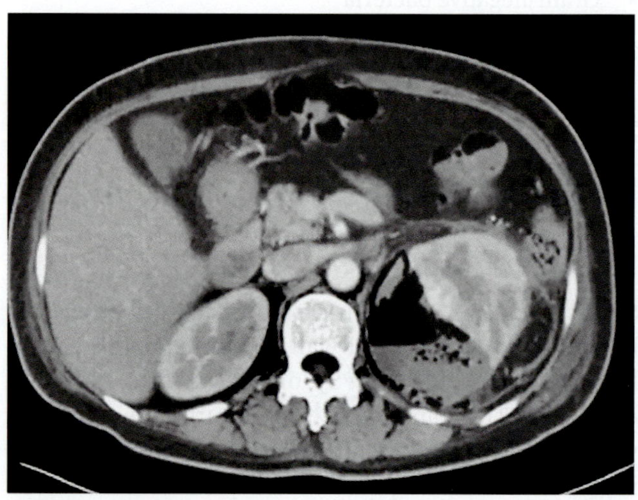

Fig. 1: Computed tomography scan.

TABLE 1: Huang and Tseng emphysematous pyelonephritis (EPN) classification.

Class	*Subclass*	*Computed tomography scan findings*	*Management plan*
Class I	–	Gas in collecting system only	Percutaneous procedures and antibiotics
Class II	–	Parenchymal gas only	Percutaneous procedures and antibiotics
Class III	Class IIIA	Extension of gas into perinephric space	*Less than two risk factors:* 85% survival rate with percutaneous drainage and antibiotics
	Class IIIB	Extension of gas into pararenal space	*Two or more risk factors:* 92% failure rate with percutaneous drainage and antibiotics
Class IV	–	EPN in solitary kidney, or bilateral disease	*Two or more risk factors:* 92% failure rate with percutaneous drainage and antibiotics

relieved either by an internal double J stent or by placing a percutaneous nephrostomy (PCN). Image-guided USG or CT percutaneous drainage (PCD) is the definitive management on most cases of EPN. In extreme scenario, wherein the patient is very toxic with CT showing extensive gas with destruction of renal parenchyma, nephrectomy is advised as a life-saving procedure.

Prognosis

Despite aggressive management, EPN remains to be an extreme form of urosepsis with mortality rates still as high as 40%. Poor prognostic factors include hypoalbuminemia, shock at presentation, thrombocytopenia, need for hemodialysis, and altered mental status.

FOURNIER'S GANGRENE

Fournier's gangrene refers to necrotizing fasciitis of the perineum and genital region caused by synergistic polymicrobial infection. It can lead to fulminant soft-tissue infection and can spread along fascial planes, resulting in necrosis of skin and subcutaneous tissue, as well as systemic sepsis. It can lead to significant morbidity and mortality if not treated aggressively.

Incidence

Fournier's gangrene accounts for 1–2% of urologic admissions.

Etiology

The common source of origin for this could be any condition where there is a virulent polymicrobial infection of the subcutaneous tissue of the perineum. It could be of urogenital, anorectal, retroperitoneal, or cutaneous origin.

Most of these patients have an underlying vascular disease or an immunosuppressing condition which makes them vulnerable to polymicrobial infection.

Underlying disorders in patients with Fournier's gangrene:
- Diabetes mellitus
- Malnutrition
- Obesity
- Poor personal hygiene
- *Immunosuppression:*
  - Chronic steroid use
  - Chemotherapy for malignancy
  - Organ transplantation
  - Human immunodeficiency virus (HIV)/acquired immunodeficiency syndrome (AIDS)
- Tuberculosis
- Syphilis

Microbiology

Fournier's gangrene is a polymicrobial infection.

Most common causative organisms:
- *Gram-negative:*
  - *E. coli*
  - *Proteus mirabilis*
  - *Pseudomonas aeruginosa*
  - *Klebsiella pneumoniae*
  - Enterobacteria
- *Gram-positive:*
  - *Staphylococcus aureus*
  - *Streptococcus faecalis*
  - Beta-hemolytic streptococci
  - *Staphylococcus epidermidis*
- *Anaerobes:*
  - *Bacteroides fragilis*
  - *Fusobacterium*
  - *Peptococcus*
  - *Clostridium perfringens*

Mixed spectrum of microbes has a synergistic action causing fulminant necrotizing fasciitis. Anaerobes produce subcutaneous gas, which produces characteristic crepitus on palpation.

Pathogenesis

Aerobic organisms induce platelet aggregation leading to vascular thrombosis. This leads to hypoxia in tissues forming oxygen free radicals, which in turn cause disruption of cell membrane and cell death causing tissue necrosis. This favors growth of anaerobic organisms, which in turn release various enzymes like lecithinase, collagenase, and hyaluronidase leading to digestion of fascial planes and production of gases like hydrogen and nitrogen.

Clinical Presentation

Fournier's gangrene is a clinical diagnosis. Prodromal symptoms such as fever, vomiting, and perineal discomfort is seen about a week before actual skin changes. Genital pain, redness, and swelling is noted eventually leading to skin necrosis. Purulent discharge may occur. Palpation may reveal crepitus in the affected area. Patients may present with high-grade fever, tachypnea, and sometimes, with frank septic shock. High index of suspicion is essential, especially in patients presenting with perineal discomfort with systemic symptoms. A delay in diagnosis may have catastrophic effects **(Figs. 2A and B).**

Investigations

Complete blood counts, renal and liver function tests, arterial blood gas (ABG), clotting profile, and serology are routinely done in patients with suspected Fournier's gangrene. Leukocytosis with neutrophilia is observed in severe infection. Coagulation profile may be altered with raised prothrombin time (PT) and activated partial thromboplastin time (APTT) in severe sepsis.

Urine, blood cultures, and wound swab pus cultures are obtained before starting on antibiotics.

X-ray abdomen and pelvis reveal the presence of gas in subcutaneous fascial layers.

Ultrasound of scrotum and perineum show hyperacoustic shadows, which is diagnostic of gas in fascial planes.

Management

The three major goals in management of Fournier's gangrene are: (1) Aggressive resuscitation, (2) administration of appropriate antibiotics, and (3) aggressive debridement of infected tissue.

Aggressive fluid resuscitation, strict glycemic control with insulin, and correcting altered coagulation parameters are mandatory. Broad-spectrum antibiotics is must with gram positive, gram negative, and anaerobic coverage. Antibiotics does not penetrate dead tissue, and hence, debridement is very essential for eradicating the source of infection.

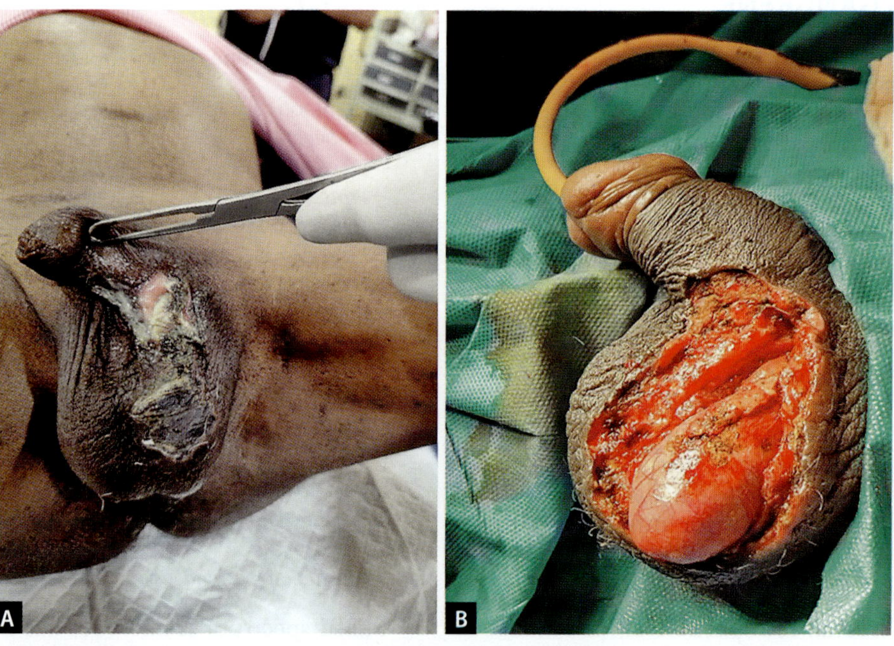

Figs. 2A and B: Fournier's gangrene.

Early and aggressive surgical debridement is of paramount importance. Its preferably done under general anesthesia and in dorsal lithotomy position. Necrotic skin and underlying necrotic subcutaneous tissue are aggressively debrided and extended till the wound edges have normal bleeding. Usually, testes are not involved and are preserved. Suprapubic cystostomy may be needed if patient has a urethral stricture. Colostomy may be needed in patients with fecal incontinence in cases where the anal sphincters were involved. If needed revision debridement are to be done 24–48 hours later.

Hyperbaric oxygen therapy has been used as an adjunct in these patients, and it is proven to reduce the hospital stay and improve wound healing.

After adequate wound healing, these patients require reconstructive procedures in the form of skin grafts or myocutaneous flaps for better cosmetic results.

Postoperative Management

Fournier's gangrene has a mortality rate of 20–40% and its much higher in patients with comorbid conditions such as poorly controlled diabetes, advanced age, heart failure, cirrhosis, and renal failure.

It is a true urological emergency and it requires high index of suspicion, early diagnosis, and aggressive treatment to reduce mortality.

SCROTAL EMERGENCIES

Torsion Testis

Any patient who presents with acute onset scrotal pain and tender swelling is considered to have an acute scrotum. The common differential diagnoses are testicular spermatic cord torsion, torsion of appendages, or epididymo-orchitis.

Torsion testis refers to a clinical condition wherein twisting of spermatic cord results in cessation of arterial blood flow to the testis resulting in ischemia, which may eventually result in gangrene and testis loss if not timely intervened.

Its prevalence is about 8 per 1 lakh males.

Predisposing Factors

Bell clapper deformity is a condition that happens because of high investment of tunica vaginalis with the spermatic cord resulting in excess mobility of testis within predisposing to intravaginal twisting of cord and testicular torsion.

Undescended testis is another predisposing factor and they are more prone for torsion.

Clinical Presentation

Most commonly occurs in the pubertal age 12–16 years. Typical presentation includes acute onset hemiscrotal pain and mild swelling, which is tender on palpation. They may also have nausea and vomiting. Clinical examination may reveal absent cremasteric reflex and high riding and horizontally oriented testis caused by shortening of cord due to torsion **(Figs. 3A and B)**.

Investigations

Torsion testis is usually a clinical diagnosis.

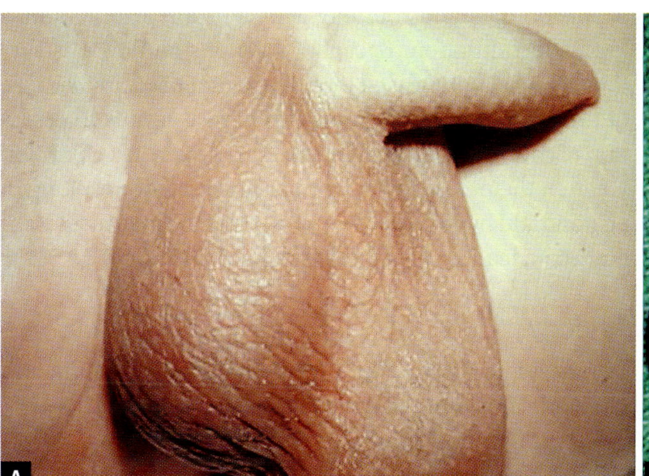

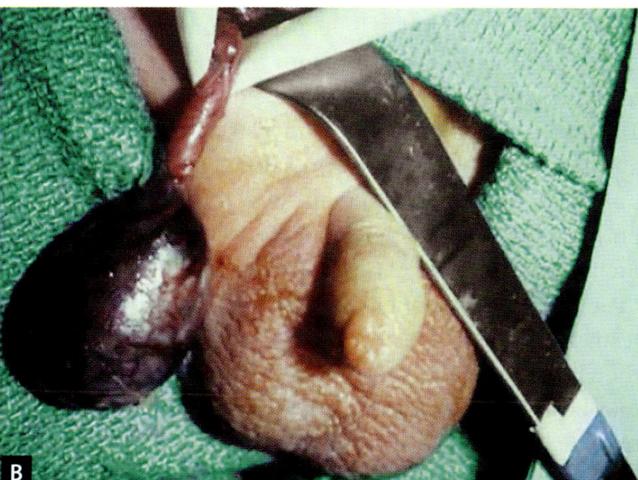

Figs. 3A and B: Bell clapper deformity.

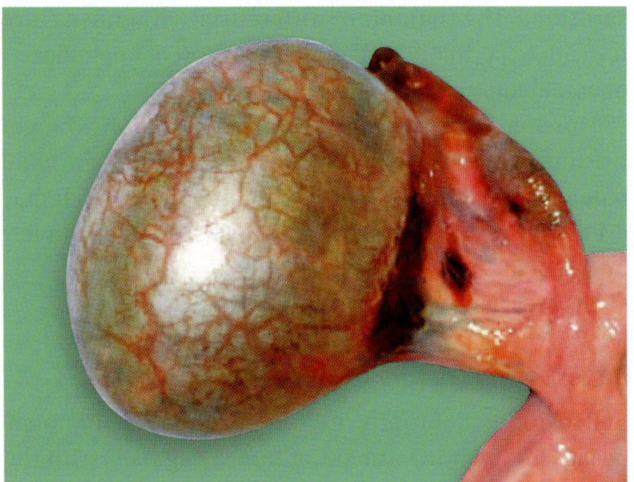

Fig. 4: Extravaginal testicular torsion.

Ultrasound scrotum with color Doppler: It offers assessment of testicular architecture and intraparenchymal blood flow. Torsion usually presents with parenchymal heterogeneity with reduced or absent waveforms in color Doppler. Color Doppler ultrasound (CDUS) has 100% sensitivity and 75% specificity. However, whenever there is a clinical suspicion of torsion and there is a delay in obtaining Doppler ultrasound, it is advisable to go for scrotal exploration rather than delaying for want of an USG, as unwanted delay may result in loss of testis due to ischemia **(Fig. 4)**.

Management

Testicular torsion is a true urological emergency because the viability of testis is inversely related to the duration of torsion. Various series show that the risk of orchidectomy is over 80% if exploration is delayed beyond 24 hours.

Surgical exploration is done through transverse or midline scrotal incision. Affected side is addressed first. The testis is delivered out and untwisted. Tunica is opened and testis is covered by warm saline soaked gauze and observed for the improvement in color. If testis regains normal pinkish color after detorsion, it can be retained and orchidopexy is done by 3-point fixation technique wherein the testis is fixed on medial, lateral, and inferior aspect of testis to scrotal wall using a nonabsorbable suture. When the viability of testis is doubtful, intraoperative Doppler may be helpful in assessing it. If testis remained dusky and necrotic, orchidectomy is completed. Often, these patients have same bell clapper deformity and contralateral testis as well, which predisposes to torsion. Hence, contralateral orchidopexy is done using 3-point fixation technique in the same sitting.

Extravaginal Torsion of Testis

Extravaginal torsion of testis is also called as perinatal torsion, and it is common in infants in the perinatal period (prenatal or during delivery or postpartum). It is called extravaginal torsion because it happens outside the tunica vaginalis, and it occurs before the fixation of tunica vaginalis and dartos. Prenatal torsion results in vanishing testis and often, a nubbin testis is noted in scrotum or in the inguinal region.

PRIAPISM

Priapism is defined as a condition wherein persistent penile erection lasts >4 hours and is not associated with sexual stimulation.

Priapism is of two types:
1. Ischemic
2. Nonischemic

Ischemic Priapism

Ischemic priapism is also termed as venous or low-flow priapism. Most of these patients present with persistent painful penile erection, which worsens over period of time. It is a surgical emergency as a delay in treatment may lead to irreversible penile ischemia and corporal fibrosis leading to permanent erectile dysfunction.

Pathophysiology of Ischemic Priapism

It is similar to a compartment syndrome. It begins with occlusion of venous outflow with constant arterial inflow for a short duration. Because of venous outflow obstruction, it leads to increased intracavernosal pressure because of tough tunica albuginea, which in turn results in cessation of cavernosal arterial inflow. This results in a condition wherein the penis is filled with stagnant blood resulting in acidotic and hypoxia to cavernosal tissues. This causes ischemic pain leading to painful prolonged erection.

Etiology

Hematological disorders such as sickle cell anemia and leukemia are common causes.

Other causes include:
- Recreational use of oral phosphodiesterase type 5 (PDE 5) inhibitors

- Alcohol or cocaine abuse
- *Drug induced:* Hydralazine and prazosin
- Total parenteral nutrition (TPN)
- Idiopathic
- Penile metastasis **(Table 2)**.

Clinical Presentation

Patient presents with painful penile erection with increasing intensity of pain over period of time. On examination, penis look bluish or dusky with tense tenese corporal bodies but with a soft glans.

In contrast, patients with nonischemic priapism present with painless semierect penis and are much comfortable at rest. They usually give a recent history of perineal trauma.

TABLE 2: Etiology of ischemic priapism.

Medications	
Intracavernosal agents	Papaverine, prostaglandin 1, phenoxybenzamine, and phentolamine
Central nervous system (CNS) agents	Trazodone, benzodiazepines, and phenothiazines
Phosphodiesterase type 5 (PDE-5) inhibitors	Sildenafil, tadalafil, and vardenafil
Antihypertensives	Prazosin, phenoxybenzamine, calcium channel blockers, beta blockers, and hydralazine
Anticoagulants	Heparin and warfarin
Hormones	Testosterone, gonadotropin-releasing hormone, and antiestrogens (tamoxifen)
Illicit drugs	Cocaine and marijuana
Parenteral nutrition	High concentration lipid infusions
Hematologic disorders:	
• Hyperviscous and hypercoagulable states • Hemoglobinopathies	• Polycythemia vera, protein-C deficiency, protein-S deficiency • Sickle cell disease and thalassemias
Immunologic diseases	Lupus and protein C deficiencies
Metabolic diseases	Gout, diabetes, nephrotic syndrome, renal failure, amyloidosis, Fabry's disease, and hypertriglyceridemia
Neurologic diseases	Spinal cord injuries, autonomic neuropathy, and spinal stenosis
Neoplastic disorders	Leukemia, multiple myeloma, and prostate/bladder/rectosigmoid/kidney cancers
Idiopathic	—

Investigations

Penile Doppler ultrasound (PDUS): It is a very sensitive investigation and ischemic priapism reveals absent cavernosal arterial inflow. On contrast, nonischemic priapism reveals a ruptured cavernosal artery with unregulated inflow and poloing of blood within corporal bodies. PDUS reveals either absence of flow in the cavernosal arteries or peak systolic velocity (PSV) <50 cm/sec and a lack of diastolic flow. In contrast, PSV >50 cm/sec is most consistent with nonischemic priapism.

Corporal blood aspiration and analysis: It is both diagnostic and therapeutic. It differentiates ischemic from nonischemic priapism. Ischemic priapism reveals hypoxic and acidotic blood content with "cranckcase-oil" appearance **(Table 3)**.

Management of Ischemic Priapism

The ultimate goal in management of ischemic priapism is to relieve pain, attain penile detumescence, and prevent damage to corporal bodies. A stepwise approach is done starting from less invasive to more invasive treatments **(Table 4)**.

- *Corporal aspiration:* It is the first line. 21 G butterfly needle is inserted into the base of penis and corporal bodies are aspirated till bright red blood appears in aspirate. This removes the hypoxic blood, relieves the intracavernosal pressure, and causes detumescence.
- *Intracavernosal injection of alpha agonist:* If mere aspiration is not successful, then diluted alpha agonist can be injected into the corporal bodies; phenylephrine is the usual drug of choice. Initial hypoxic blood is aspirated and 500 µg phenylephrine is injected and observed for detumescence. If erection persists,

TABLE 3: Corpus cavernosal blood gas parameters—ischemic versus nonischemic priapism.

Parameter	*Ischemic priapism*	*Mixed venous blood (flaccid penis)*	*Nonischemic priapism*
Color	Dark red	Medium red	Bright red
pH	<7.25	7.35	7.4
pO_2 (mm Hg)	<30	40	>90
pCO_2 (mm Hg)	>60	50	<40

then this procedure is repeated every 5 minutes until detumescence occurs. One has to watch for some adverse effects of phenylephrine such as headache, palpitations, hypertension, and arrythmia **(Figs. 5A and B)**.

Surgical Management of Ischemic Priapism

If the earlier mentioned conservative options fail, one has to resort to surgical options. The main goal of surgical correction involves creation of a fistula between obstructed corpus cavernosum with either glans or corpus spongiosum or dorsal penile vein or great saphenous vein thereby creating an alternate drainage for the corpus cavernosum and relieving the intra corporal pressure causing detumescence.

TABLE 4: Stepwise approach in management of ischemic priapism.

Step	*Ischemic priapism emergency*
1	Determine ischemic vs. nonischemic
2	Treat priapism, then underlying disorder if present
3	Aspiration and irrigation
4	Injection of sympathomimetic agent, repeat if needed; phenylephrine preferred (Dose: 100–500 µg every 3–5 minutes for up to 1 hour)
5	Observe for side effects
6	Consider shunt if injections fail
7	Shunt should be distal (cavernoglanular). Use proximal shunt only if distal fails
8	Oral systemic therapy is not warranted

These procedures are termed as shunt procedures and they are classified into:
- Distal and
- Proximal shunts

Distal shunts
- *Winter shunt* **(Fig. 6)**: It is the least invasive shunt procedure. It can be done under local anesthesia. A tru-cut biopsy needle is inserted through the glans into the corpus cavernosum and a core tissue of tunica albuginea separating them is removed creating a fistula between both. Sometimes, one has to remove multiple core of tissues to create adequate drainage causing successful detumescence.
- *Ebbehoj procedure* **(Fig. 7)**: In this modification, instead of a tru-cut needle, a 11 blade is inserted vertically through glans into cavernosum and rotated 90° laterally, thereby creating a bigger T-shaped shunt. It can be performed under local anesthesia.
- *Al ghorab shunt:* In this procedure, a transverse incision is made on the dorsal aspect of glans about 1 cm distal to coronal sulcus. About 1 cm incision is made on the corpus spongiosum and cavernosum and an elliptical-shaped tissue is removed creating a bigger fistula between them.

Proximal shunts: These are attempted when the distal shunts fail to relieve the erection.
- *Quackels cavernoso-spongiosal shunt:* It is done under regional anesthesia. Patient is placed in lithotomy position and longitudinal perineal incision is made.

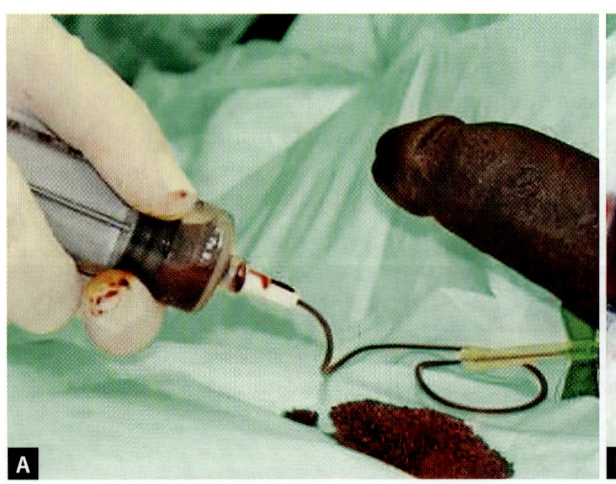

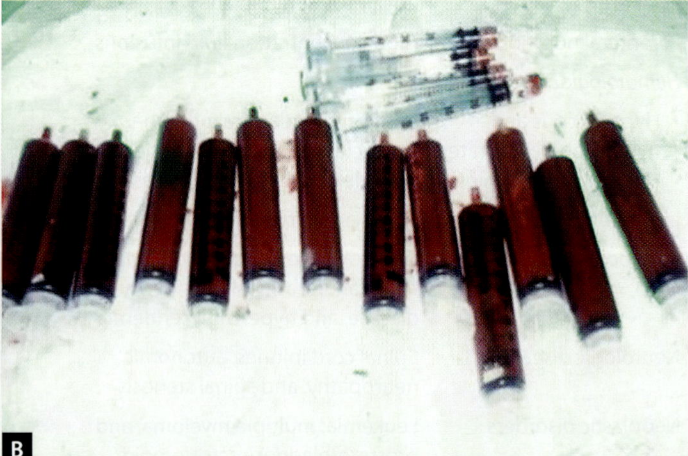

Figs. 5A and B: Initial corporal aspirate in ischemic priapism shows dark, deoxygenated blood. Subsequent aspirations will show brighter blood.

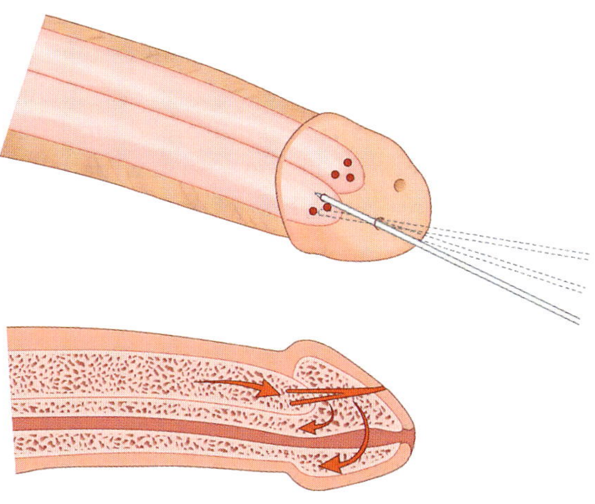
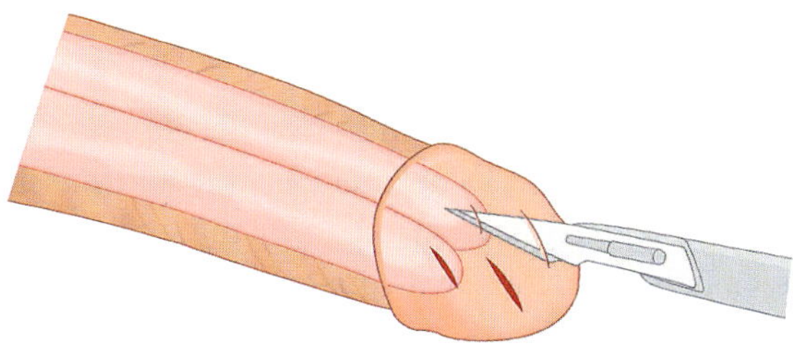

Fig. 6: Winter shunt.

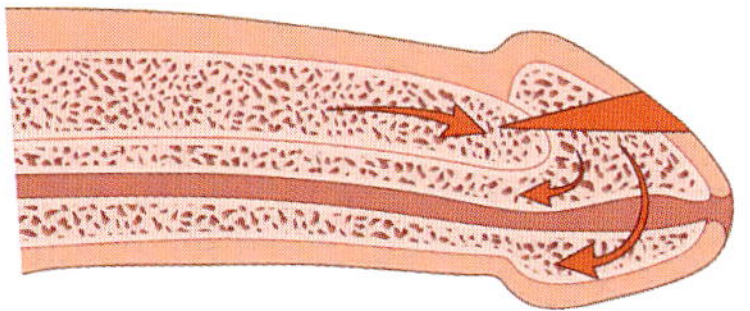

Fig. 7: Ebbehoj procedure.

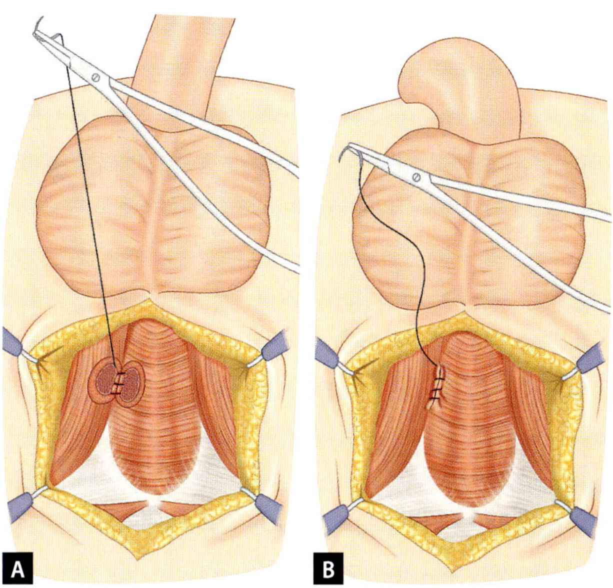

Figs. 8A and B: Cavernosospongiosal shunt (Quackels). It is important that the shunt is created in the perineum between the urethral bulb and aura. If placed too distal, it will not be effective and will carry a higher risk of urethral injury.
Source: Hohenfellner et al. (2007).

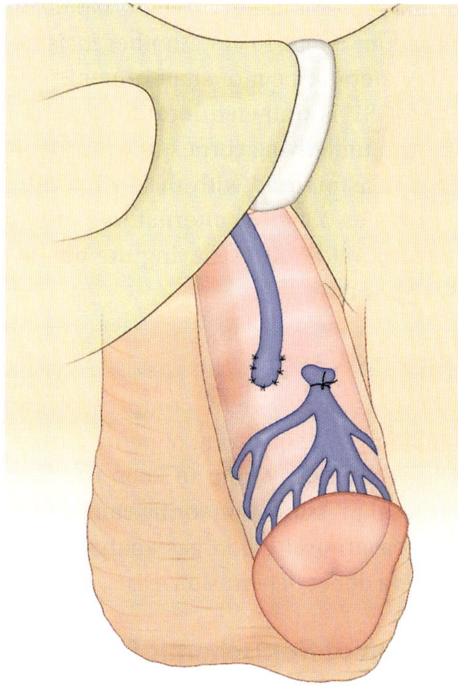

Fig. 9: Cavernoso-dorsal vein shunt (Barry). The dorsal vein is sutured to a window in the corpus cavernosum to provide shunting.
Source: Hohenfellner et al. (2007).

Bulb of corpus spongiosum is exposed and adjacent corpus cavernosum is also dissected. About 1 cm incision is made on them close to each other. An elliptical-shaped tissue is removed creating a bigger fistula between them and the walls are sutured using 5-0 PDS. It is usually done on one side. If it fails, it can be done on the contralateral side cavernosum as well **(Figs. 8A and B)**.

- *Barry Cavernoso-dorsal vein shunt:* In this procedure, incision is made over the base of penis. Dorsal vein of penis is mobilized and appropriate size incision is made through tunica albuginea into the corpus cavernosum. It is anastomosed with dorsal vein of penis using 5-0 PDS **(Fig. 9)**.

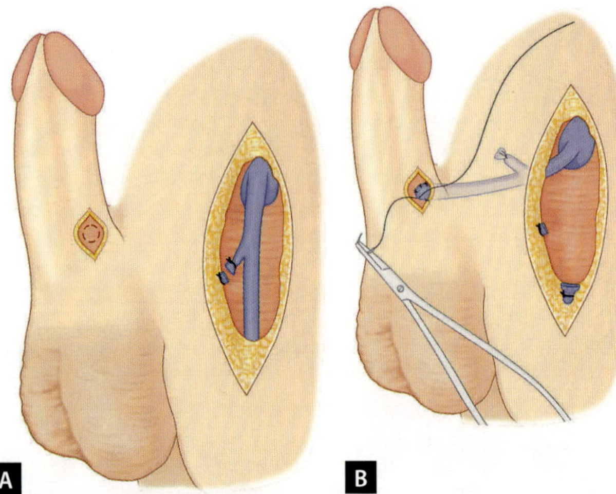

Figs. 10A and B: Cavernoso-saphenous vein shunt (Grayhack). The saphenous vein is mobilized by dividing and ligating the tributaries. It is crucial that the saphenous vein is passed without tension, torsion or angulation.

Source: Hohenfellner et al. (2007).

- *Grayhack Cavernoso-Saphenous vein shunt:* Patient is placed in supine frog leg position. Transverse incision is made over the saphenofemoral junction below the inguinal ligament. Great saphenous vein is mobilized for about 10 cm. Another incision is made over the lateral aspect of shaft of penis close to the root and GSV is tunneled into it. Small segment of tunica with underlying corpus cavernosum is excised and it is anastomosed with the GSV using 5.0 PDS. This provides a better alternate venous drainage of the corporal bodies relieving the penile erection **(Figs. 10A and B)**.

Postoperative Care

It is advised to avoid tight compressive dressings. Manual milking and squeezing of penis during first few postoperative days may help to keep the shunt open. Intracavernosal pressure monitoring can be done. Penile Doppler or cavernosal blood gas analysis can be done when there is a doubt of perfusion exists.

Management of Nonischemic Priapism

It occurs following a perineal trauma resulting in rupture of cavernosal artery leading to unregulated cavernosal arterial inflow. It is not an emergency. These patients have painless erection and corporal blood gas aspirate reveals bright blood and analysis reveals well oxygenated blood. Penile Doppler confirms it and identifies site of arterial rupture.

Treatment remains conservative and most patients improve over a period of time. In few patients, the conservative measures fail, selective embolization or surgical ligation of the fistula usually corrects the priapism.

URO TRAUMA

Renal Injuries

Epidemiology and Etiology

Renal injuries contribute to 10% of all abdominal trauma and it is the most common genitourinary organ to be involved in trauma. Most common mode of injury is blunt injury arising from motor vehicle accidents (MVA).

Pathophysiology

Renal injury occurs following rapid deceleration injury following MVA. It results in kinetic energy transmission to kidneys, which may have an impact on the surrounding rib cage. Children and those with pre-existing renal anomalies are more prone to injury.

Clinical Presentation

History of sudden deceleration injury or direct blow to lower thorax or upper abdomen should raise the suspicion of renal trauma. Clinical examination may reveal gross hematuria, flank hematoma, and renal angle tenderness.

Initial Management

Patient should be assessed for hemodynamic instability and if any, it has to be corrected with IV crystalloids and blood transfusion, if necessary. Basic blood investigations such as creatinine, complete hemogram, urine analysis, blood grouping, and matching should be done.

Radiological Evaluation

American Urological Association (AUA) and European Association of Urology (EAU) has proposed guidelines for evaluation of renal trauma.

- All patients with penetrating trauma presenting with likelihood of renal injury:
  - Flank ecchymosis
  - Entry or exit wound to lower chest or upper abdomen
  - Ipsilateral rib fracture

- Any patient with suspected blunt injury abdomen, especially with history of sudden deceleration injury or fall from a height
- Blunt trauma presenting with any one of the following should be evaluated for renal injury.
  - Gross hematuria
  - Shock (systolic BP <90 mm Hg) at presentation with microscopic hematuria
- All pediatric patients presenting with shock and microscopic hematuria (>5 RBC/HPF)

Contrast-enhanced computed tomography urogram: Contrast-enhanced CT abdomen pelvis with immediate and delayed images is the investigation of choice in patients with suspected renal trauma. Early arterial and venous phase visualizes the renal parenchyma whereas the delayed images taken 10–15 minutes after contrast delineates the pelvicalyceal system and the ureters **(Fig. 11)**.

Renal injuries are graded by the American Association for Surgery of Trauma (AAST) **(Table 5)**.

Single shot intravenous pyelogram: It is less sensitive than CECT urogram and is not routinely done. It is done in very selective situations where CECT could not be done because the patient was hemodynamically unstable and wheeled into operation theater (OT) from explorative laparotomy. It is done in cases where a perinephric hematoma is noted intraoperatively or when renal injury is suspected due to gross hematuria primarily to confirm the presence of contralateral kidney.

2 mL/kg body weight of IV contrast is injected and a single X-ray abdomen was taken 15 minutes later. Presence of contrast excretion in renal fossa indicates the presence of kidneys.

Management

Nonoperative management: Most patients with renal trauma who are hemodynamically stable can be managed conservatively with good outcome. It involves ICU admission, continuous vitals monitoring, strict bed rest, serial hematocrit monitoring, and watching for resolution of hematuria. Patient is usually catheterized to closely monitor urine output.

Most minor urinary extravasations are managed conservatively and most of them resolve without any active intervention. If there were any signs of infection or enlarging urinoma causing paralytic ileus, an attempt to place a double J (DJ) stenting or percutaneous nephrostomy is done along with percutaneous drainage of the collection.

Indications for repeat imaging and reassessment:

- All patients with high-grade renal trauma AAST grade IV and V
- Any patients on conservative management who shows signs of complications such as dropping hematocrit, worsening of pain, and hemodynamic instability

Operative management: Any patients with renal trauma and hemodynamic instability must be explored.

Indications for renal exploration:

- *Absolute indications include:*
  - Hemodynamic instability with no or transient response to resuscitation
  - Expanding or pulsatile renal hematoma (indicating renal artery laceration)
  - Suspected renal vascular pedicle avulsion
  - Pelviureteric junction avulsion.
- *Relative indications are:*
  - Urinary extravasation with significant renal parenchymal devascularization
  - Renal injury together with pancreatic or colon injury (these patients have a higher complication rate if their renal injury is not repaired at the time of colon/pancreatic injury)
  - Arterial thrombosis
  - Urinary extravasation from parenchymal injury

Renal Exploration

The best approach in suspected renal injury is the transabdominal approach because it allows thorough evaluation of all intra-abdominal organs. The first step in renal exploration is to have a renal hilar control and renal vessels are isolated and controlled before Gerota's fascia is opened. The inferior mesenteric vein is identified, and an incision is made medial to it over the mesentery extending upward till the ligament of Teitz. This exposes the anterior surface of aorta and left renal vein is identified as it crosses over the aorta. The renal arteries are then identified posterior to the renal veins and are looped. The right renal vein is identified anterior to the right renal artery. Once the renal vessels are isolated and controlled, the colon is reflected medially and the kidneys are exposed. Gerota is opened and kidneys are inspected for the extent of injury. The bleeder vessels can be suture ligated, nonviable tissue is debrided, and parenchymal defects are reapproximated using gel foam bolsters. Collecting system injuries if any are closed in a water-tight manner using absorbable sutures. In reno-vascular injuries, in case of small segmental

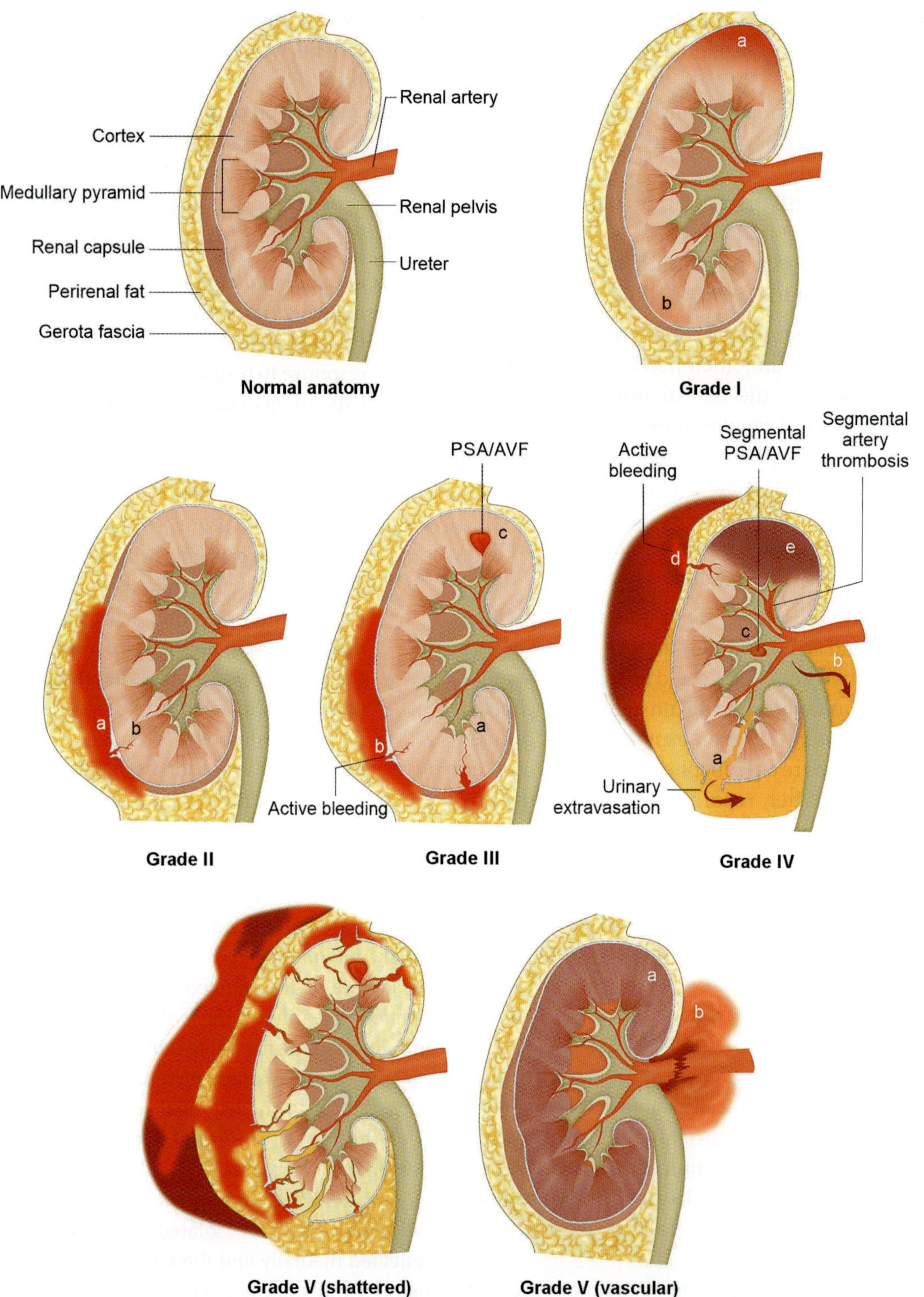

Fig. 11: Classification of renal injuries by grade illustrated based on 2018 AAST revision. (AVF: arteriovenous fistula; AAST: American Association for the Surgery of Trauma; PSA: prostate specific antigen)

TABLE 5: American Association for the Surgery of Trauma (AAST) organ injury severity scale for the kidney (2018 revision).

Grade	*AIS severity*	*Imaging criteria*	*Operative criteria*	*Pathological criteria*
I	2	• Subcapsular hematoma and/or parenchymal contusion without laceration • Parenchymal contusion without laceration	Nonexpanding subcapsular hematoma	Subcapsular hematoma or parenchymal contusion without parenchymal laceration
II	2	• Perirenal hematoma confined to Gerota's fascia • Renal parenchymal laceration ≤1 cm depth without urinary extravasation	• Nonexpanding perirenal hematoma confined to Gerota's fascia • Renal parenchymal laceration ≤1 cm depth without urinary extravasation	• Perirenal hematoma confined to Gerota's fascia • Renal parenchymal laceration ≤1 cm depth without urinary extravasation
III	3	• >1 cm parenchymal depth of renal cortex without collecting system rupture or urinary extravasation • Any injury in the presence of a kidney vascular injury or active bleeding contained within Gerota's fascia	Renal parenchymal laceration >1 cm depth without collecting system rupture or urinary extravasation	Renal parenchymal laceration >1 cm depth without collecting system rupture or urinary extravasation
IV	4	• Parenchymal laceration extending into urinary collecting system with urinary extravasation • Renal pelvis laceration and/or complete ureteropelvic disruption • Segmental renal vein or artery injury • Active bleeding beyond Gerota's fascia into the retroperitoneum or peritoneum • Segmental or complete kidney infarction(s) due to vessel thrombosis without active bleeding	• Parenchymal laceration extending into urinary collecting system with urinary extravasation • Renal pelvis laceration and/or complete ureteropelvic disruption • Segmental renal vein or artery injury • Segmental or complete kidney infarction(s) due to vessel thrombosis without active bleeding	• Parenchymal laceration extending into urinary collecting system • Renal pelvis laceration and/or complete ureteropelvic disruption • Segmental renal vein or artery injury • Segmental or complete kidney infarction(s) due to vessel thrombosis without active bleeding
V	5	• Main renal artery or vein laceration or avulsion of hilum • Devascularized kidney with active bleeding • Shattered kidney with loss of identifiable parenchymal renal anatomy	• Main renal artery or vein laceration or avulsion of hilum • Devascularized kidney with active bleeding • Shattered kidney with loss of identifiable parenchymal renal anatomy	• Main renal artery or vein laceration or avulsion of hilum • Devascularized kidney • Shattered kidney with loss of identifiable parenchymal renal anatomy

branches, it can be ligated. In case of major renal arteries or vein, they are repaired using 5-0 prolene sutures. If the damage is beyond repair of if the patient is very unstable, nephrectomy is to be done as a life-saving procedure **(Figs. 12 and 13)**.

Complications

The mortality following a major renal injury is about 4.6–8%. The common complications following a renal trauma is a transient acute kidney injury (AKI), urinoma and perinephric abscess, delayed bleeding, and systemic hypertension.

Ureteral Injuries

Ureteral injuries are quite rare because of its anatomical location. It constitutes only about 1% of all genitourinary trauma. The most common form of ureteric injuries are iatrogenic.

Etiology of Ureteric Injuries

- *External trauma:* These are generally rare and could be blunt or penetrating trauma. Blunt trauma is common in children following rapid deceleration injury and penetrating injuries are common following bullet or stab wounds.

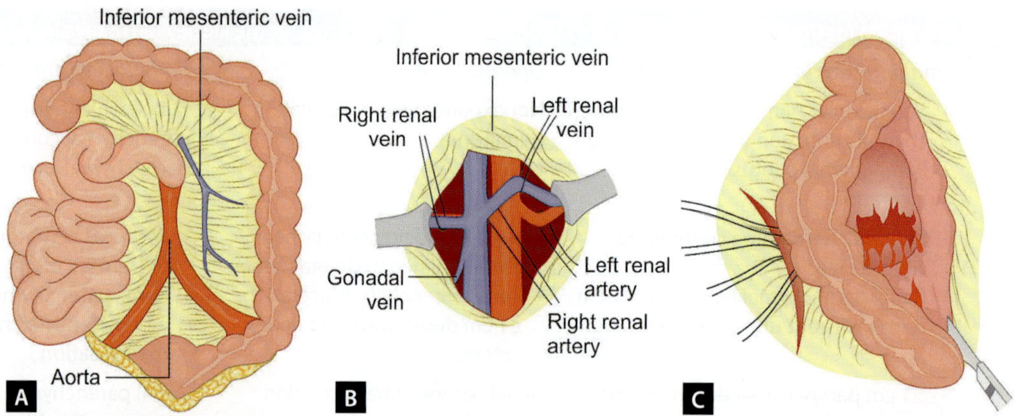

Figs. 12A to C: Surgical approach to renal vessels and hilum. (A) Relationship between the aorta, posterior peritoneum, and inferior mesenteric vein; (B) Window in posterior peritoneum made between aorta and inferior mesenteric vein demonstrating each renal artery and vein; (C) After vascular exposure and isolation, exploration of Gerota's fascia is obtained by incising the peritoneum lateral to the descending colon (for a left-sided injury).
Source: Wein et al. (2011).

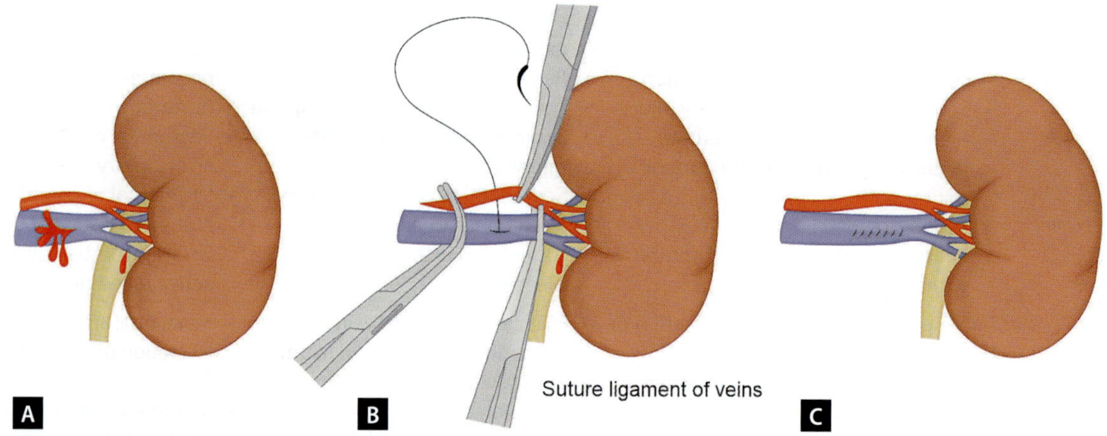

Figs. 13A to C: Surgical management of vascular injuries. (A) Schematic showing injury to different portions of the renal vein; (B) Injuries are repaired; (C) or divided, depending on location and size.
Source: Wein et al. (2011).

- *Iatrogenic trauma:* This is the most common form of ureteric injuries. It usually occurs following an open or laparoscopic procedure or following ureterorenoscopy. It is more common following gynecological procedures and has a rough incidence of 0.02–1.5%.

Ureteric injuries can happen because of any one of the following mechanisms:

- Inadvertent suture ligation
- Crushing while applying clamps
- Partial or complete transection
- Ischemic injuries to ureter following electrocoagulation
- Too much of stripping of ureteric adventitia

The pelvic portion of ureter is more likely to be injured because it runs in close approximation with the uterine and ovarian vessels and cervix. A thorough knowledge of the anatomic relations and proper evaluation of preoperative imaging will aid in avoiding this mishappening **(Figs. 14 and 15)**.

Investigations

High index of suspicion and a prompt diagnosis of ureteric injuries helps in successful outcome.

- *CECT urogram:* It is the investigation of choice. Delayed excretory images help in delineating the pelvicalyceal system and the ureters. Extravasation

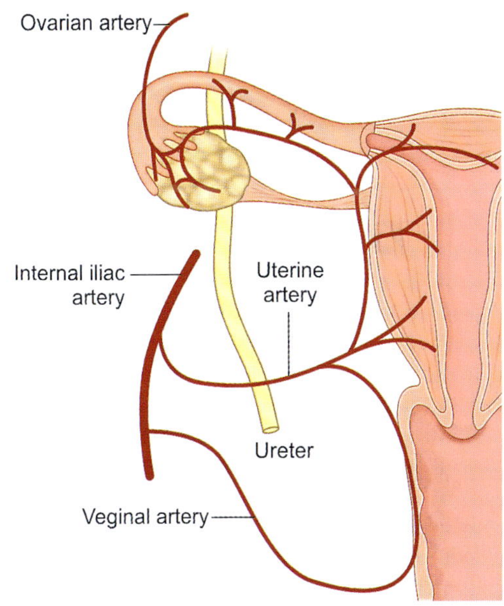

Fig. 14: Ureteral anatomy showing relationship to fallopian tube and uterine artery.

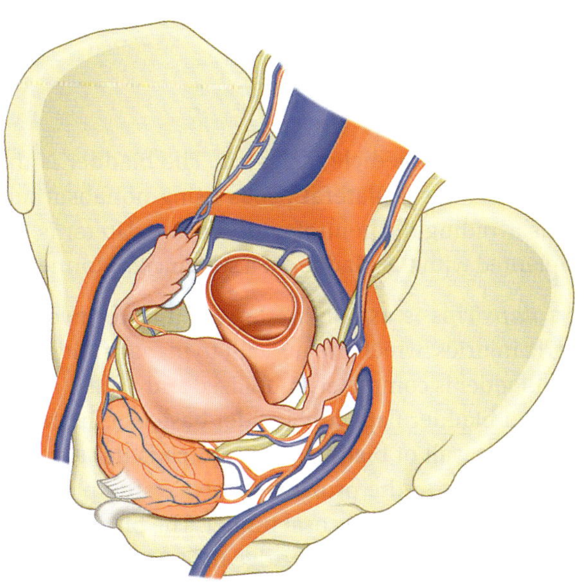

Fig. 15: Relation of the ureter to nearby structures.

of contrast in the medial perirenal space is the most common finding observed in ureteric injuries. In cases of complete ureteric obstruction, there may be significant hydroureteronephrosis with absence of contrast in the distal ureter.

- *Intravenous urogram (IVU):* It was used in the past to delineate the ureters. With the advent of CT urogram, its been used rarely these days.

TABLE 6: American Association for the Surgery of Trauma (AAST) organ injury severity scale for the ureter.

Grade	*Description of injury*
I	Hematoma only
II	Laceration 50% of circumference
III	Laceration >50% of circumference
IV	Complete tear ≤2 cm of devascularization
V	Complete tear >2 cm of devascularization

BOX 2: Principles of repair for grade III–V injuries.

Principle of reconstruction of complete ureteral injuries:
- Debridement of ureteral ends to fresh and bleeding tissue
- Spatulation of the ureteral ends
- Internal stenting of the ureter
- Watertight and tension-free anastomosis with absorbable suture
- External, retroperitoneal, and nonsuction drainage
- Protection of the anastomosis by omental or peritoneal flap

- *Cystoscopy and retrograde pyelogram:* If the CT is inconclusive, this can be done for accurate diagnosis. Cystoscopy is done and ureteric orifices are canulated and radio opaque contrast is injected in the retrograde manner and the extent of injury, especially the segment of ureter distal to the injury, can be accurately assessed.

Intraoperative Diagnosis

Direct visual inspection of ureter is the most reliable method of assessing the ureteric integrity and the extent of injury. Presence of urinary extravasation, contusion, and decreased ureteric peristalsis are subtle finding that may suggest an ureteric injury.

Severity of ureteric injuries is assessed by AAST **(Table 6)**.

Surgical Principles of Ureteric Repair

It depends on patients' general condition, time of diagnosis, site, and extent of injury. If the patient is stable, one can plan for a formal ureteric reconstruction. If the patient is unstable then diverting urine by placing a percutaneous nephrostomy and definitive ureteric repair can be done after stabilizing the patient.

The following general principles should be strictly adhered to while planning for a ureteric reconstruction **(Box 2)**.

The type of reconstructive procedure depends on the site and extent of the ureteric injury **(Fig. 16)**.

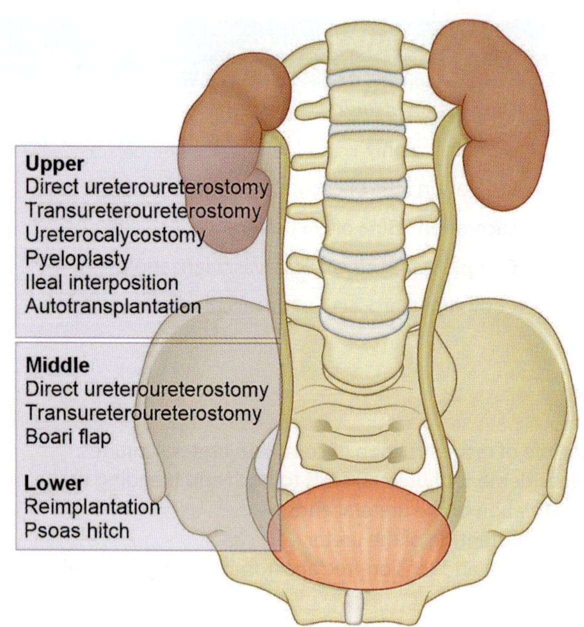

Fig. 16: Options for ureteral repair of complex injuries based on its location.
Source: Hohenfellner et al. (2007).

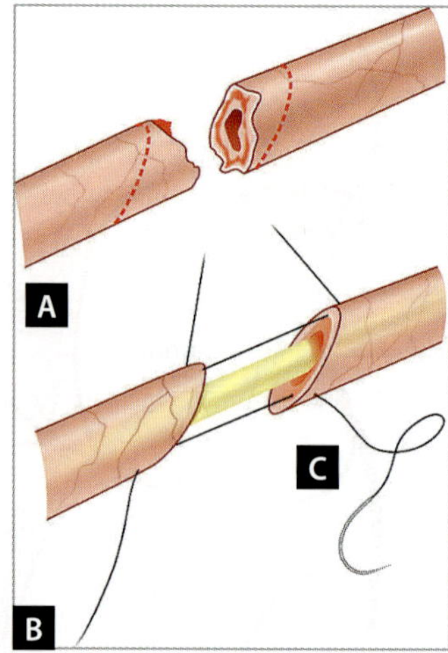

Figs. 17A to C: Ureteroureterostomy, end-to-end anastomosis of the ureter. Careful debridement is indicated to avoid later complications caused by delayed tissue breakdown. (A) The well-vascularized ureteral ends are spatulated, (B) a stent is inserted, (C) and an anastomosis is performed with a thin (e.g., 5-0 or 6-0) monofilament (e.g., Monocryl or PDS) suture. The stent should be removed 6 weeks postoperatively and a follow-up renogram and intravenous urogram (IVU) should be obtained after 3 months to assess the patency of the repair.

Ureteroureterostomy and primary repair: It is usually preferred in short segment ureteric injuries usually following stab injuries. This should not be attempted in gunshot injuries or delayed thermal injuries, because they are notorious to have extensive microvascular destruction of adjacent healthy looking ureteric ends, which may later develop ischemia and slough out.

It is an end-to-end anastomosis and is preferred in upper and mid ureteric injuries. Ureters are spatulated and repaired using absorbable sutures over a DJ stent in a tension free manner. Avoid stripping of ureter and too much mobilization of the ureters during this procedure **(Figs. 17A to C)**.

Transureteroureterostomy: These are usually reserved in distal ureteric injuries and those with small capacity bladder, which precludes the use of bladder for ureteric reconstruction. In this procedure, the injured ureter is debrided and transposed to contralateral ureter and anastomosed in an end-to-side fashion. The course of ureter is usually fashioned in such a way that acute angulation is avoided.

Ureteric reimplant and psoas hitch: It is the preferred technique in patients with distal one-third ureteric injuries. In this procedure, the bladder is fully mobilized and often the contralateral pedicle is ligated. The bladder is then anchored to the ipsilateral psoas using nonabsorbable sutures avoiding the genitofemoral nerve. Ureter is then reimplanted with the bladder in a submucosal tunnel.

Boari flap: This is usually preferred in lower two-third ureteric injuries, which are difficult to manage with psoas hitch. Bladder is completely mobilized and a full thickness U-shaped bladder flap with a wider base is fashioned on the anterior wall of bladder. Psoas hitch is done and the flap is brought to the proximal ureteric stump and it is reimplanted in a sub mucosal tunnel. The bladder is then closed in 2 layers. This can bridge defects up to 15 cm in length **(Figs. 18 and 19)**.

Intestinal replacement of the ureter: This is done in cases with near complete loss of ureter. An isoperistaltic segment of bowel usually the ileum with its pedicle is chosen and it is anastomosed with renal pelvis proximally and with the bladder distally. These patients are likely to develop hyperchloremic metabolic acidosis and has to be adequately managed in the postoperative period.

Autotransplantation of kidney: This is done in cases with complete ureteric loss and who are not suitable for ileal

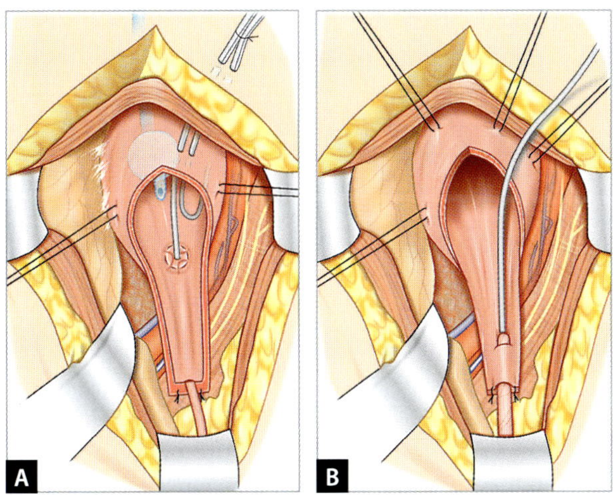

Figs. 18A and B: *Source:* Hohenfellner et al. (2007).

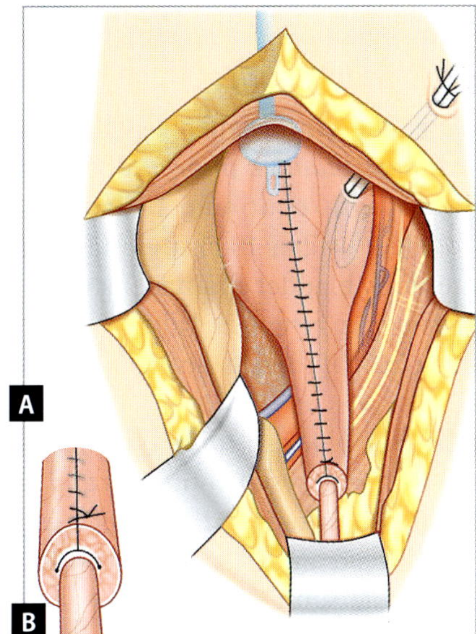

Figs. 19A and B: (A) Opened bladder with raised Boari flap and submucosal ureteral implantation; (B) Tabularized bladder after bladder closure.

Source: Hohenfellner et al. (2007).

ureteric interposition. In this procedure, kidney is removed with its renal pedicle and it is transplanted in the iliac fossa close to bladder. Renal vessels are reanastomosed with the external iliac vessels and remnant ureter or renal pelvis is anastomosed directly to the bladder **(Fig. 20)**.

Bladder Injuries

Incidence of bladder injuries is relatively low. However, missed ladder injuries can cause significant morbidity.

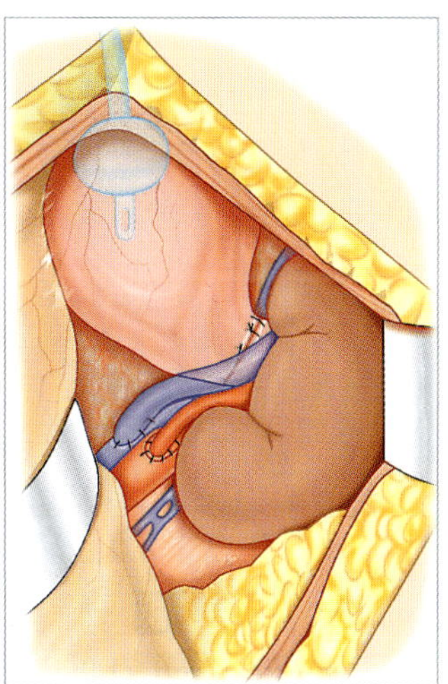

Fig. 20: Autotransplantation can be indicated in cases with a solitary kidney and a complete ureteral avulsion or compromised kidney function. The affected kidney is transplanted into the iliac fossa in a classical fashion with vascular anastomosis and with a pyelovesicostomy. The bladder catheter can be removed after 3 weeks. A follow-up renogram and intravenous urogram (IVU) should be obtained after 3 months to assess the patency of the repair.

Etiology

- *External trauma:* Road traffic accidents (RTA) are a major cause of bladder injuries. They are often associated with pelvic fractures. Many times, bladder injuries are associated with multiorgan injury.
- *Iatrogenic trauma:* Urinary bladder is the most common genitourinary organ to be involved in iatrogenic injury. They are common following pelvic surgeries or during transurethral procedures such as transurethral resection of bladder tumors.

Classification (Figs. 21A to D)

Usually, bladder injuries are classified based on the anatomical site into intraperitoneal or extraperitoneal **(Table 7)**.

Clinical Presentation

Most of the patients may present with gross hematuria. The combination of gross hematuria with concomitant pelvic fracture is an absolute indication for cystogram to look for bladder injuries. Patients may also present with lower abdominal contusion, tenderness, inability to pass urine without any palpable bladder, and features suggestive of peritonitis.

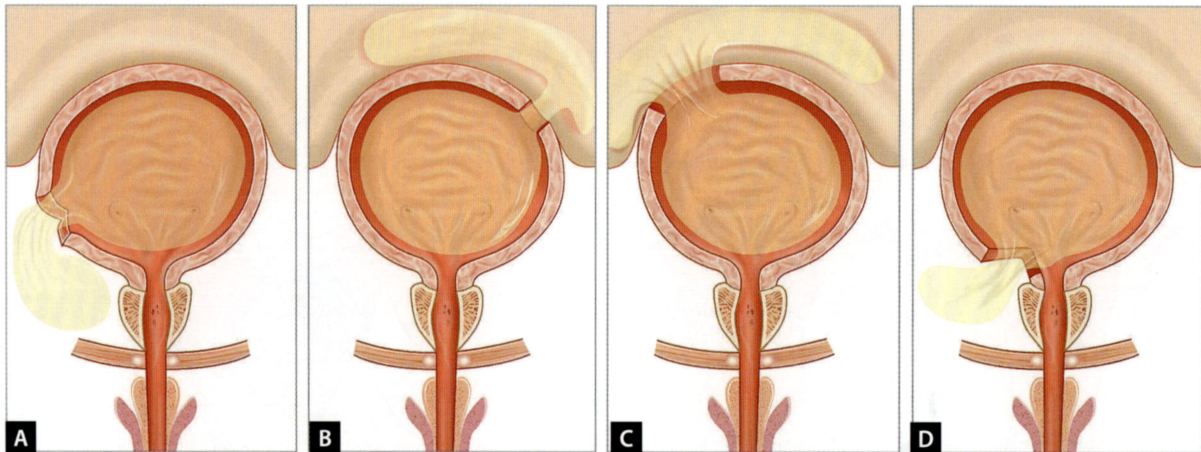

Figs. 21A to D: American Association for the Surgery of Trauma (AAST) classification of bladder injury. (A) Grade 3—extraperitoneal laceration of the bladder wall >2 cm; (B) Grade 3—intraperitoneal laceration of the bladder wall <2 cm; (C) Grade 4—intraperitoneal laceration of the bladder wall >2 cm; (D) Grade 5—intraperitoneal or extraperitoneal laceration of the bladder wall extending into the bladder neck or trigone.

TABLE 7: American Association for the Surgery of Trauma (AAST) organ injury severity scale for the bladder injury.

Grade	*Injury type*	*Description of injury*
I	Hematoma	Contusion and intramural hematoma
I	Laceration	Partial thickness
II	Laceration	Extraperitoneal bladder wall laceration <2 cm
III	Laceration	Extraperitoneal (>2 cm) or intraperitoneal (<2 cm) bladder wall laceration
IV	Laceration	Intraperitoneal bladder wall laceration >2 cm
V	Laceration	Intraperitoneal or extraperitoneal bladder wall laceration extending into the bladder neck or ureteral orifice (trigone)

Investigations

Computed tomography cystogram: It is considered to be the investigation of choice. It involves retrograde filling of bladder with contrast for about 350 mL in a gravity-dependent manner from a height of 40 cm followed by CT screening of abdomen and pelvis. Presence of contrast extravasation implies the presence of bladder injury. If the contrast is confined to pelvis in the extraperitoneal space, it shoes extraperitoneal bladder injury. If the contrast is seen in the paracolic gutters within the peritoneal cavity, it implies intraperitoneal injury **(Figs. 22A to D)**.

Treatment of Bladder Injuries

Treatment depends on the extent of bladder injury.

- *Extraperitoneal bladder injury:* Most of these can be managed with continuous bladder drainage. Usually, a larger caliber 18 Fr urethral foley is placed and continuous bladder drainage is done for about 14 days. Cystogram is repeated after 2 weeks to look for any contrast leak. If there is no leak, catheter is safely removed.
- *Intraperitoneal bladder injuries:* These are often associated with features of peritonitis and hence, they must be aggressively repaired. Bladder is explored and edges are trimmed and closed primarily in two layers using absorbable sutures. In case of a large injury, a suprapubic cystostomy (SPC) can be placed. Bladder is catheterized for 7–10 days. Cystogram is done after 10 days to assess bladder healing before catheter removal. Most of the bladder injuries heal well without much complications.

Traumatic Penile Injuries

Penile injuries are uncommon. These account for 10% of all genitourinary injuries. Prompt diagnosis and treatment is essential to avoid long term physical, functional, and psychological sequelae of penile injuries.

Pathophysiology

Penile fracture is a form of blunt injury to erect penis. It refers to a condition where there is a breach in the tunica

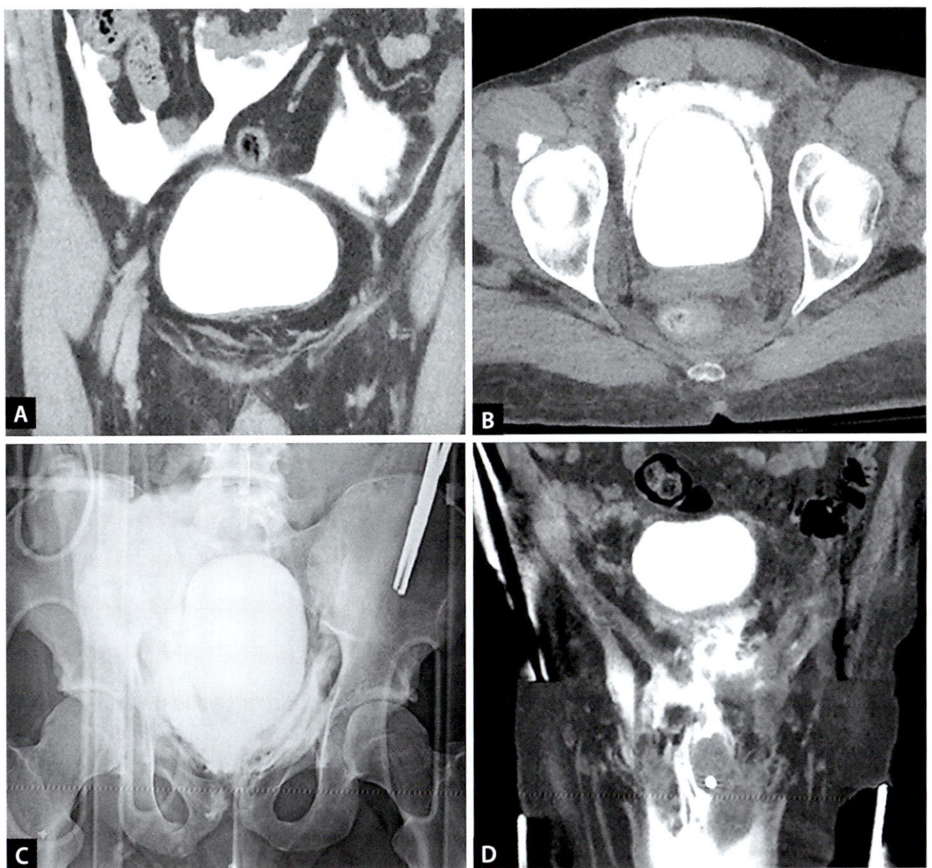

Figs. 22A to D: Computed tomography (CT) and fluoroscopic imaging of bladder rupture including: (A) Coronal view of CT cystogram showing an intraperitoneal (IP) rupture with extravasated contrast outlining loops of bowel; (B) Axial view of CT cystogram showing an extraperitoneal (EP) bladder rupture with molar tooth extravasation pattern; (C) Fluoroscopic cystogram showing an EP rupture with extravasation into the soft tissues of the pelvis; and (D) Coronal view of CT cystogram showing an EP rupture with extensive extravasation tracking into the scrotum.

albuginea of the penis and it is often seen following a coital trauma. During erection, the intracavernosal pressures are high and tunica is thin especially at the ventral aspect, which can predispose to tunical tear following coital trauma.

Clinical Presentation

Patient typically presents with history of coital trauma, cracking, or snapping sound during intercourse followed by sudden detumescence, penile swelling, and ecchymosis. They may present with classic eggplant deformity because the hematoma is confined within bucks fascia of penis.

Diagnosis

Diagnosis is usually clinical. In doubtful cases, ultrasound or MRI can aid in clinching diagnosis.

Ultrasonography: It can help in assessing the integrity of tunica and can locate the site of tunical breach.

Magnetic resonance imaging: It accurately demonstrates the presence, exact location, and the extent of the tunical tear. It can also pick up any associated urethral injury if any **(Figs. 23A to C)**.

Management of Penile Fracture

Prompt surgical exploration and primary repair should be done if the tunica is the treatment of choice. It can be done through a circumferential degloving or ventral penile midline incision. The corpus cavernosum is thoroughly inspected, hematoma is evacuated, and tunica is closed with nonabsorbable sutures. If there is a suspected urethral injury, flexible urethrocystoscopy is performed and

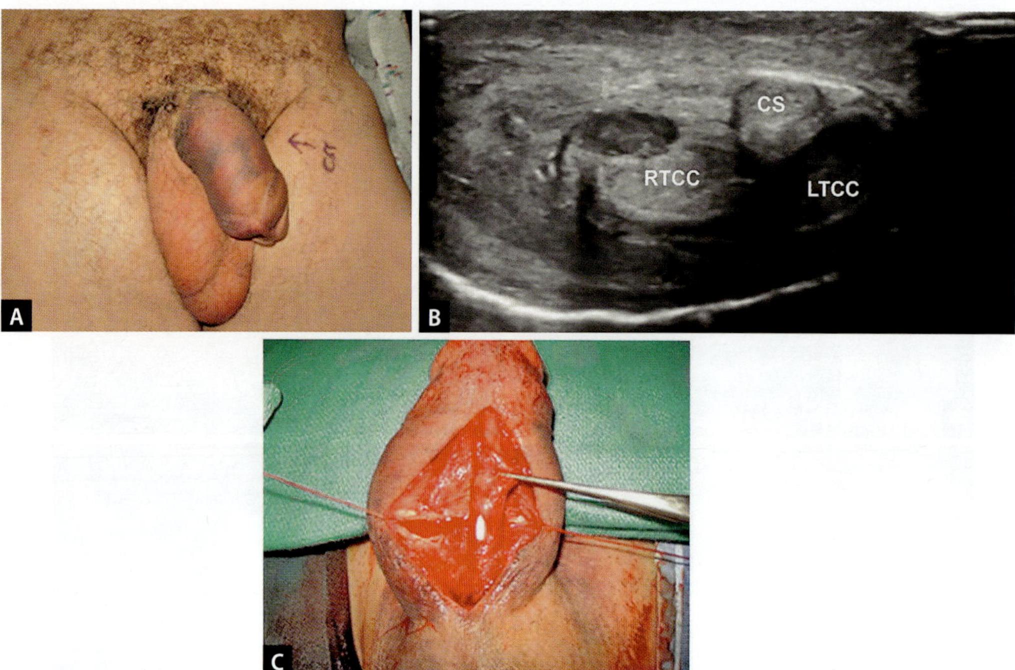

Figs. 23A to C: Penile fracture. (A) Ecchymosis and eggplant deformity; (B) Ultrasound of penile fracture. Note hypoechoic focus of hematoma arising out of the right corpus cavernosum (RTCC), intact corpus spongiosum (CS), and left corpus cavernosum (LTCC); (C) Ventral tunica rupture in a different patient crossing midline with associated urethral injury exposing urethral catheter.

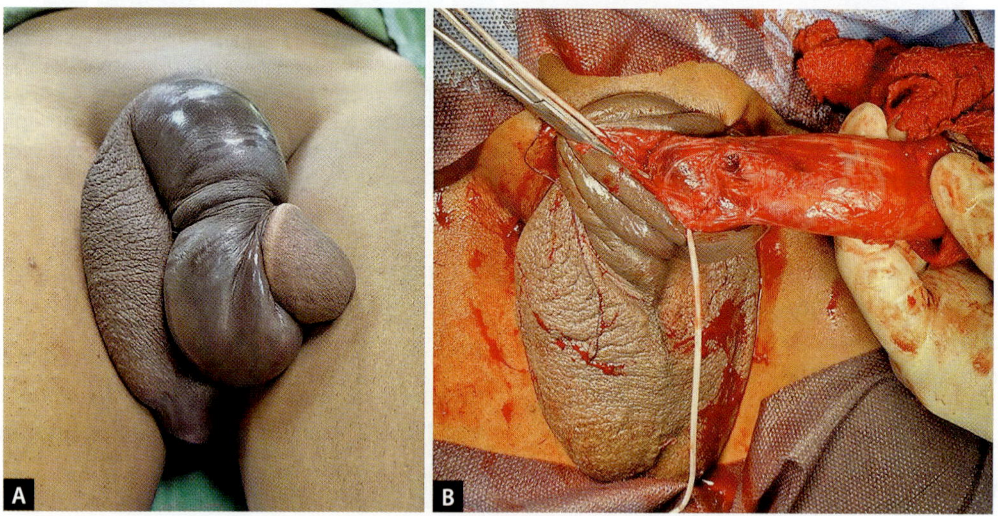

Figs. 24A and B: Penile fracture.

urethral injuries are closed primarily using an absorbable suture over a Foley catheter **(Figs. 24A and B)**.

Traumatic Urethral Injuries

Urethral injuries are not common and they occur more commonly in a polytrauma setting, especially with a pelvic fracture. High index of suspicion, prompt diagnosis, and timely treatment is the key to success.

Etiology

Anatomically, male urethra is divided into anterior and posterior urethra by the urogenital diaphragm. Penile

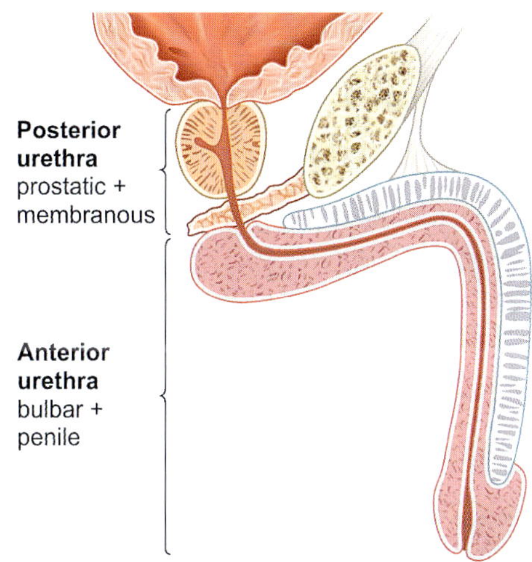

Fig. 25: Anatomy of the male urethra.
Source: Hohenfellner et al. (2007).

and bulbar urethra constitutes the anterior urethra while the membranous and prostatic urethra constitutes the posterior urethra **(Fig. 25)**.

Posterior Urethral Injuries

Posterior urethral injuries are most commonly associated with pelvic fractures following RTA or fall from a height. The severe shearing force that causes pelvic fracture also causes disruption of the prostatomembranous junction resulting in posterior urethral injuries. Hence, they are also termed as pelvic fracture urethral distraction defects.

American Association for the Surgery of Trauma has proposed the following classification for posterior urethral injuries **(Table 8)**.

Anterior Urethral Injuries

They are more common following blunt injury to perineum, the most common being the straddle bulbar urethral injury. In this form of trauma, the bulbar urethra is trapped and compressed by the blunt force against the inferior aspect of pubic symphysis resulting in urethral injury.

Other common causes of anterior urethral injury include iatrogenic injury during faulty catheterization or urethral instrumentation, coital injury, or penetrating injuries.

Clinical Presentation

The classical presentation includes blood at meatus, inability to pass urine, and clinically palpable bladder.

TABLE 8: Organ injury scaling III classification of urethral injuries.

Type	*Description*	*Appearance*
I	Contusion	Blood at the urethral meatus; normal urethrogram
II	Stretch injury	Elongation of the urethra without extravasation on urethrography
III	Partial disruption	Extravasation of contrast at injury site with contrast visualized in the bladder
IV	Complete disruption	Extravasation of contrast at injury site without visualization in the bladder; <2 cm of urethral separation
V	Complete disruption	Complete transection with >2 cm urethral separation or extension into the prostate or vagina

Source: Moore EE, Cogbill TH, Jurkovich GJ, McAninch JW, Champion HR, Gennarelli TA, et al. Organ injury scaling. III: Chest wall, abdominal vascular, ureter, bladder, and urethra. J Trauma. 1992;33(3):337-9.

There can be associated hematoma and other associated injuries such as pelvic fracture.

Radiological Evaluation

Retrograde urethrography ***(Figs. 26A to C)****:* This is the gold standard investigation of choice in a suspected case of urethral injury. This is done by placing the patient in 30° oblique position and injecting about 20 mL of radio opaque contrast within the urethra. This delineates the entire anterior urethra. When an SPC is placed, it can be combined with cystogram, which also gives information about the status of bladder neck and the posterior urethra.

Management of Urethral Injuries

Whenever a urethral injury is suspected, retrograde urethrography is performed to rule out urethral injury. If it is normal, a gentle attempt of catheterization is done. If it fails or the retrograde urethrography shows an extensive urethral injury with acute urinary retention, then a SPC is placed and planned for a delayed urethral repair. It is difficult to assess the exact extent of urethral injuries in acute setting, and hence, it is better to wait for 3–6 months by which time, it may have healed with fibrosis and stricture, a formal repair is far easier in this setting.

In cases of posterior urethral injuries, SPC is placed in the initial setting and usually wait is done for 3–6 months for complete resolution of the pelvic hematoma and

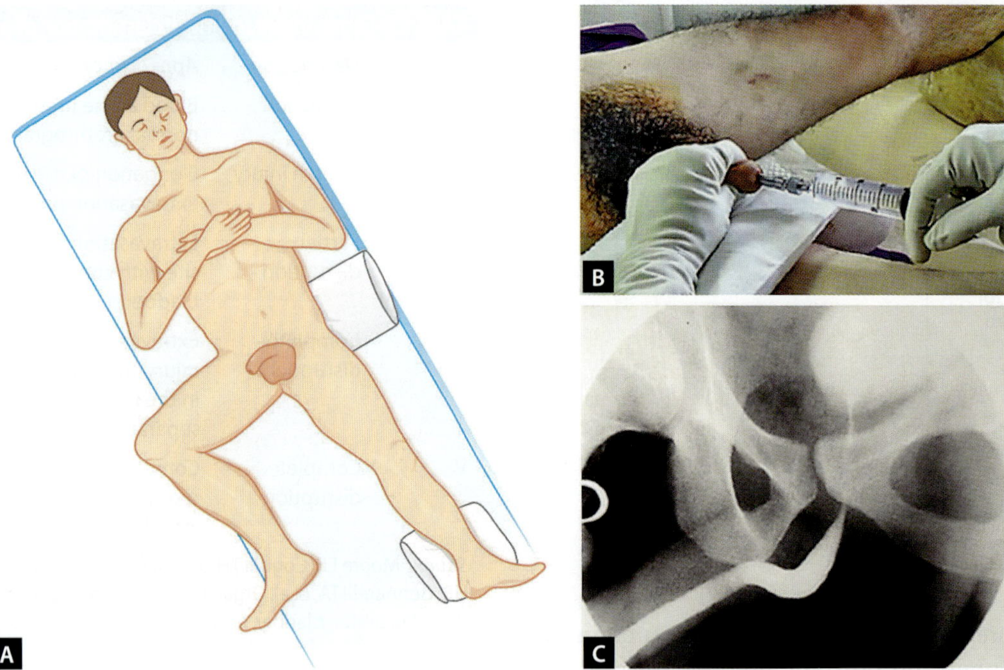

Figs. 26A to C: Retrograde urethrography. (A) Patient positioning; (B) Cone-tip syringe injecting the urethra; (C) Normal retrograde urethrography (RUG), penile, bulbar, and posterior urethra demonstrated without extravasation; note elongation of the posterior urethra and bladder displaced by perivesical hematoma.

completion of the fibrosis. Then a progressive perineal anastomotic urethroplasty is performed wherein the scar fibrous tissue between the cut ends of urethra are excised and end-to-end anastomotic urethroplasty is done over a urethral catheter. It involves the following steps, which have to be done in a progressive manner till one achieves a tension-free anastomosis.

1. Urethral mobilization
2. Crural separation
3. Inferior pubectomy
4. Supracrural urethral rerouting

SECTION

6

Vascular Emergencies

CHAPTER 19

Vascular Emergencies

M Murali

ACUTE LIMB ISCHEMIA

Etiology

- Embolism
  - *Cardiac source:* Valvular pathology, ischemic heart disease, and atrial myxoma
  - *Noncardiac source:* Aneurysm and penetrating aortic ulcer
  - Paradoxical embolus from deep vein thrombosis (DVT) with patent foramen ovale
- Thrombosis
  - Native vessel pathology
  - Aortic dissection and intramural hematoma
  - Trauma

Presentation

6Ps: Pain, pulseless limb, pallor, poikilothermia, paresthesis, and paralysis.

Earliest symptom: Pain

Earliest sign: Absent pulse

Sign of progressing ischemia: Neurological deficit (sensory loss—paresthesia followed by motor dysfunction—paralysis).

Sign of advanced irreversible ischemia: Gangrenous changes (also sign of nonsalvageable limb)—nerves are most sensitive to ischemia followed by muscles and skin dies last **(Figs. 1 to 3)**.

Rutherford Classification of Acute Limb Ischemia

Rutherford classification of acute limb ischemia is given in **Table 1**.

Not imminently threatened—Class IIa: Incomplete sensory deficit

Imminently threatened—Class IIb: Motor and sensory deficit

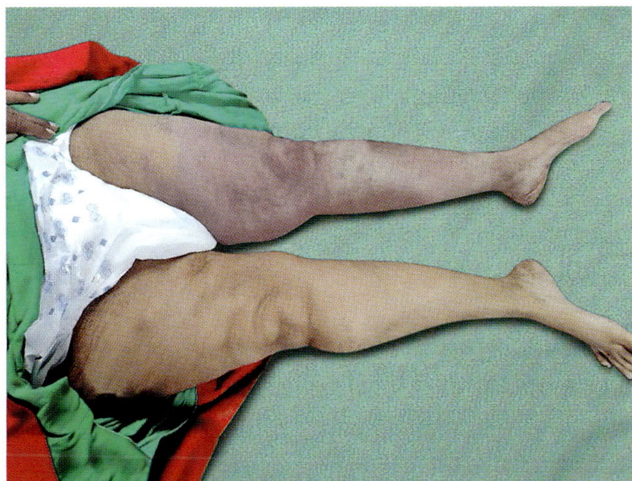

Fig. 1: Color changes in the left leg in comparison to right leg showing profound ischemia presented late—class III ischemia.

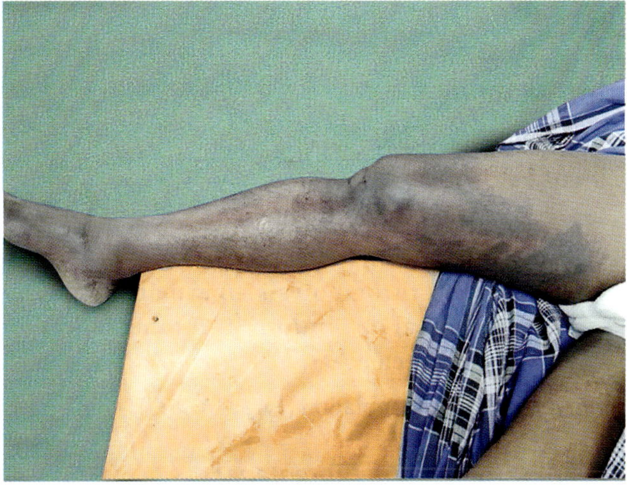

Fig. 2: Right leg gangrenous changes of skin till mid-thigh, sign of advanced ischemia—class III ischemia. Patient had a hip disarticulation.

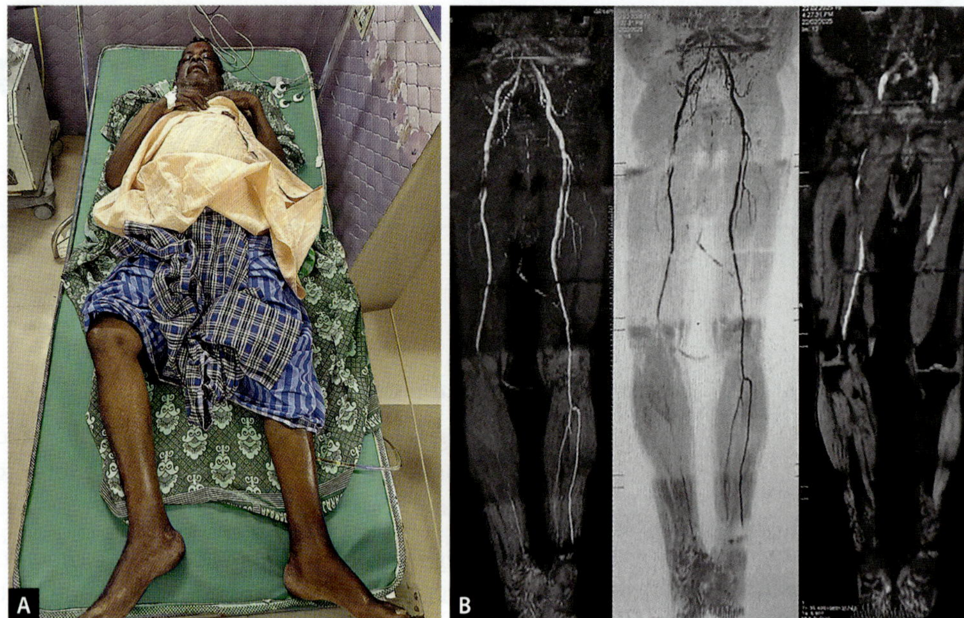

Figs. 3A and B: (A) Patient having foot drop on right leg and it can be compared to the neutral position of feet on left side. It is a feature of progressive limb-threatening ischemia—class IIb; (B) Right limb with noncontrast magnetic resonance (MR) angiography—the right limb has acute cut-off at knee level and no flow beyond suggesting severe progressing disease.

TABLE 1: Rutherford classification.

Limb ischemia classification			
Description	***Class I: Viable***	***Class II: Threatened***	***Class III: Irreversible***
Clinical description	Not immediately threatened	Salvageable if promptly treated	Major tissue loss and amputation unavoidable
Capillary return	Intact	Intact and slow	Absent (marbling)
Muscle weakness	None	Mild and partial	Profound, paralysis (rigor)
Sensory loss	None	Mild and incomplete	Profound anesthetic
Arteriovenous Doppler	Audible	Inaudible or audible	Inaudible

Management

Class I—Viable and Class IIa—Not Imminently Threatened

- Preoperative imaging
- Revascularization with thrombolysis (catheter-directed thrombolysis/pharmacomechanical/mechanical aspiration thrombectomy) or thromboembolectomy

Unfit patient: Anticoagulation **(Figs. 4A to C)**

Class IIb—Imminently Threatened

- *Operating room:* On table imaging
- Thromboembolectomy or bypass or endovascular management (pharmacomechanical/mechanical aspiration thrombectomy)

Class III—Irreversible

Amputation.

Complications in Management of Acute Ischemic Limb

- Compartment syndrome
- Ischemic neuropathy
- Muscle necrosis
- Recurrent thrombosis

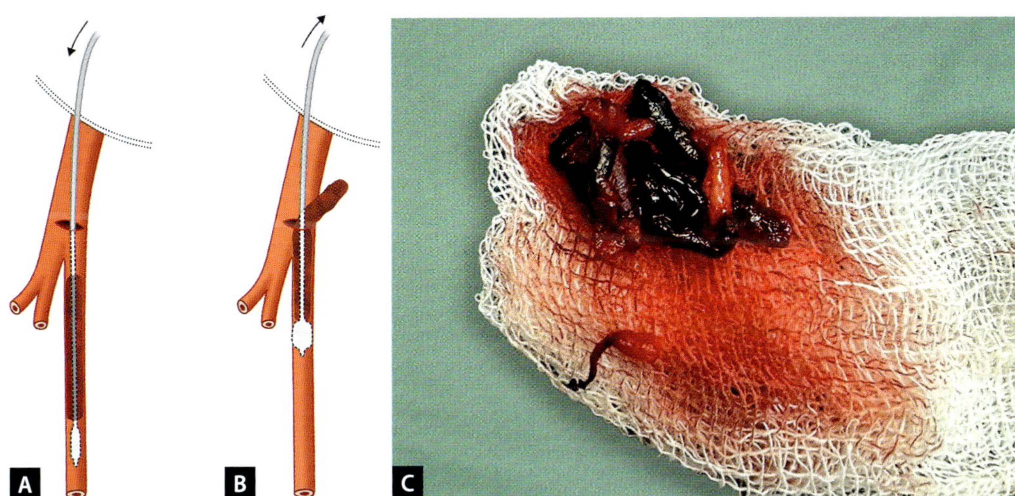

Figs. 4A to C: Pictorial representation of femoral artery embolectomy with Fogarty catheter. (A) Fogarty balloon is passed beyond the clot from arteriotomy; (B) Inflated balloon is used to trap and fish it out; (C) The clots retrieved after an embolectomy—the dark color clots are also called secondary thrombosis after occlusion of vessel and lack of outflow vessel.

- Limb swelling
- *Reperfusion syndrome:* Hypotension, hyperkalemia, myoglobinuria, and renal failure

Contraindications for Thrombolysis Necessitating Open Surgery

Contraindications to Thrombolytic Therapy

- *Absolute contraindications:*
  - Established cerebrovascular events (including transient ischemic attack) within last 2 months
  - Active bleeding diathesis
  - Recent (<10 days) gastrointestinal bleeding
  - Neurosurgery (intracranial or spinal) within last 3 months
  - Intracranial trauma within last 3 months
  - Intracranial malignancy or metastasis
  - Relative major contraindications
  - Cardiopulmonary resuscitation within last 10 days
  - Major nonvascular surgery or trauma within last 10 days
  - Uncontrolled hypertension (>180 mm Hg systolic or >110 mm Hg diastolic)
  - Puncture of noncompressible vessel
  - Intracranial tumor
  - Recent eye surgery
  - Minor contraindications
  - Hepatic failure, particularly with coagulopathy
  - Bacterial endocarditis
  - Pregnancy
  - Diabetic hemorrhagic retinopathy

COMPARTMENT SYNDROME

- Manifested immediately or delayed to 12–24 hours after reperfusion.
  - *Inadequate fasciotomy after revascularization:* Most common cause of preventable limb loss
- *Pain and loss of light touch sensation:* Earliest sign
- Suspected in any patient complaining of increasing pain after injury **(Figs. 5 and 6)**
- *Presentation:*
  - Tense compartment
  - Pain on passive range of motion
  - Progressive loss of sensation
  - Weakness
  - Loss of arterial pulses: *Late finding*—associated with poor prognosis
- *Safest approach:* Fasciotomy when compartment pressure (CP) >25 mm Hg
- Low threshold for fasciotomy
  - Trauma patient after prolonged ischemia before reperfusion
  - Children
  - Psychiatric patients
  - Head injury/comatose patients

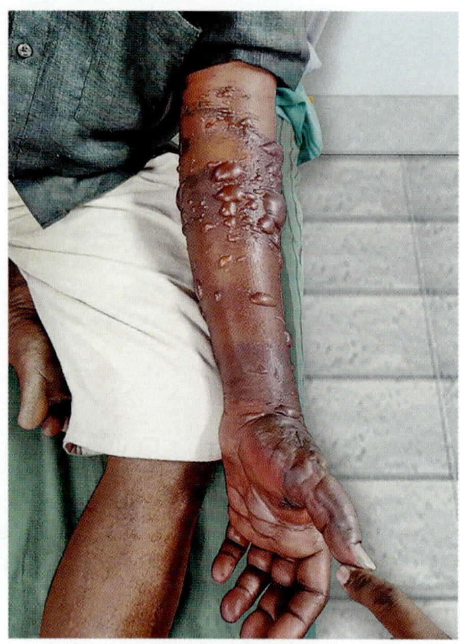

Fig. 5: Patient with elbow dislocation managed with native treatment presenting with delayed compartment syndrome.

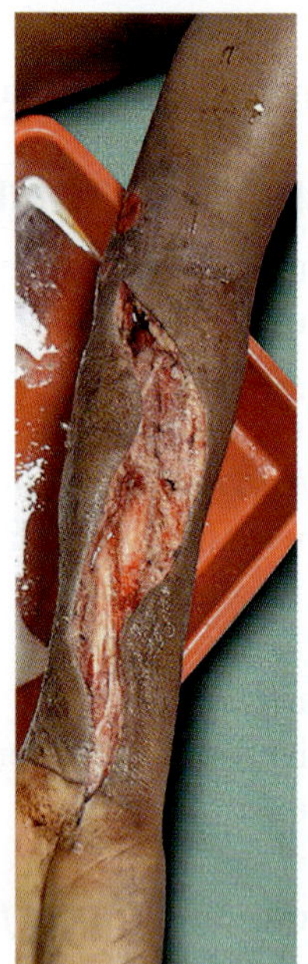

Fig. 6: Status of limb after few days of *"fasciotomy"*—a timely limb-saving procedure.

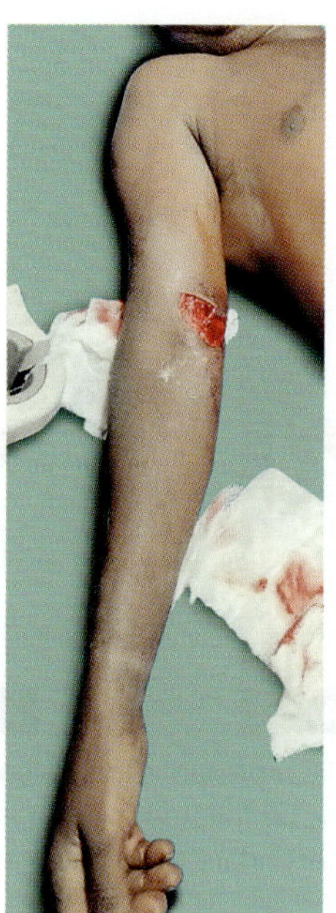

Fig. 7: Puncture laceration at distal arm with history of bleeding and absent pulses.

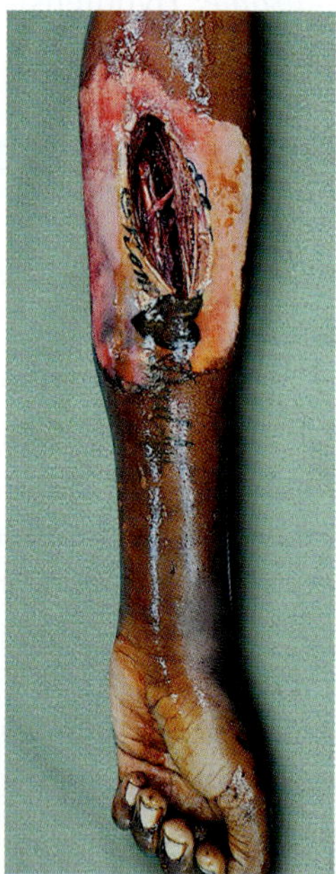

Fig. 8: Injury at workplace during farming—ploughing machine causing high-velocity injury.

VASCULAR EXTREMITY TRAUMA

Hard Signs of Vascular Injury

- Loss of pulses
- Severe arterial bleeding
- Active uncontrolled hemorrhaging
- Rapidly expanding pulsatile hematoma
- Palpable thrill or bruit **(Figs. 7 to 16)**
- Signs of distal ischemia (pain, pallor, paresthesia, paralysis, and poikilothermia)

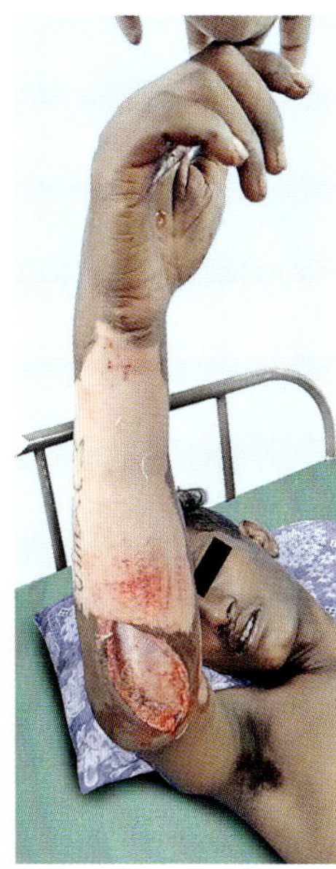

Fig. 9: Patient with extensive injury but has good neurological function—holding the examiner's hand against gravity.

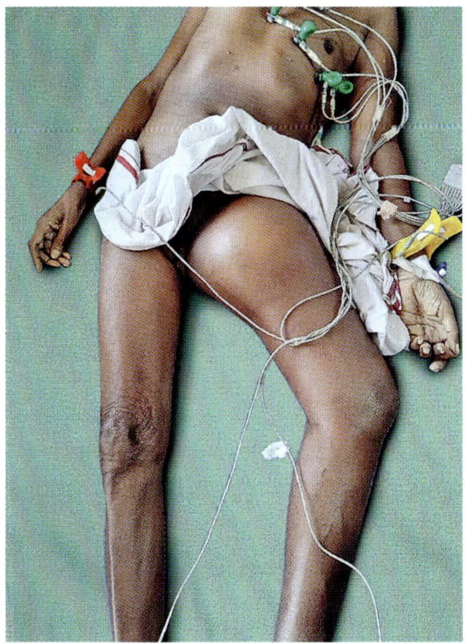

Fig. 10: Swelling in proximal left thigh—fracture femur causing injury to femoral artery and presenting with femoral artery pseudoaneurysm.

Soft Signs

- Small nonexpanding hematoma
- Subjectively decreased pulse
- Peripheral nerve deficit
- History of pulsatile or significant hemorrhage at time of injury

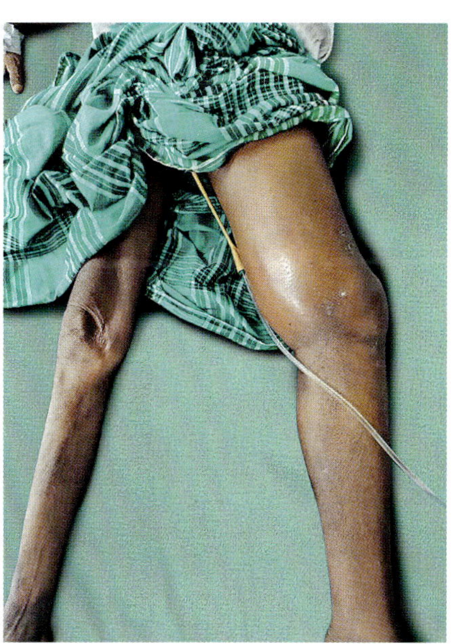

Fig. 11: Swelling in distal left thigh—patient has knee dislocation and popliteal artery injury causing popliteal artery pseudoaneurysm.

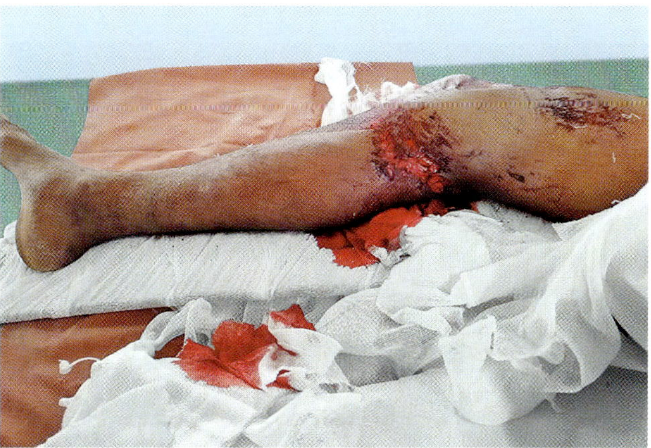

Fig. 12: Bleeding from popliteal fossa—patient having proximal both bone fracture with open wound in popliteal fossa causing extravasation.

- Unexplained hypotension
- High-risk orthopedic injuries (fracture, dislocation, and penetration)

Algorithm

- *Hard signs (>90% risk of arterial injury; 50% require intervention)*
  - Immediate arterial exploration without further investigation

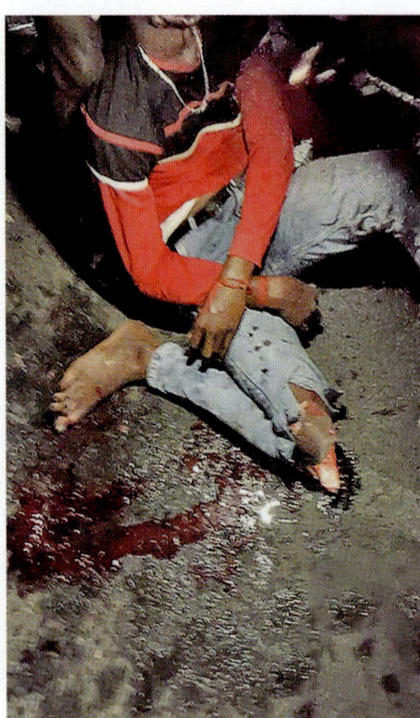

Fig. 13: High velocity trauma—proximal tibia protruding out of skin and patient has exsanguination due to arterial injury in the accident site.

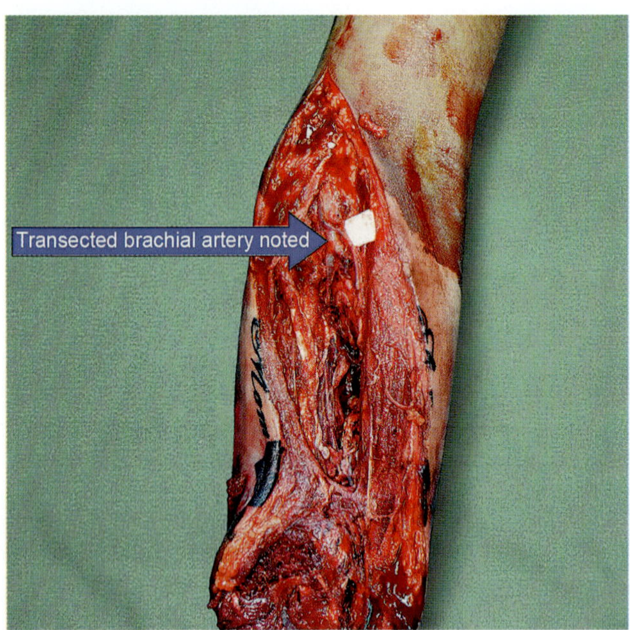

Fig. 14: Transected brachial artery as marked by arrow of the same patient in Figure 8.

- *Soft signs (30% risk of arterial injury)*
    - Perform ankle brachial pressure index (ABPI)
    - Doppler ultrasound (U/S)
    - Computed tomography (CT) angiogram
    - Evaluation of compartment pressures

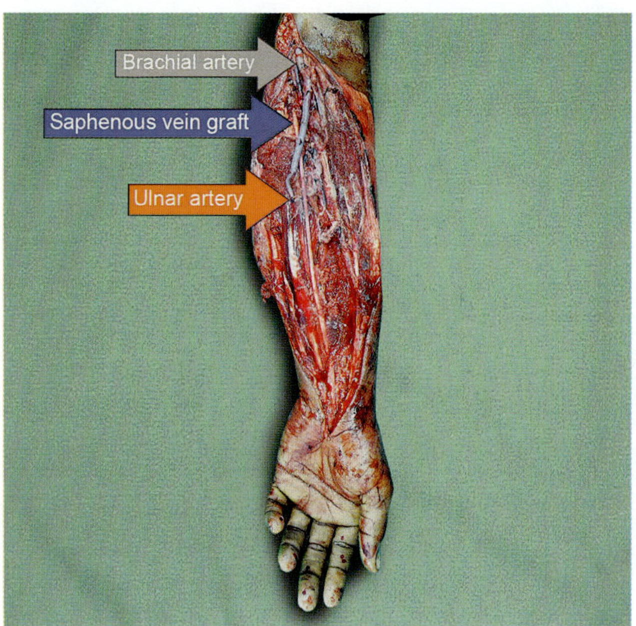

Fig. 15: Intraoperative image after fasciotomy, debridement, and reconstruction by brachial artery-to-ulnar artery bypass with saphenous vein graft.

Management

- Fasciotomy is done to assess the muscle status and to prevent revascularization-induced compartment syndrome **(Figs. 14 and 15)**.
- Identify and control bleeding vessels.
- Restore circulation to limb by thrombectomy or bypass.
- If limb is non salvageable, consider amputation.
- In unstable patient, do temporary shunting to get time.

RUPTURED ABDOMINAL AORTIC ANEURYSM

- Patient presents with new abdominal and/or back pain, cardiovascular collapse, or loss of consciousness **(Tables 2 and 3)**
- Patient may not be aware of the aneurysm **(Table 4)**.
- Risk of rupture is related directly to aneurysm size—Laplace law **(Fig. 16)**
- *>0.5 cm/year:* Relative indication for early repair
- *Unless ruptured/symptomatic:* Prophylactic repair
- *Risk of aneurysm rupture exceeds risk of all cause deaths in the patient:* Intervention **(Figs. 17 to 20)**

TABLE 2: Size of ascending, descending, and infrarenal aorta in men and women.

Wannheim et al.	*Men*	*Women*
Ascending aorta	4.7 cm	4.2 cm
Descending aorta	3.7 cm	3.3 cm
Infrarenal aorta	3.0 cm	2.7 cm

TABLE 3: Recommended size for intervention of asymptomatic aortic aneurysm.

Location	*Size criteria*	*Comment*
Ascending/root	≥55 mm	All patients, including BAV
	≥50 mm	Patients with Marfan syndrome
		BAV with risk factors for dissection
	≥45 mm	Selected patients with Marfan syndrome
	>45 mm	When aortic valve is being intervened on
	>27.5 mm/m^2	For patients with a small body size
Arch	≥55 mm	All patients
	Any size	Signs or symptoms of local compression
Descending	≥55 mm	When TEVAR possible
	≥60 mm	Open repair (less for Marfan syndrome)
Abdominal	≥55 mm	All patients

(BAV: bicuspid aortic valve; TEVAR: thoracic endovascular aneurysm repair)

TABLE 4: Annualized risk of rupture of abdominal aortic aneurysm (AAA) based on size.

Description	*Diameter of aorta (cm)*	*Estimated annual risk of rupture (%)*	**Estimated 5-year risk of rupture (%)**
Normal aorta	2–3	0	0 (unless AAA develops)
Small AAA	4–5	1	5–10
Moderate AAA	5–6	2–5	30–40
Large AAA	6–7	3–10	>50
Very large AAA	>7	>10	Approaching 100

*The estimated 5-year risk is more than 5 times the estimated annual risk because over that 5 years, the AAA, if left untreated, will continue to grow in size.

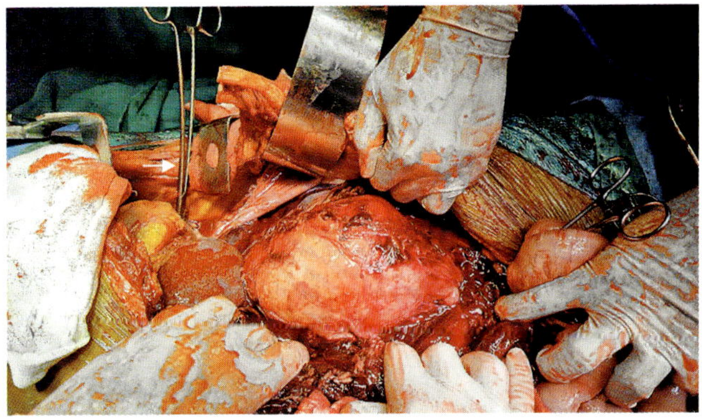

Fig. 16: Case of ruptured type-V thoracoabdominal aortic aneurysm (TAAA)—thoracolaparotomy. Arrow shows clamp in descending thoracic aorta to stop exsanguinating.

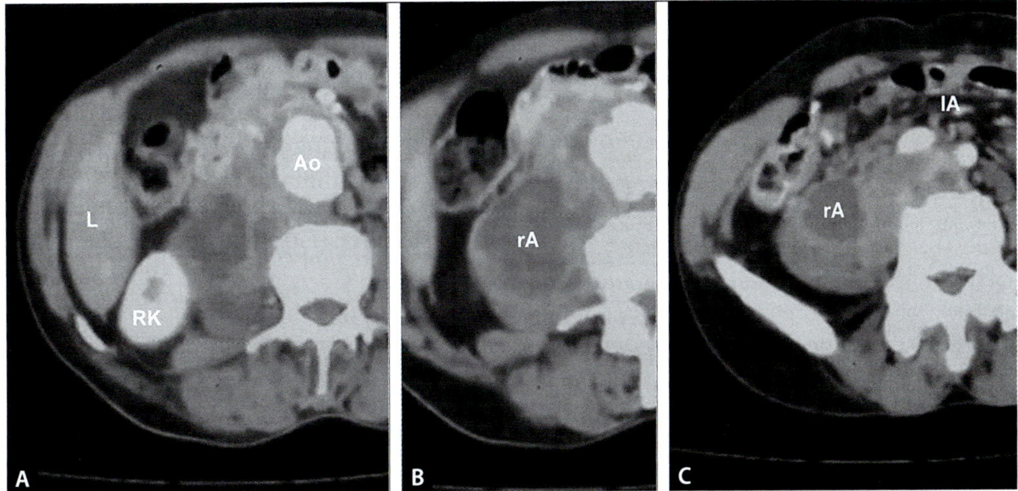

Figs. 17A to C: Ruptured abdominal aortic aneurysm (rAAA) in a gentleman who was identified in CECT abdomen when evaluating for abdominal and back pain. (Ao: aorta; IA: normal sized Iliac arteries; L: liver; rA: ruptured aortic segment; RK: right kidney)

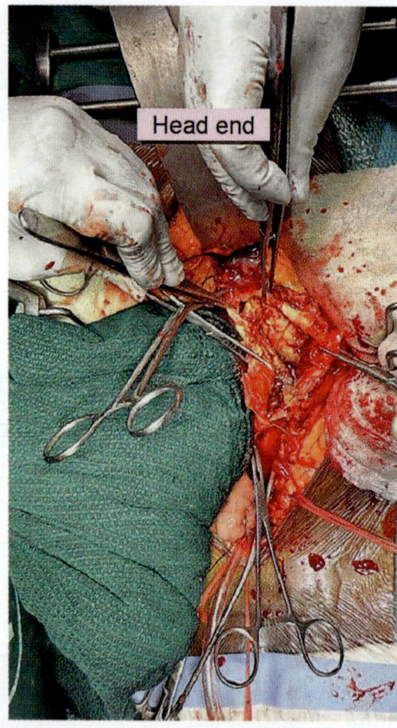

Fig. 18: Aneurysm sac opened after proximal and distal control.

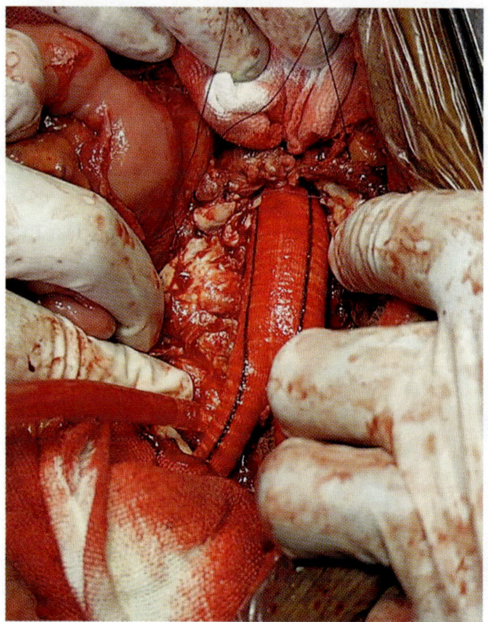

Fig. 19: Polyester (Dacron) bifurcated graft sewn to normal aorta at top excluding flow from aneurysm and two limbs perfusing each leg arteries—silk sutures are on the wall of aneurysm sac.

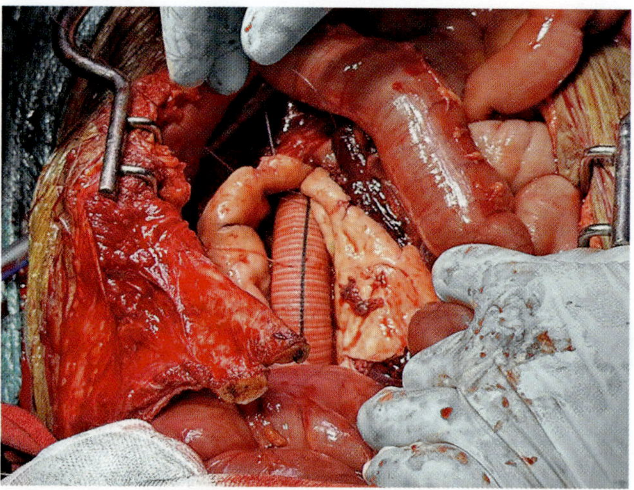

Fig. 20: Aneurysm sac is closed over the graft and completion of endoaneurysmorrhaphy.

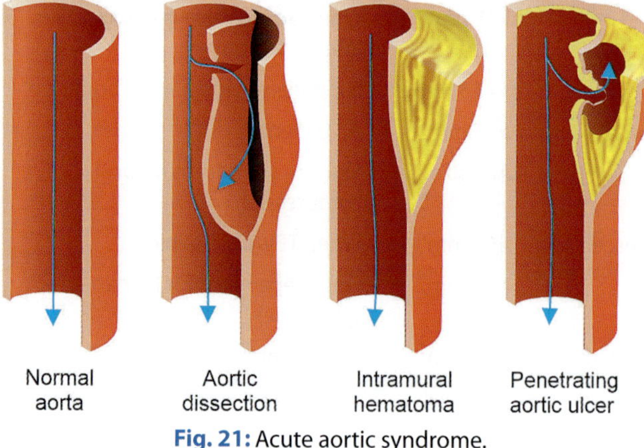

Fig. 21: Acute aortic syndrome.

AORTIC DISSECTION

Acute aortic syndrome is shown in **Figures 21 to 23**.

- Same disease within a spectrum and in fact may occur together
- Based on level of involvement of the aortic wall
- Significant overlap between the three conditions.
  1. Aneurysmal disease involves all three layers of the aorta.
  2. Penetrating atherosclerotic ulcer (PAU) is a disease of the intima and media.
  3. Aortic dissection (AD) and intramural hematoma (IMH) are diseases of the media.

Classification

See **Figures 22 and 23.**

Management

Type A: Aortic Dissection

Frozen elephant trunk (FET)/surgical repair: Mortality increases by 1–2% for every hour after initial event—risk of myocardial infarction (MI), stroke, and pericardial tamponade.

Type B: Aortic Dissection

- *Medical management:* Unless there is evidence of rupture or malperfusion
- *Selective β-blockade:* Preferred first line
  - Lowers blood pressure
  - Reduces aortic tension from the pressure impulse (dP/dt)

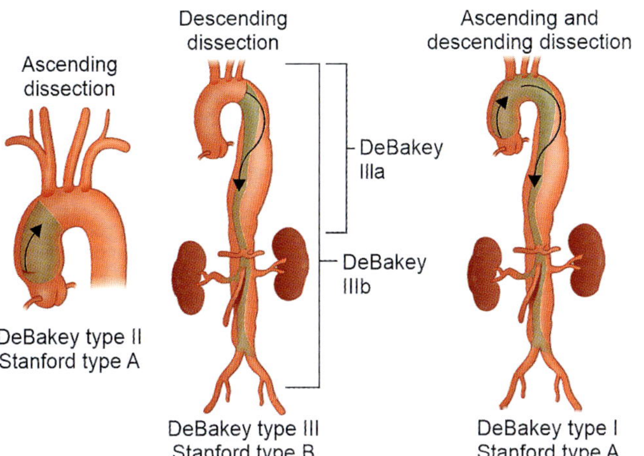

Fig. 22: Acute aortic syndrome.

  - *Goal:* Reduction of pulse pressure while maintaining end-organ perfusion—anti-impulse therapy.
- *Thoracic endovascular aneurysm repair:* Treatment of choice for complicated dissections (rupture or malperfusion) and as an option for noncomplicated dissection.
  - *Goals:* Coverage of the primary intimal tear and obliteration and/or thrombosis of the false lumen.

VENOUS THROMBOEMBOLISM

Wells model: Accounts the main risk factors—bed immobilization, surgery, or trauma; clinical signs or swelling, and edema; as well as another diagnosis being possible:

- Lower limb trauma, surgery, or plaster—risk of vessel damage and more
- Immobilization for >3 days or surgery within last month—blood stagnation risk
- Tenderness along femoral or popliteal veins
- Entire limb swelling
- Nonvaricose dilatation of collateral superficial veins
- Calf >3 cm bigger circumference, 10 cm below tibial tuberosity—specific DVT sign
- Pitting edema—specific DVT symptom
- History of confirmed DVT—patient or family history increase risk

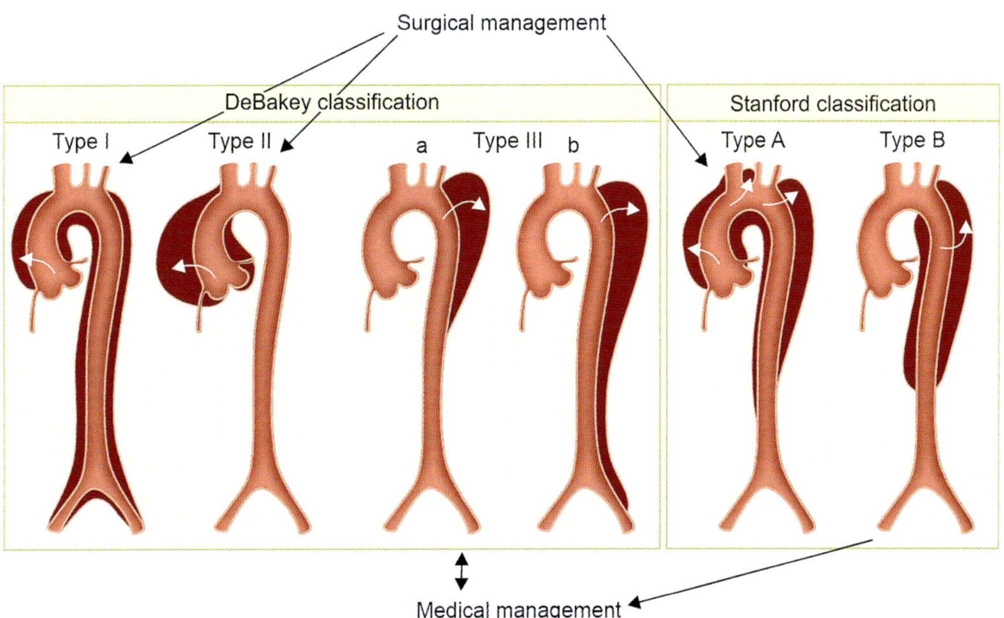

Fig. 23: Management of acute aortic syndrome.

TABLE 5: Clinical decision guide for suspected deep vein thrombosis (DVT) based on Wells score, D-dimer, and ultrasound requirement.

Wells score	*Interpretation*	*Pretest DVT probability*	*D-dimer*	*Ultrasound*
<1	DVT unlikely	5%—low probability	Negative	Not necessary
<1	DVT unlikely	5%—low probability	Positive	Necessary
1–2	DVT unlikely	17%—moderate probability	Negative	Not necessary/necessary upon clinical decision
1–2	DVT unlikely	17%—moderate probability	Positive	Compulsory
>2	DVT likely	35%—high probability	Negative	Necessary
>2	DVT likely	35%—high probability	Positive	Compulsory

- Malignancy—in treatment or not for the past 6 months is considered a risk factor
- Intravenous drug use, particularly involving groin injection
- Alternative diagnosis more likely than DVT, such as external venous compression, superficial venous thrombosis, postphlebitic syndrome, inguinal lymphadenopathy, muscle damage, or cellulites **(Table 5)**.

Investigations

Investigations are given in **Flowchart 1**.

Flowchart 1: Investigations.

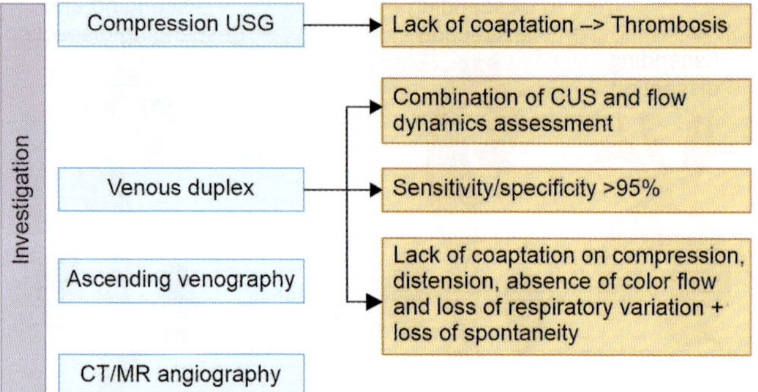

(CUS: combining conventional ultrasound; CT: computed tomography; MR: magnetic resonance; USG: ultrasound)

Inferior Vena Cava Filters (Figs. 24A and B)

- Prevent pulmonary embolism (PE)
- *Indication:* DVT patients who have—
  - Contraindication for anticoagulation
  - Having complications of anticoagulation
  - Patients with recurrent venous thromboembolism (VTE) not achieving adequate anticoagulation with portal hypertension (PHT).
- *Complications:* Thrombosis, migration, kinking, and erosion of filter
- Retrievable filters are indicated now **(Table 6)**.

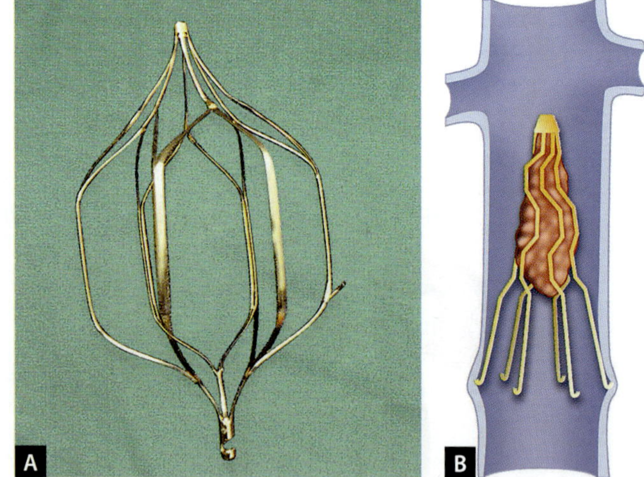

Figs. 24A and B: Inferior vena cava (IVC) filter—real life image and pictorial diagram of how it is placed in infrarenal IVC to trap clot.

Treatment

- *Anticoagulation:* Heparin, low-molecular-weight heparin (LMWH), warfarin, newer oral anticoagulants
- Inferior vena cava (IVC) filter placement
- Thrombolysis
- Amputation for venous gangrene

Phlegmasia Alba Dolens

Phlegmasia alba dolens is also colloquially known as *milk leg* or *white leg*.

- Acute progression of DVT
- After DVT, leg must rely on the superficial venous system for drainage **(Fig. 25)**.
- The superficial system is not adequate to handle the large volume of blood being delivered to the leg via the

TABLE 6: Modified Wells criteria for predicting pulmonary embolism (PE).

Variable	*Score*
Clinical signs and symptoms of deep vein thrombosis (DVT) (minimum of leg swelling and pain on palpation of deep veins)	3
Alternative diagnosis less likely than PE	3
Heart rate >100 bpm	1.5
Immobilization >3 days or surgery within past 4 weeks	1.5
Previous DVT or PE	1.5
Hemoptysis	1
Malignancy (treatment or palliation within past 6 months)	1
A score of <4 means PE is *unlikely* (12.4%), >4 is *suggestive* of PE (37.1%)	

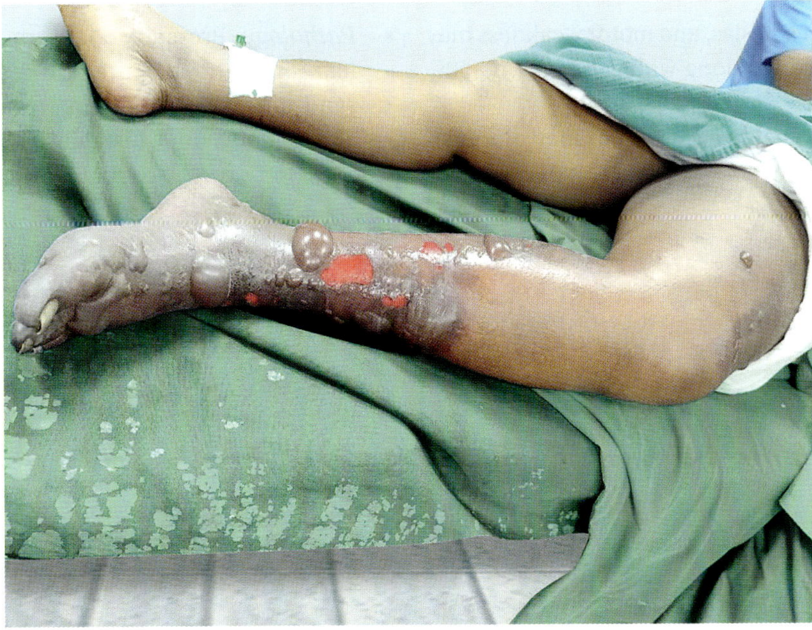

Fig. 25: Case of left iliofemoral deep vein thrombosis (DVT) after native treatment presenting with compartment syndrome—venous gangrene.

arterial system—edema, pain, and a white appearance (alba) of the leg.

- Phlegmasia alba dolens is distinguished, clinically, from phlegmasia cerulea dolens in that there is no ischemia and congestion.
- In severe cases of venous obstruction, the arterial pulse may gradually disappear, and venous gangrene may ensue.

Phlegmasia Cerulea Dolens

Phlegmasia cerulea dolens literally means "painful blue inflammation".

- Uncommon severe form of lower extremity DVT **(Figs. 26 and 27)**
- Edema, tight shiny skin, cyanosis (inadequate blood oxygenation), petechiae or purpura, and sudden severe pain

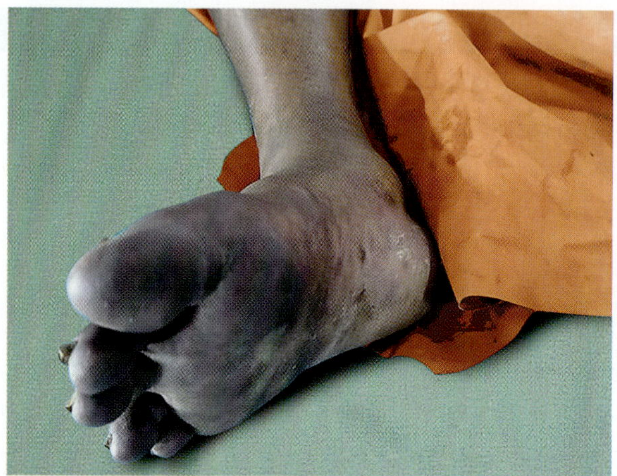

Fig. 26: Case of neglected right iliofemoral deep vein thrombosis (DVT) with forefoot gangrene.

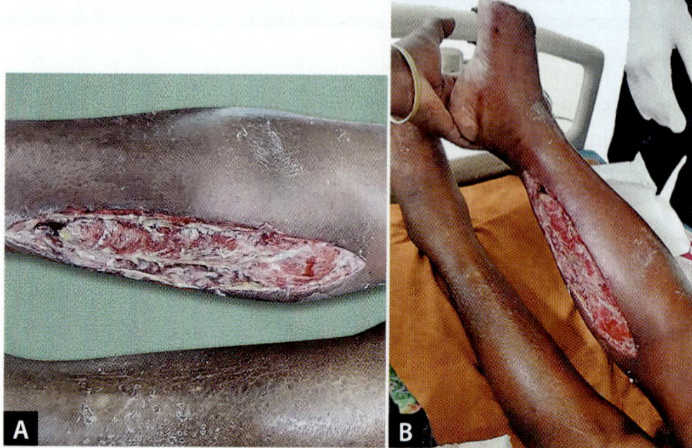

Figs. 27A and B: Same patient as in **Figure 6** postfasciotomy and anticoagulation image along with right forefoot amputation being done.

- Blisters, bullae, paresthesias, and motor weakness may develop in severe cases, along with gangrene in ~50% of cases
- Distal pulses are palpable early on but may diminish over time
- *Pathology:* Pressure raises up in the veins, plasma leak out into the interstitial space, compartment syndrome, acute ischemia, gangrene, hypovolemia, and hemodynamic instability.

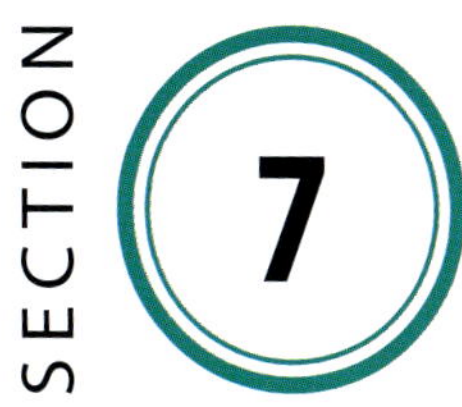

SECTION 7 Emergencies in Plastic Surgery

Surgical Emergencies in Patients with Facial Trauma

Vijay Jaganathan

INTRODUCTION

The three salient emergencies in facial trauma are:

1. Airway compromise
2. Life-threatening hemorrhage
3. Reversible structural injury to the eye or optic nerve.

AIRWAY COMPROMISE

Airway compromise usually happens in combined mandibular-maxillary trauma due to hemorrhage and soft-tissue swelling.

Management

- Endotracheal intubation—attempted initially
- Cricothyroidotomy and tracheostomy after the patient has been stabilized (if unable to intubation)
- Nasotracheal intubation is contraindicated in *severe naso-orbitoethmoid and skull base fractures.*

LIFE-THREATENING HEMORRHAGE

Life-threatening hemorrhage is considered if:

- There is 3 or more units of blood loss *or*
- *If hematocrit is below 29%.*

Management

If there is significant soft-tissue avulsion:

- Pressure packing
- Rapid placement of *temporary bolster sutures*
- Attempts to clamp and ligate vessels are avoided.

In case of penetrating trauma:

- Vessel identification and ligation *or*
- Angiographic selective embolization

If bleeding in blunt trauma:

- *Bleeding associated with midfacial fractures:* Fracture reduction and stabilization by *IMF using fixation screws.*
- *Bleeding associated with skull base and nasoethmoid fractures:* Anteroposterior nasal packing and selective angiography, if these measures fail.
- *In unstable patients:* Fracture reduction and nasal packing may be attempted during the angiography time to be followed immediately with embolization.

INJURIES TO ORBIT AND CONTENTS

- Increased intraocular pressure
- Globe rupture
- Optic nerve impingement
- *Increased intraocular pressure*
- *Acute increased intraocular pressure*
- Manifested by pain and vision loss
- Retrobulbar hematoma or decreased orbital volume.

Treatment

- *Lateral canthotomy*
- *Administration of*
  - Mannitol
  - Acetazolamide
  - Steroids

COMPRESSION OF OPTIC NERVE

Vision loss may result from mechanical compression of the optic nerve.

- Diagnosis by computed tomography (CT orbit)
- *Treatment:* Prompt emergent surgical decompression to preserve vision (usually by endoscopic methods by cranial base surgery specialist).

EXTRAOCULAR MUSCLE ENTRAPMENT

- Extraocular muscle entrapment presents as the inability to move the eye on the trajectory controlled by the entrapped muscle (restriction of upward gaze if inferior rectus entrapped in orbital floor fractures)

- Pain on attempted motion
- *Forced duction test done:* Eyeball does not move on forced movement with surgical forceps (done in theatre after anaesthetising)
- *CT scan coronal cuts:* Tear-drop sign
- *Treatment:* Surgical release of the entrapped contents and orbital floor reconstruction with bone graft or titanium mesh implants **(Fig. 1)**.

EMERGENCY AIRWAY MANAGEMENT IN PIERRE ROBIN SEQUENCE

Pierre Robin sequence (PRS) is the most common syndrome associated with cleft palate. Concerning for:

- Isolated cleft palate (U- or V-shaped)
- Glossoptosis
- Retrognathia

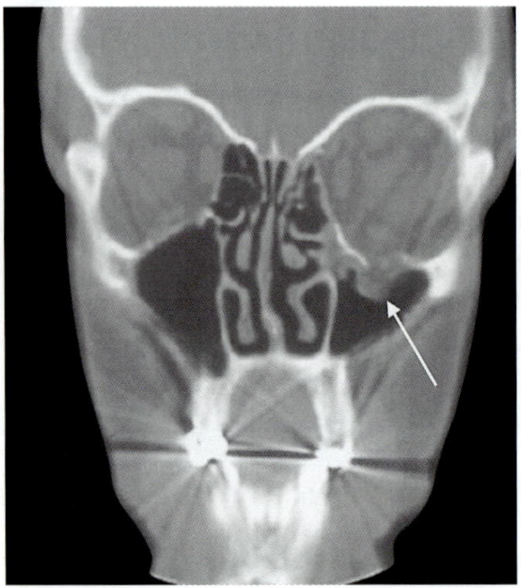

Fig. 1: Hemorrhage.

- Respiratory difficulty
- Feeding difficulty **(Fig. 2)**.

Pathophysiology

Pierre Robin Sequence is described as a "sequence" because primary problem is micrognathia. Glossoptosis is secondary to inability of tongue to accommodate in a small floor of the mouth.

Cleft palate is secondary to protruding tongue preventing the fusion of lateral palatine shelves.

Diagnosis

Diagnosis is primarily clinical and based on the triad of features—micrognathia, glossoptosis, and cleft palate.

Management

Conservative Management

Mild cases often respond to nonsurgical measures:

- *Positioning:*
  - Prone or lateral positioning
  - Gravity aids to pull the tongue forward
  - 70% of cases become better
- Nasopharyngeal stenting
- Continuous positive airway pressure (CPAP).

Surgical Management

It is indicated in severe cases, syndromic PRS, or when conservative measures fail.

- *Tongue-lip adhesion (labioglossopexy):*
  - Sutures the tongue to the lower lip to keep it in an anterior position

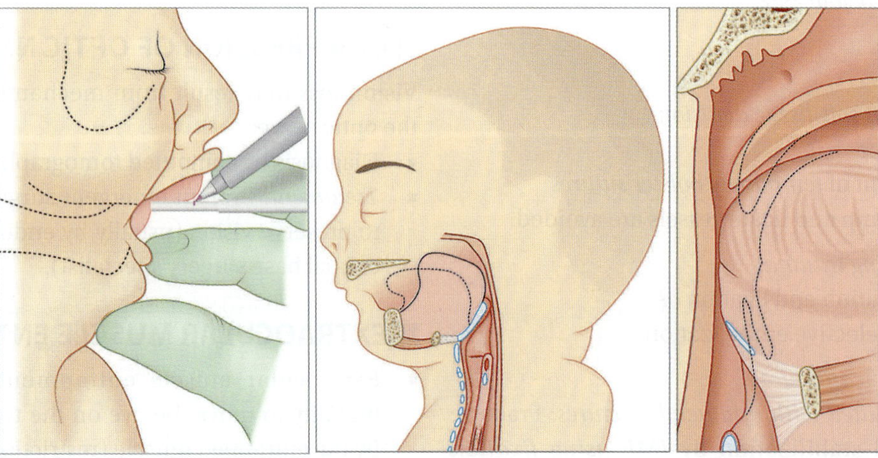

Fig. 2: Emergency airway management.

- *Mandibular distraction osteogenesis:*
    - Advances and elongates the jaw
    - The three phases of distraction osteogenesis are:
        1. *Latency (postosteotomy rest)*
        2. *Activation (incremental lengthening of the jaw)*
        3. *Consolidation (bone healing and formation)*
- *Tracheostomy:*
    - Used in cases with multilevel airway obstruction
    - It is the gold standard for airway protection.

TEMPOROMANDIBULAR JOINT DISLOCATIONS AND MANAGEMENT

Anatomy

- The temporomandibular joint (TMJ) is a bilateral synovial joint.
- It is protected by an articular capsule, temporomandibular ligaments, and an articular disc.
- The disc acts as a cushion between condyle and the temporal bone.
- Dislocations occur when the mandibular condyle is displaced from its position in the glenoid fossa.
- Most common dislocation is anterior dislocations (condyle moves forward in front of the articular eminence).

Risk Factors

Hypermobile syndromes (e.g., Marfan and Ehlers-Danlos), weak or torn temporomandibular ligaments or overstretched joint capsule, and preexisting TMJ injuries or recurrent dislocations.

Clinical Presentation

- Pain
- *Locked open jaw:* Inability to close the mouth
- Forward displacement of mandible in anterior dislocations
- *Malocclusion*
- Visible and palpable indentation in front of the ear by the anteriorly displaced condyle
- *Deviation:* In unilateral dislocations, jaw deviating toward the unaffected side.

Diagnosis

- *Physical examination:*
    - Observe for an open mouth with a protruding jaw and pain localized to the TMJ.
    - Palpate displaced mandibular condyle in the preauricular area.
- *Imaging studies:*
    - Radiographs (Panorex view)
    - *CT scans:* Necessary if there is suspicion of associated injuries, such as basilar skull fractures or intracranial trauma.

Management

Management is divided into nonsurgical reduction and adjunct therapies.

Patient Preparation

- Pain relief and muscle relaxation
- Essential for successfully reducing a TMJ dislocation
- Parenteral analgesics, sedatives, or muscle relaxants given
- Manipulation of the mandible is easier into its correct anatomical position
- An alternative is the administration of a *local anesthetic injection into the TMJ space.*

Reduction Techniques

- *Bimanual intraoral traction technique:*
    - Stand or sit in front of the patient.
    - Place thumbs on the patient's posterior molars or mandibular ridge.
    - Wrap fingers around the mandible to stabilize it.
    - Apply downward (inferior) and backward (posterior) pressure to release the condyle from the articular eminence and guide it back into the glenoid fossa.
- *Alternative reduction techniques:*
    - *Posterior intraoral technique:*
        - Clinician standing behind the patient
        - Place thumbs on the lower molars and press downward (inferiorly) and backward (posteriorly) and apply pressure.

Adjunct Measures and Aftercare

- *Supportive devices:*
    - *Barton's bandage:* It secures the mandible and prevents wide opening, often used for chronic dislocations.
    - *Soft cervical collar:* It provides support and serves as a reminder to limit jaw movement.

- *Medications:*
  - *Nonsteroidal anti-inflammatory drugs (NSAIDs):* Alleviate pain and inflammation.
  - *Muscle relaxants:* Reduce spasm and tension.
- *Patient education:*
  - Avoid excessive jaw opening (>2 cm) and activities that strain the TMJ.
  - Adopt a soft diet, avoiding hard or gummy food for 3 weeks.
  - Support the mandible with the hand during yawning to prevent redislocation.

PYOGENIC FLEXOR TENOSYNOVITIS

Tenosynovitis is caused by an infection of the tendon sheath, can lead to swelling along the tendons of the fingers and wrist, with patients reporting difficulty in moving the affected digit.

Synovial sheaths in flexor tendons gives fluid filling planes to glide inside a closed compartment that helps in execution of flexor actions.

The sheath extends from midpalmar crease to A1 pulley just proximal to distal interphalangeal (DIP).

Thumb flexor sheaths extend along the radial bursa of palm.

Little finger sheath extends along ulnar palmar bursa.

Clinical Features

Kanavel's four cardinal signs of flexor tenosynovitis:

1. Fusiform swelling in the finger
2. Posture of digit is partially flexed
3. Entire flexor tendon sheath tenderness
4. Pain on passive extension in a dispropriate manner.

The last sign is the one most consistently present and the one seen earliest in the infection process.

Management

- Within the first 24 hours, treat with parenteral antibiotics.
- Unsuccessful or patient seen after 48 hours surgical drainage.

Surgical Approach

- Two separate incisions.
  1. One on the midaxial incision—*between the A3 and A4 pulleys; synovium is incised.*
  2. A second on the *palm over the tendon to drain the cul-de-sac.*

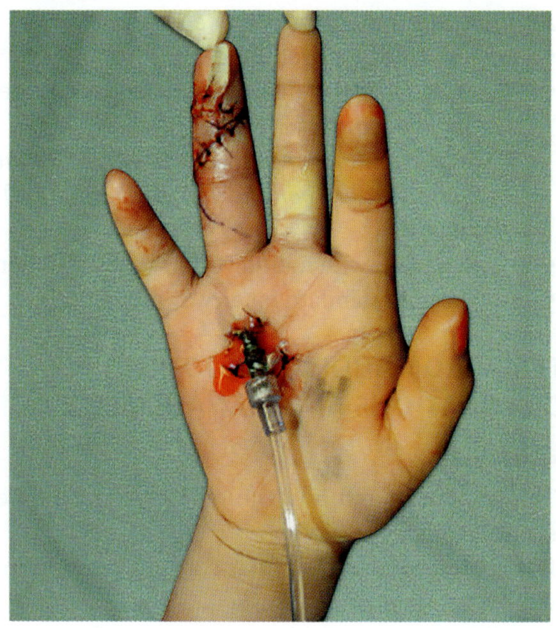

Fig. 3: Pyogenic flexor tenosynovitis.

- *Polyethylene catheter beneath the A1 pulley into the sheath,* flushed *every 2 hours after surgery* ***(Fig. 3)***.

REPLANTATION

Malt and McKhann performed the first replantation at midhumeral level in 1962.

Kleinert performed first vascular repair in fingers the next year.

- *Replantation:* Reattachment of completely amputated part
- *Revascularization:* Reconstruction of vessels in severely injured limb to make it viable but some soft tissue is still intact.
- *Minor replantation:* Reattachment at the wrist, hand, or digital level.
- *Major replantation:* At level proximal to the wrist.

Contraindications for Replantation

- Severe *crush or multilevel injury* of the amputated part
- A psychotic patient has *willfully self-amputated.*
- Amputation in patients with severely atherosclerotic arteries
- *Amputation of a single digit proximal to the flexor digitorum superficialis (FDS) distal insertion* (zone 2), (except in children or adults in demanding profession (musician).

Indications for Replantation of Amputated Parts

- Whenever possible, for a thumb amputation
- Single digits amputated distal to the FDS insertion
- Multiple injured digits
- Most amputations in children, including single-digit
- Guillotine-sharp clean amputations.

Ischemia Time

- *Amputated digits:* 12 hours of warm ischemia is a relative contraindication
- *Above proximal forearm*: Contraindicated in more than 6–10 hours of warm ischemia time.

TRANSPORT OF AMPUTATED PART: BAG-IN-BAG TECHNIQUE

- The amputated part is wrapped in a lightly moistened saline gauze.
- Then it is placed in a clean, dry, plastic bag, which is sealed.
- This bag is placed on top of ice in a Styrofoam container.
- It should sufficiently cool at 4–10°C without freezing **(Fig. 4)**.

The order of repair is usually:

- Bone first
- Tendons and muscle units
- Arteries
- Nerves
- Finally, veins

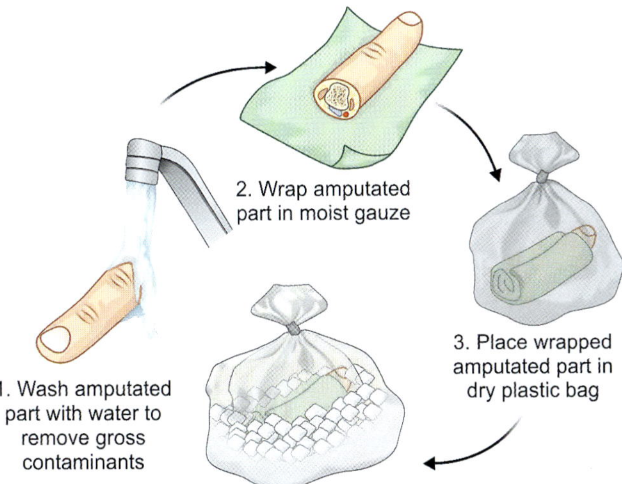

Fig. 4: Bag-in-bag technique.

COMPARTMENT SYNDROME IN UPPER LIMB REQUIRING FASCIOTOMY

Definition

Compartment syndrome is a surgical emergency characterized by increased pressure within a closed muscle compartment, leading to reduced blood flow and tissue ischemia.

The most common sites of compartment syndrome are the lower leg and forearm.

Clinical Features

Hallmark symptoms are:

- Pain out of proportion to the injury
- Tense swelling
- Diminished pulses (which may be difficult to detect due to swelling)
- Sensory deficits
- Classic signs include the "5 P's"—pain, pallor, pulselessness, paresthesia, and paralysis.

Diagnosis

- Clinical suspicion is most important.
- Rarely confirmed by measuring *intracompartmental pressure.*
- Intracompartmental pressure greater than 30 mm Hg is an indication for an urgent fasciotomy.
- Pressure difference within 20–30 mm Hg of the patient's diastolic blood pressure is an indication for compartment syndrome.
- Doppler ultrasound and radiography imaging *are not useful.*

Management

- Prompt surgical intervention is crucial.
- Fasciotomy involves making incisions in the fascial compartments to relieve the pressure and restore blood flow.
- This procedure is done emergently and requires proper postoperative wound management to prevent infection.

Procedure

Upper arm fasciotomy

- Medial incision
- Lateral incision

It is done to decompress the anterior and posterior compartments **(Fig. 5)**.

- *Volar forearm compartment release:*
    - Wide extensile exposure that starts from medial epicondyle and extends to proximal wrist crease.

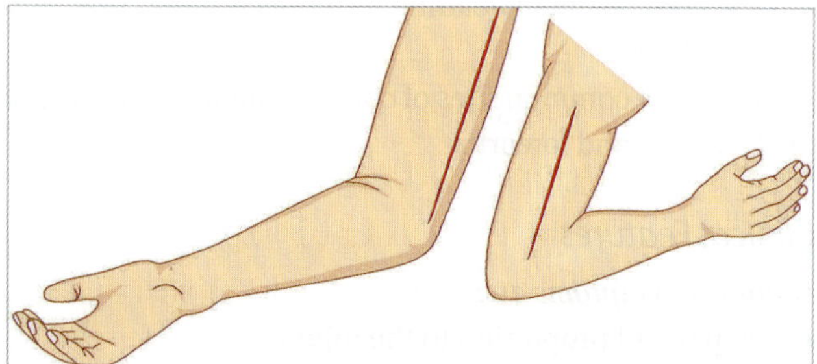

Fig. 5: Incision design for the upper arm fasciotomy.

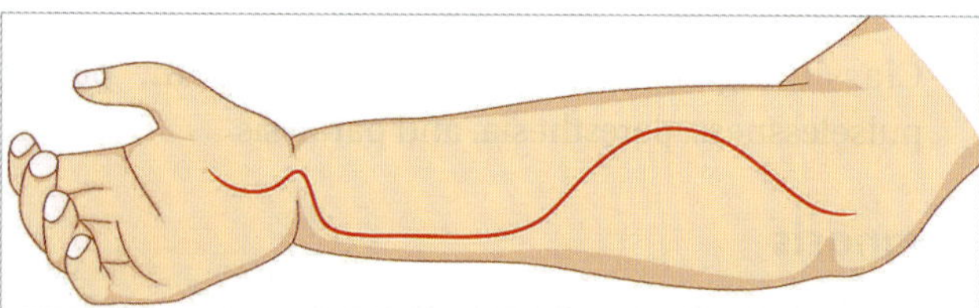

Fig. 6: Volar forearm compartment release.

    - Avoid the median nerve exposure by adequate curvature.
    - The incision enters between flexor carpi ulnaris and flexor digitorum superficialis **(Fig. 6)**.
    - *There, decompress the median nerve and deep group of flexor muscles.*
- *Dorsal forearm compartment syndrome:*
    - *On line between distal radioulnar joint and lateral epicondyle, a longitudinal incision is made.*
    - Between the extensor digitorum communis and extensor carpi radialis brevis, the fascia is approached, *and compartments are released by four incisions.*
    - Parallel and radial to second and fourth metacarpal, two incisions are made.
    - A longitudinal incision along *ulnar aspect of the hypothenar eminence releases hypothenar compartment* **(Fig. 7)**.
- Midaxial lateral incision is made along the noncontact side of the finger **(Fig. 8)**.

Complications

Complications of compartment syndrome include muscle necrosis, nerve damage, infection, and permanent functional deficits.

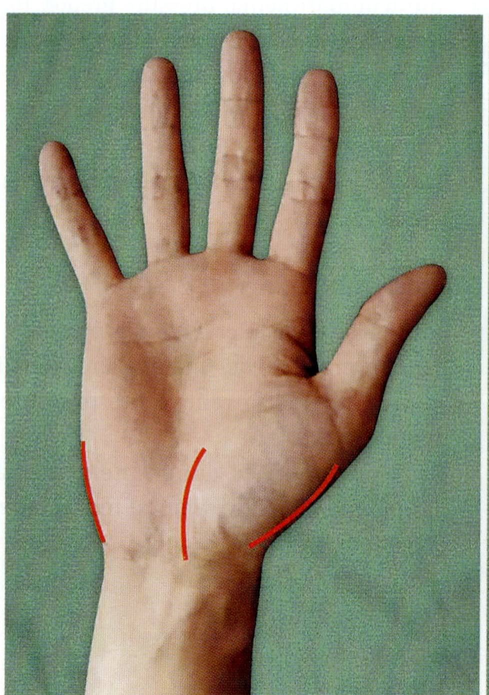

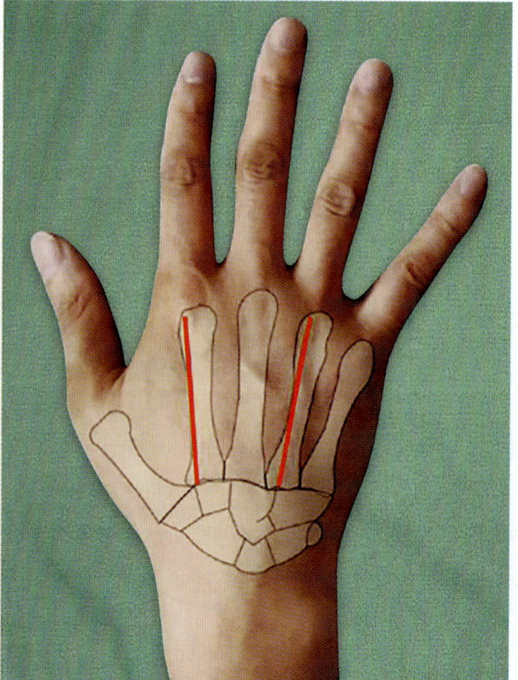

Fig. 7: Finger decompression.

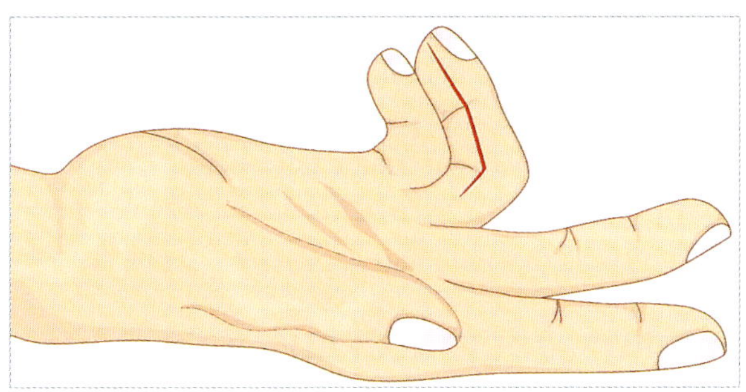

Fig. 8: Incision design for digital compartment release.

Delayed fasciotomy increases the risk of severe long-term impairment. Additionally, rhabdomyolysis can occur in cases of prolonged ischemia.

BURN INJURIES: ESCHAROTOMY

Incise the burns wound/eschar up to subcutaneous tissue.

Indications:

- Nonexpanding, inflexible eschar, which limit distal extremity perfusion or torso expansion
- Near circumference burns having partial-thickness or full-thickness at extremities.

Clinical Features

- Decrease in the neurovascular examination
- Limited chest expansion
- Elevated intra-abdominal pressures.

Escharotomy procedure:

- It is done bedside with adequate sedation.
- Diathermy is used.

After escharotomies are completed: Follow-up neurovascular examination should document return of pulses and distal perfusion.

Incision patterns:

- Extend the wound beyond the deep burn.
- Perform diathermy on any significant bleeding vessels.
- Apply hemostatic dressing and elevate the limb postoperatively.

Upper Limb

- At midaxial
- In front of the elbow medially to avoid the ulnar nerve.

Hand

- Midline at level of digits
- Release muscle compartments

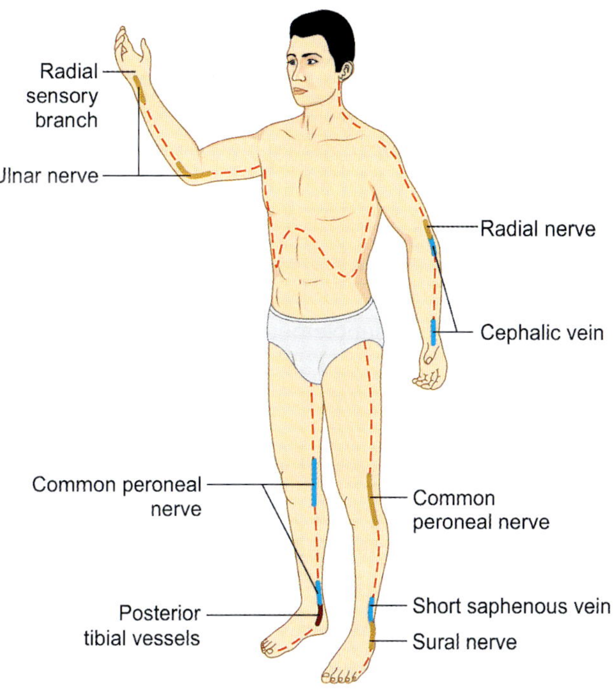

Fig. 9: Escharotomy.

Lower Limb

- At midaxial
- Medially at ankle to avoid the long saphenous vein
- Anterior fibula head to avoid the common peroneal nerve.

Chest

- Lateral to the nipples
- Below the clavicle
- At level of the xiphisternum **(Fig. 9)**.

POST FREE-FLAP VASCULAR INSUFFICIENCY

Post free-flap vascularity of flap disturbance can be due to arterial or venous problems.

Clinical Features

If decreased arterial perfusion:

- Pale flap
- Cold flap
- Decrease turgor
- Shriveled flap
- No bleeding on scratch test.

If venous congestion:

- Increase in temperature
- Swollen flap
- Darkish blue hue
- Increased bleeding (dark red blood) on scratch test.

Diagnosis

- Clinical examination is the best method.
- *Imaging techniques:* Doppler ultrasound or arteriography is done to supplement clinical findings.

Management

Arterial insufficiency:

- Thrombosis of anastomosis is the most common reason for arterial problem.
- Urgent return to operating room to revise anastomosis.
- Salvage by vascular arterial revision on table.

Venous insufficiency of a flap:

- **More common** and onset more insidious
- Low pressure of venous system is more vulnerable to extrinsic pressure.

Salvaging venous congestion:

- Release insetting sutures causing tension or kinking.
- Prick with a needle serially.
- De-epithelialization of a portion of flap.
- Remove nail plate in digit, with periodic application of heparin solution.
- *Hirudo medicinalis* or medicinal leeches.
- Cannulation of a vein with an angiocatheter and periodically draining flap.

HYDROFLUORIC ACID BURNS

- Hydrofluoric (HF) acid causes corrosion of tissue with free hydrogen ions along with dehydration.
- *Fluoride ion combines with calcium and magnesium to form insoluble salts.*
- Systemic absorption induce intravascular calcium chelation and hypocalcemia.

Treatment

- Apply copious 2.5% calcium gluconate gel (at every 15-minute intervals until the pain resolves).
- Cardiac monitoring and monitor QT interval
- Intravenous calcium chloride to maintain heart function
  - Underlying bone and soft tissue injury may happen.
  - Serum magnesium and potassium monitored closely.

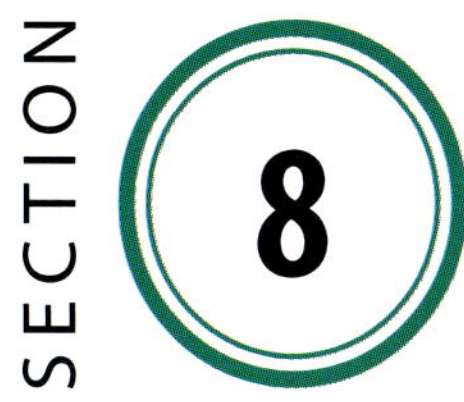

SECTION 8 Cardiothoracic Surgery Emergencies

CHAPTER 21

Cardiothoracic Emergencies

KS Saravana Krushna Raja

INTRODUCTION

- Majority of thoracic injuries (nearly 70%) occur due to blunt injury [commonly due to road traffic accidents (RTA)]
- Penetrating chest injuries are the most common causes of mortality from trauma up to the age of 40 years.

BLUNT INJURY CHEST

- Acceleration-deceleration injuries (involved in RTA)
- Accidental fall
- Sports injuries
- Assaults
- Blasts.

Blunt injury chest is shown in **Figure 1**.

Pediatric individuals: Chest wall is immature and flexible but intrathoracic injuries may occur.

Adults: Ribs were prone to injuries from even low impact and provide less protection to the underlying heart, lungs, and great vessels. Death rate is high even with minor injuries.

Penetrating chest injury is shown in **Figures 2 and 3**.

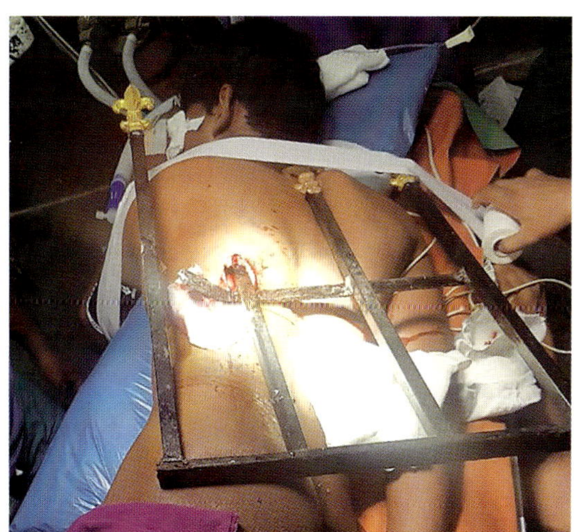

Fig. 2: Tracheal injury.

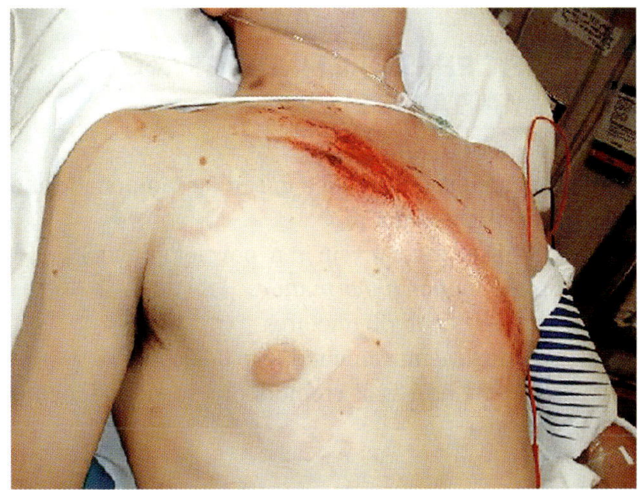

Fig. 1: Blunt injury chest.

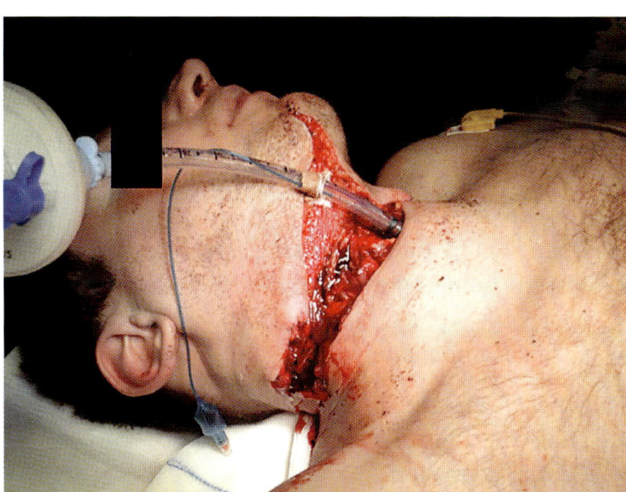

Fig. 3: Tracheal repair.

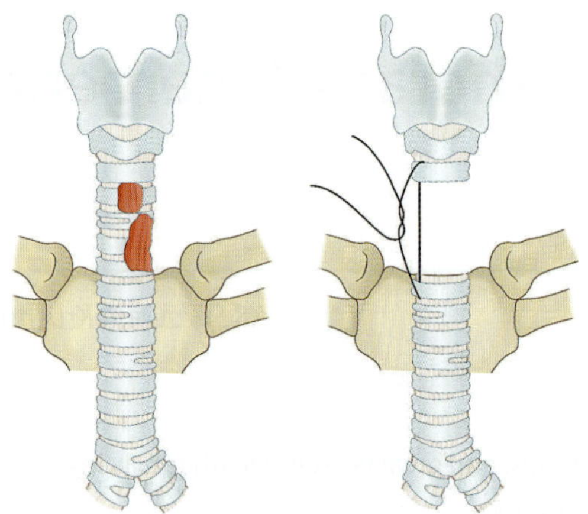

Fig. 4: Life-threatening conditions according to Advanced Trauma Life Support (ATLS).

Flowchart 1: Pathophysiology of chest trauma.

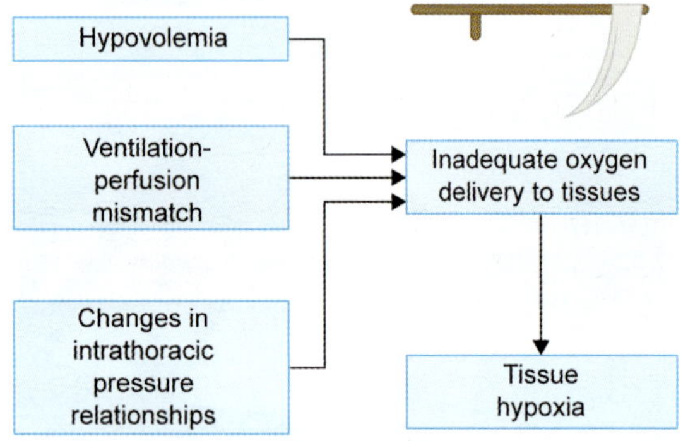

Nearly 5 cm of trachea can be safely resected for reconstruction ***(Fig. 4)****.*

- Tension pneumothorax (left or right)
- Flail chest with pulmonary contusion
- Massive hemothorax
- Open pneumothorax
- Cardiac tamponade **(Flowchart 1)**

Immediate life threats:

- Upper airway obstruction
- Tension pneumothorax
- Open pneumothorax ("sucking chest wound")
- Massive hemothorax
- Flail chest
- Cardiac tamponade

Potential life threats:

- Lung contusion
- Cardiac contusion
- Aortic rupture
- Diaphragmatic rupture

TABLE 1: Management of acute lethal chest injuries.

Injury	*Management*
Tension pneumothorax	Tube thoracostomy
Massive intrathoracic hemorrhage	Tube thoracostomy and operative repair
Cardiac tamponade	Pericardiocentesis and operative repair
Deceleration aortic injury	Operative repair
Massive flail chest with pulmonary contusion	Intubation, pain control, and fluid restriction
Upper/lower airway obstruction	Intubation, airway, and bronchoscopy
Tracheobronchial rupture	Bronchoscopy and operative repair
Diaphragmatic rupture with visceral herniation	Operative repair
Esophageal perforation	Operative repair

- Tracheobronchial tree injury—larynx, trachea, and bronchus
- Esophageal trauma

MISCELLANEOUS CHEST INJURIES (TABLE 1)

- Subcutaneous emphysema
- Traumatic asphyxia
- Simple pneumothorax
- Hemothorax
- Scapular fracture
- Chest wall rib fractures

Objects that may cause chest injuries are shown in **Figures 5A to C**.

SPECIFIC PHYSICAL FINDINGS IN CHEST TRAUMA (TABLE 2)

- *Neck veins*
    - Enlarged and distended in cardiac tamponade and tension pneumothorax
    - Collapsed jugular vein in hypovolemic shock
- *Chest wall motion abnormalities*
    - Limited due to rib fractures
    - Paradoxical movement due to flail chest
- *Palpation:* Chest wall crepitus due to subcutaneous emphysema
- *Percussion*
    - Hyperresonant in pneumothorax
    - Dull in hemothorax

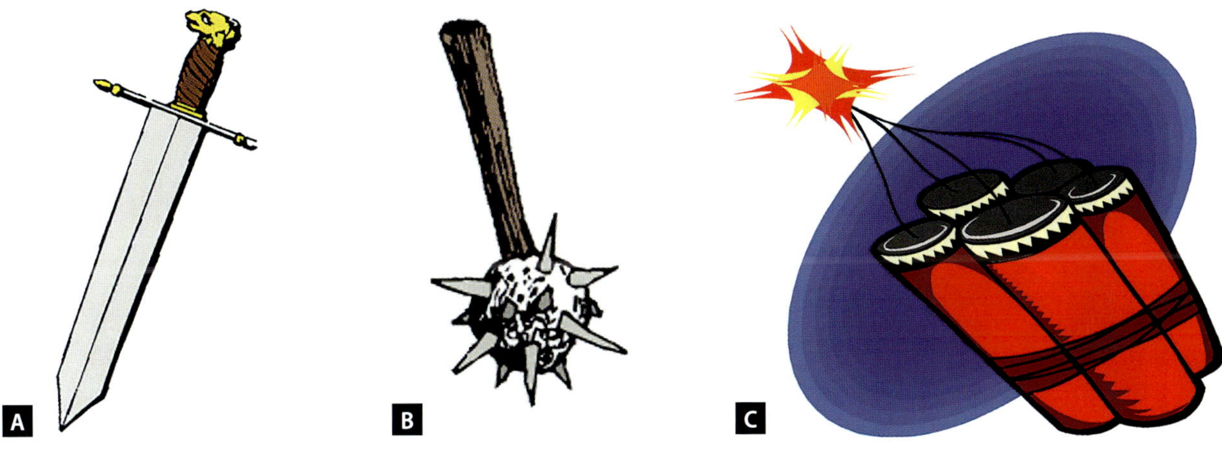

Figs. 5A to C: Objects that may cause chest injuries.

TABLE 2: Physical findings in chest trauma.

Types of trauma	*Tracheal position*	*Chest expansion*	*Breath sounds*	*Percussion*
Tension pneumothorax	Away	Decreased	Diminished or absent	Hyper resonant
Simple pneumothorax	Midline	Decreased	May be diminished	May be hyperresonant, usually normal
Hemothorax	Midline	Decreased	Diminished if large, otherwise small	Dull, especially posteriorly
Pulmonary contusion	Midline	Normal	Normal, may have crackles	Normal
Lung collapse	Toward	Decreased	May be reduced	Normal

- *Auscultation:* Decreased breath sounds in pneumothorax or hemothorax

EXTENDED FOCUSED ASSESSMENT FOR THE SONOGRAPHIC EVALUATION OF THE TRAUMA PATIENT

Extended focused assessment with sonographic in trauma (EFAST) is shown in **Figure 6**.

Tension Pneumothorax (Figs. 7A and B)

- *Immediate decompression in tension pneumothorax:* Needle thoracostomy **(Figs. 8A and B)**

Open Pneumothorax (Figs. 9 to 13)

- Difficulty in breathing
- Subcutaneous emphysema
- Decreased lung sounds on affected side
- Bubbling on exhalation from wound (sucking chest wound)

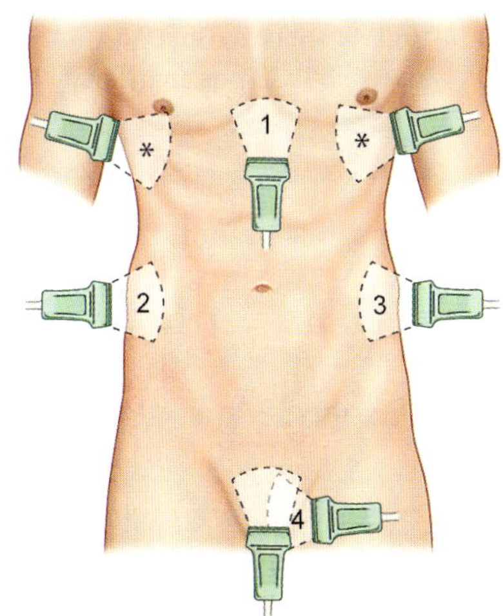

Fig. 6: Sonographic evaluation of the trauma patient.

RIB FRACTURES AND ASSOCIATED INJURIES

- 4–9 ribs fractures may cause injuries to the lung, bronchus, pleura, and heart.

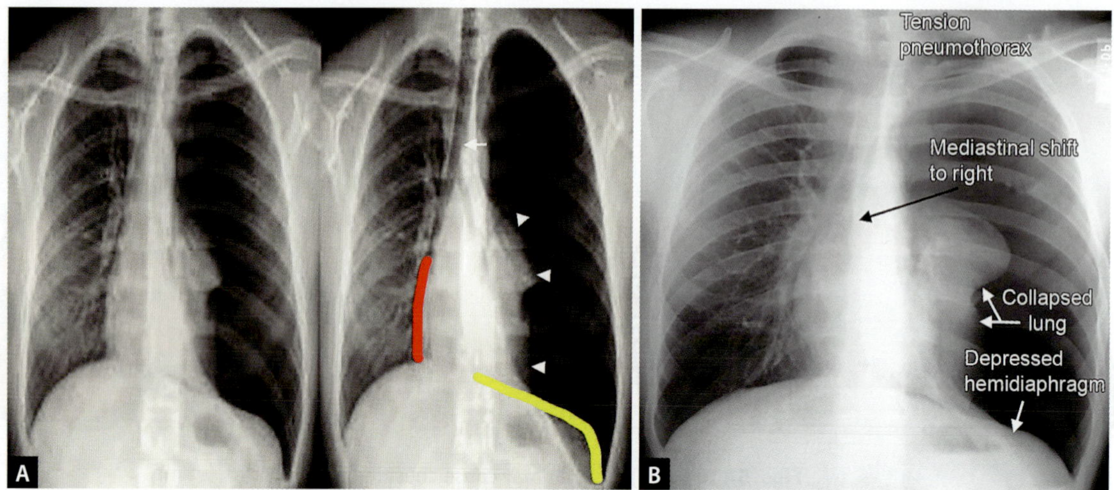

Figs. 7A and B: Tension pneumothorax.

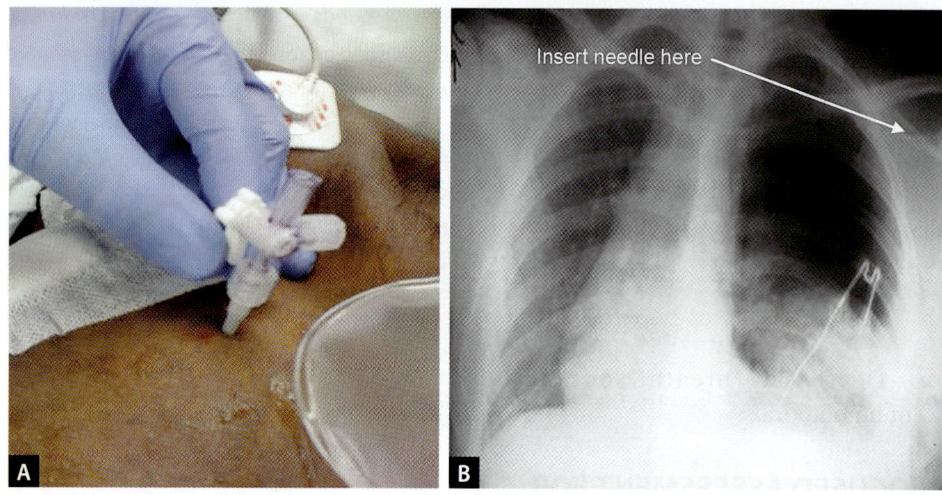

Figs. 8A and B: Needle thoracostomy.

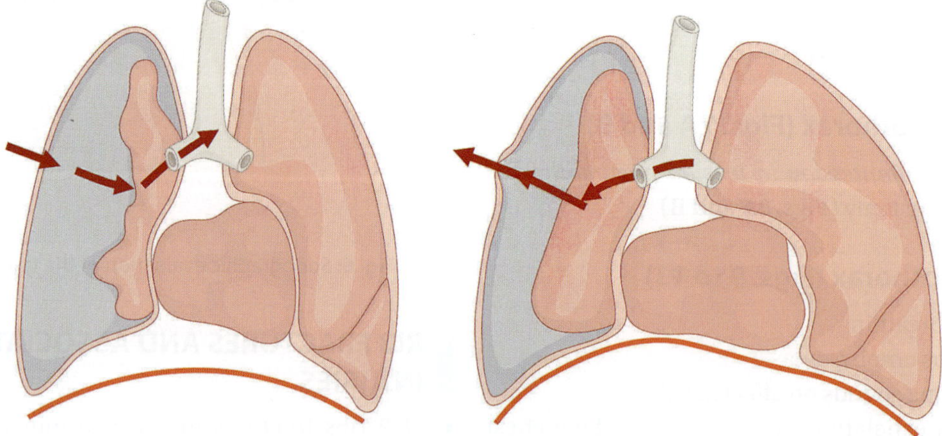

Fig. 9: Open pneumothorax.

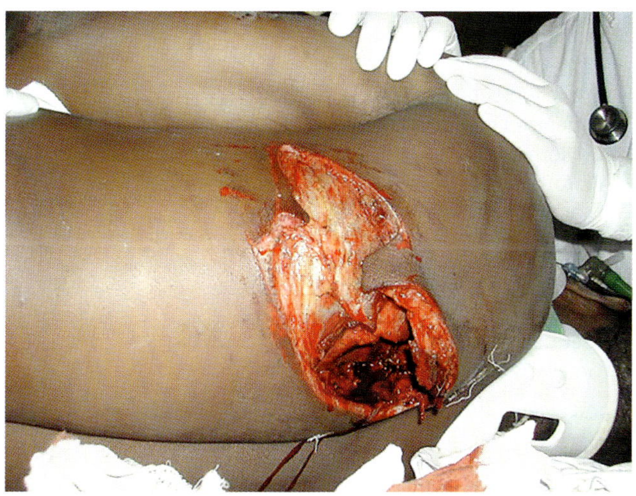

Fig. 10: Flail chest.

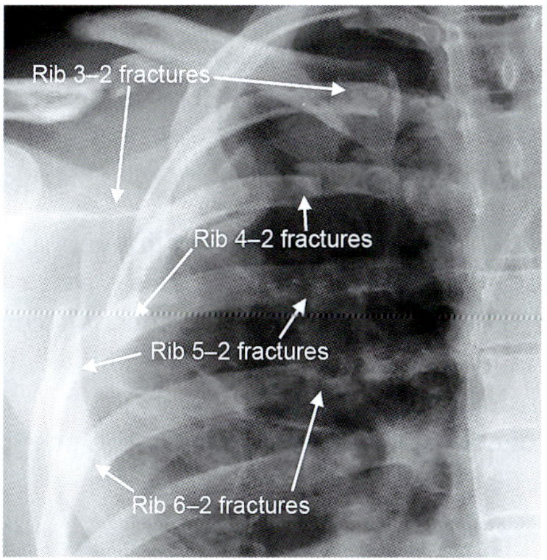

Fig. 11: Fracture of 3 or more ribs in at least two places on the same side.

- Rib fracture below ninth rib is associated with hepatic, splenic, or renal injury.
- First rib fracture commonly at subclavian sulcus or at the neck posteriorly is associated with injury to aorta, subclavian vessels and brachial plexus.

OSTEOSYNTHESIS RIBS

- It is the commonly associated injury in blunt thoracic trauma **(Fig. 15)**.
- Hemorrhage into alveolar and interstitial space
- Classical presentations include difficulty in breathing, tachypnea, hemoptysis, and hypotension
- Clinical examination shows crepitations and decreased air entry.

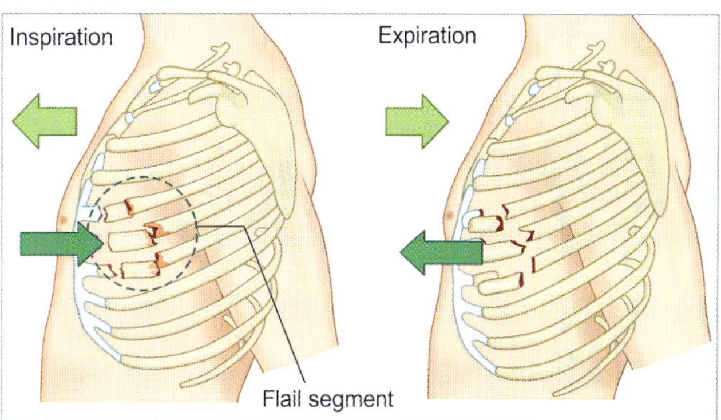

Fig. 12: Flail chest.

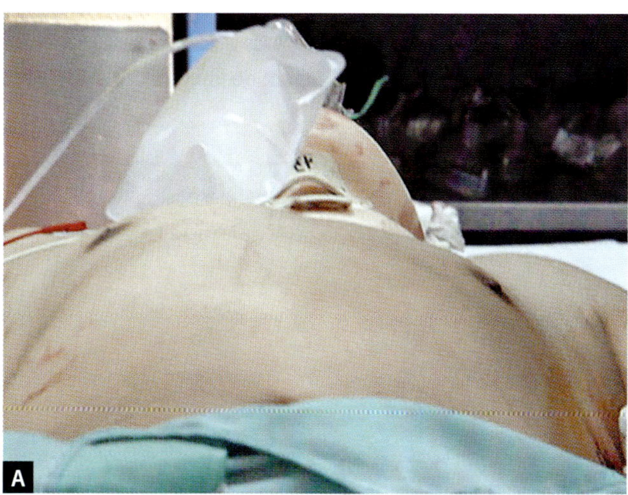

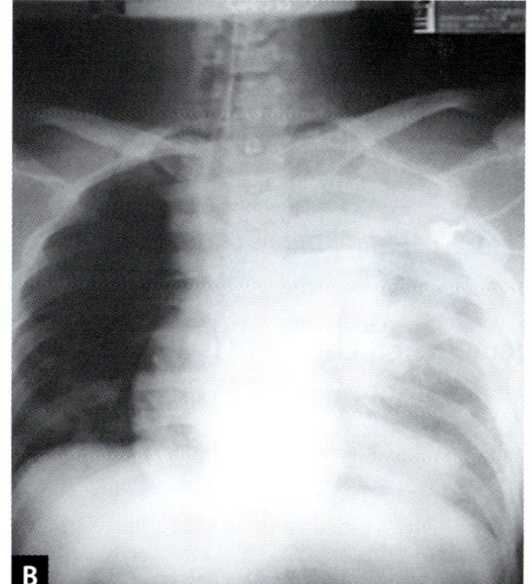

Figs. 13A and B: Left hemothorax.

- Computed tomography (CT) chest is diagnostic.
- *Complications:* Respiratory insufficiency, secondary pneumonia and systemic inflammatory response syndrome (SIRS), and acute respiratory distress syndrome (ARDS)

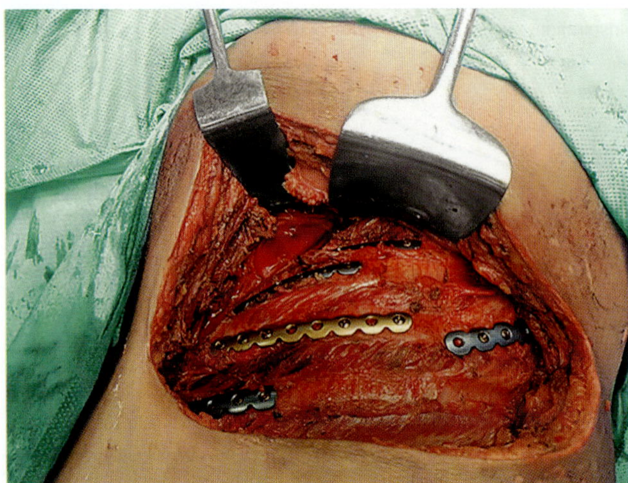

Fig. 14: Management of rib fracture.

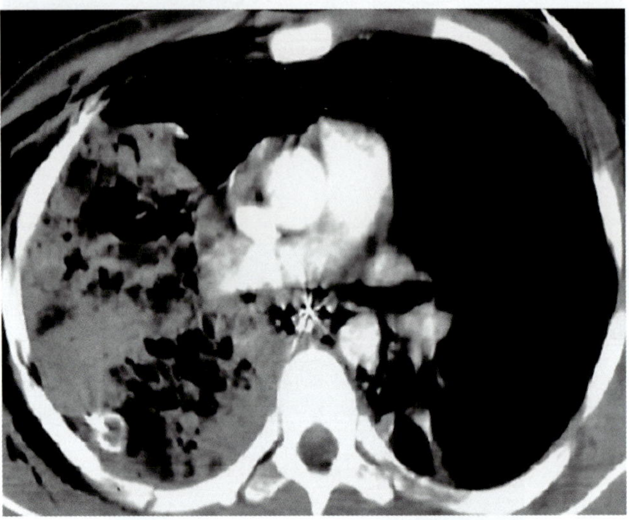

Fig. 15: Complications of thoracic trauma.

- Management of Rib fracture is now by open reduction and Internal Fixation (ORIF) **(Fig. 14)**

Pulmonary:
- Atelectasis
- ARDS
- Acute lung injury
- Pneumonia
- Infarction
- Lung abscess
- Arteriovenous fistula
- Bronchial stenosis
- Tracheoesophageal fistula

Pleural space:
- Empyema
- Bronchopleural fistula
- Organized hemothorax
- Chylothorax
- Fibrothorax
- Diaphragmatic hernias

Vascular:
- Thromboembolism
- Air embolism
- Pseudoaneurysm
- Great vessel fistula

Chest wall:
- Hernias
- Persistent pain
- *Mediastinum:*
  - Mediastinitis
  - Pericarditis

ROLE OF VIDEO-ASSISTED THORACOSCOPIC SURGERY IN THORACIC TRAUMA

Hypotension after chest injury is commonly associated with hypovolemia and it should be aggressively corrected initially with crystalloids while other possible conditions like pneumothorax, cardiac tamponade and blunt cardiac injury are to be evaluated.

Cardiac arrhythmias should raise the possibility of blunt cardiac injury.

Indications:
- Treatment for ongoing thoracic hemorrhage
- Treatment of retained hemothorax
- Treatment of persistent pneumothorax
- Diagnosis and treatment of diaphragmatic injuries
- Pericardial window for relief of cardiac tamponade
- Management of thoracic duct injuries
- Treatment of posttraumatic empyema
- Removal of foreign bodies

Relative contraindications:
- Coagulopathy
- Prior thoracotomy

Absolute contraindications:
- Hemodynamic instability
- Suspected cardiac injury
- Suspected great vessel injury
- Inability to tolerate single lung ventilation
- Inability to tolerate lateral decubitus position

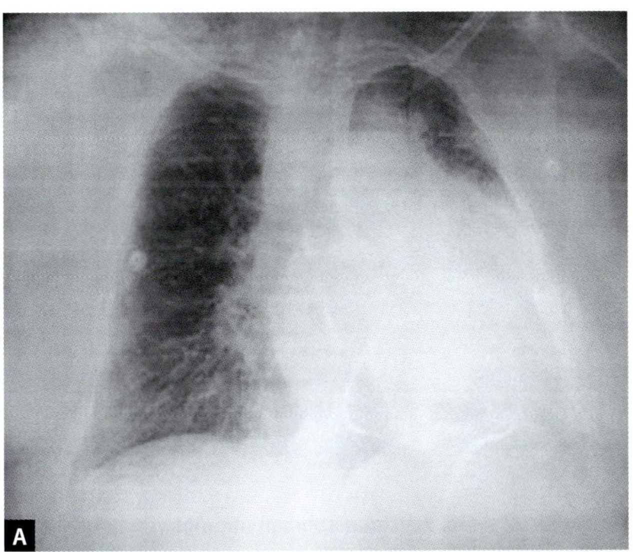

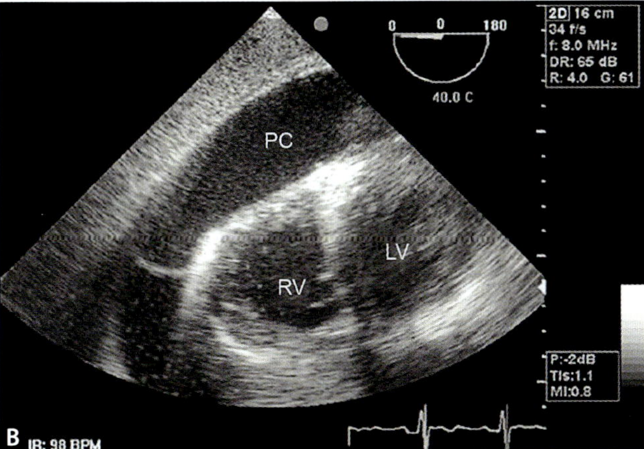

Figs. 16A and B: (A) Enlarged cardiac silhouette; (B) Pericardial effusion.

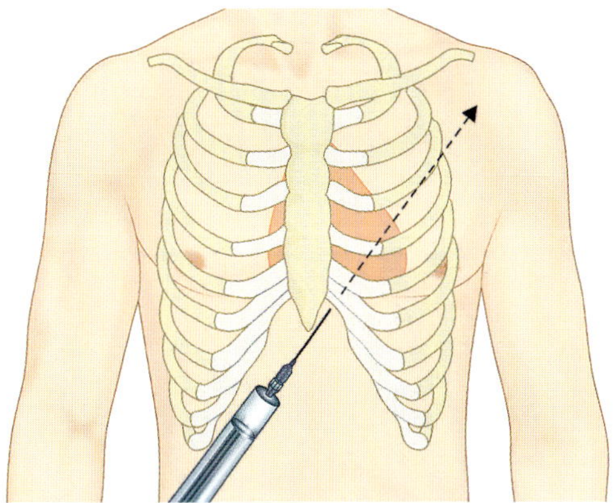

Fig. 17: Subxiphoid pericardiocentesis.

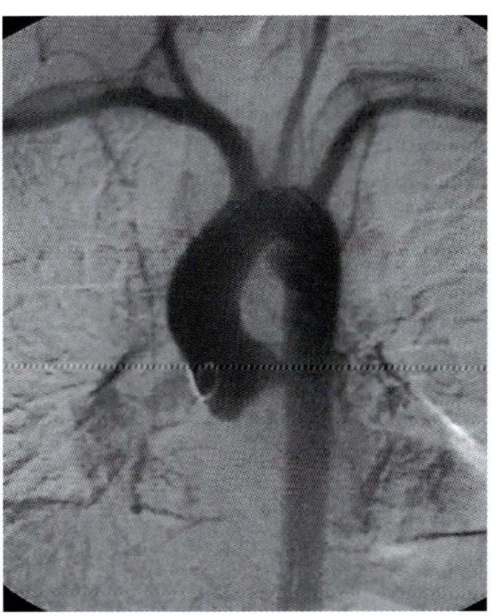

Fig. 18: Traumatic aortic injury distal to the left subclavian artery.

CARDIAC TAMPONADE

- Commonly from penetrating injuries
- "Beck's triad"
  1. Raised venous pressure—neck veins
  2. Decreased arterial blood pressure
  3. Muffled (muted) heart sounds
- Due to the presence of blood in the pericardial cavity, it inhibits cardiac activity.
- Commonly associated with "pulsus paradoxus"—a decrease of systolic blood pressure of 10 mm Hg or more during inspiration
- *Electrocardiogram (ECG):* Sinus tachycardia, low voltage complexes, and electrical alternans
- E*chocardiogram (ECHO):* Pericardial effusion
- *Chest X-ray anteroposterior (AP) view:* Enlarged cardiac silhouette **(Figs. 16A and B)**

SUBXIPHOID PERICARDIOCENTESIS

- 18-gauge needle is inserted in the left xiphoid costal cartilage angle directed toward posterior aspect of the left shoulder.
- Needle is at 45° angle to frontal and sagittal plane **(Fig. 17)**.

GREAT VESSEL INJURY

Aortic Injury

- Descending thoracic aortic injury is mostly lethal and it results in >40% of mortalities after blunt chest trauma.
- Site of injury is usually at ligamentum arteriosum, caused by shearing force at the point of fixation.
- Plain chest X-ray has nearly 95% of negative predictive value for diagnosing blunt traumatic aortic lesions **(Fig. 18)**.

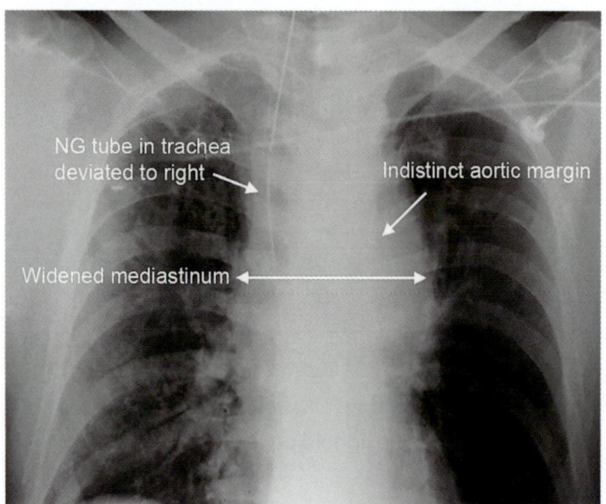

Fig. 19: Aortic injury on X-ray. (NG: nasogastric)

- Spiral CT scan with angiography has about 96% sensitivity and nearly 99% specificity

Traumatic Aortic Rupture

Radiological signs:

- Widened mediastinum (>8 cm)
- Fractured first and second rib
- Obliteration of aortic knob
- Trachea deviated to right
- Pleural capping
- Elevated left main stem bronchus
- Obliterated "aortic window"
- Esophagus shifted to right (Ryle's tube at T4) **(Fig. 19)**
- Depressed right mainstem bronchus

Traumatic Diaphragmatic Injury

- More common on left side
- Herniation of abdominal contents into chest
- Strangulation of bowel through diaphragm has a mortality >50%
- Ryle's tube seen in chest on X-ray is diagnostic **(Fig. 20)**

Left Diaphragmatic Injury

Left diaphragmatic injury is shown in **Figure 20**.

EMERGENCY ROOM THORACOTOMY

Indications:

- Cardiac tamponade
- Persistent intra-thoracic hemorrhage
- For internal cardiac massage **(Figs. 21A and B)**

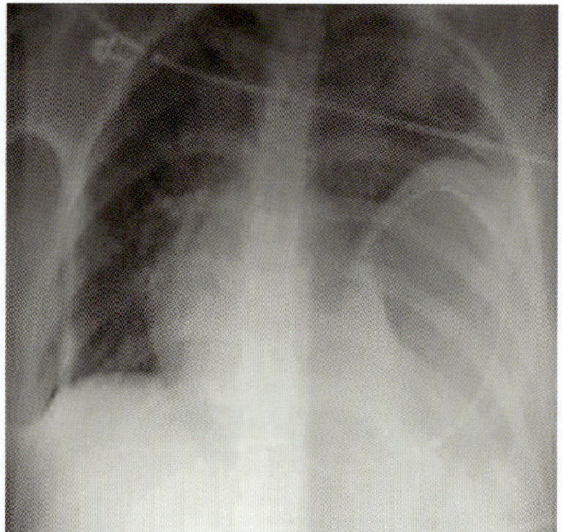

Fig. 20: Left diaphragmatic injury.

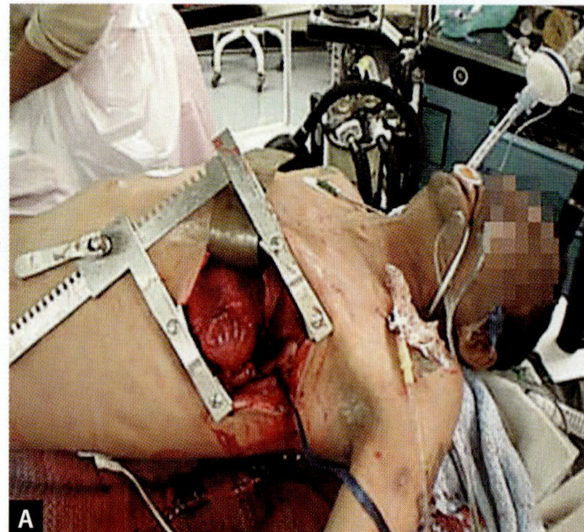

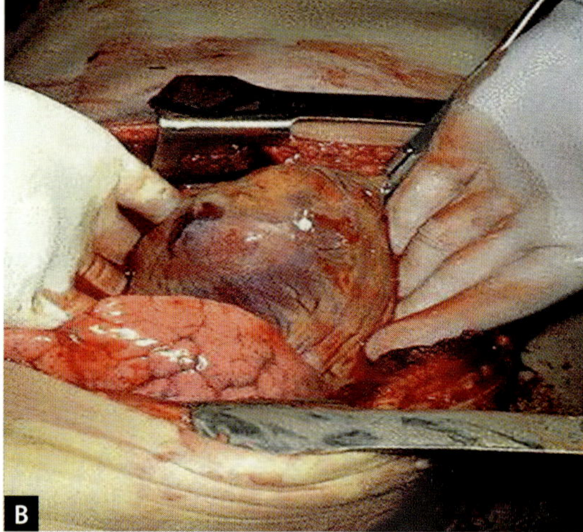

Figs. 21A and B: (A) Left anterolateral thoracotomy; (B) Left thoracotomy extended toward right by clam-shell incision.

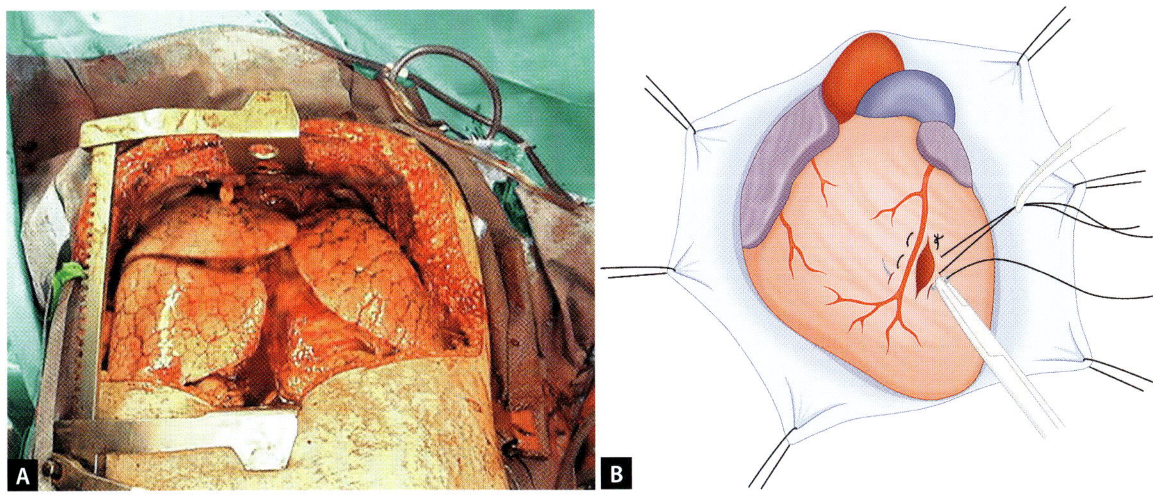

Figs. 22A and B: Ventricular repair.

URGENT THORACOTOMY

Indications:

- Persistent intercostal drainage of >1,500 mL or more than 200 mL per hour drainage for subsequent 3 hours.
- Hemothorax with large blood clot
- Development of cardiac tamponade
- Massive air leak or incomplete lung expansion despite of adequate drainage
- Suspicious injury to the great vessels **(Figs. 22A and B)**.

SECTION 9

Pediatric Emergencies

Pediatric Surgery Emergencies

Raghul M

TRACHEOESOPHAGEAL FISTULA

Definition and Epidemiology

Tracheoesophageal fistula (TEF) is a congenital abnormality characterized by an abnormal communication between the trachea and esophagus, often associated with esophageal atresia. It is a critical condition frequently diagnosed in neonates **(Fig. 1)**.

Clinical Features

Clinical signs include excessive drooling, choking during feeds, and respiratory distress.

Diagnosis

Diagnosis is established through a combination of clinical observation and imaging studies (such as chest X-ray demonstrating coiling of nasogastric (NG) tube in the upper esophageal pouch).

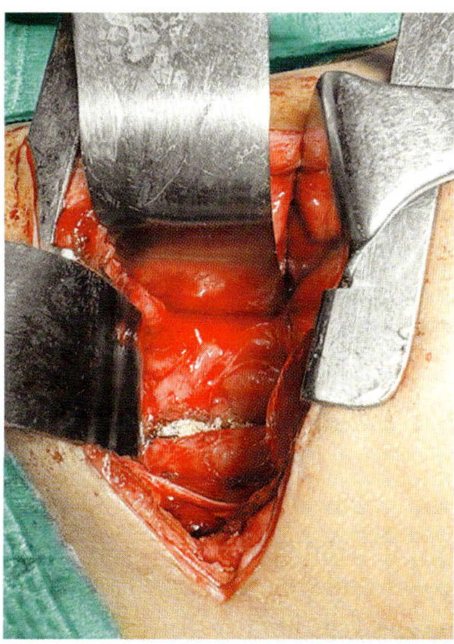

Fig. 1: Anastomosed esophageal ends.

Management

- Immediate stabilization is crucial, often involving airway management and nutritional support via parenteral means.
- Definitive surgical repair is necessary to correct the anomaly, typically within the first 48 hours of life.
  - Right posterolateral thoracotomy + fistula ligation esophago-esophageal anastomosis is the treatment.
  - Long segment pure esophageal atresia would need an gastrotomy and esophagostomy with a definitive repair at a later date.
- Postoperative care focuses on monitoring for complications such as aspiration pneumonia and esophageal stricture.

FOREIGN BODY ASPIRATION

Definition and Epidemiology

Foreign body aspiration (FBA) refers to the inhalation of an object into the respiratory tract, leading to airway obstruction. It is particularly prevalent in children aged 1–3 years.

Clinical Features

- Symptoms can vary from acute respiratory distress, wheezing, and stridor, to more chronic presentations such as persistent cough and recurrent respiratory infections.
- Acute presentations occur immediately after the incident, while chronic cases may lead to failure to thrive in children.

Diagnosis

Diagnosis is based on clinical history, physical examination, and imaging studies, typically chest X-rays or computed tomography (CT) scans, along with bronchoscopy, which can provide direct visualization.

Management

- Management involves immediate removal of the foreign body, often through bronchoscopy.
- Close monitoring for respiratory complications and addressing any underlying issues that may cause recurrent aspirations are also important.

CONGENITAL DIAPHRAGMATIC HERNIA

Congenital diaphragmatic hernia (CDH) is a developmental defect in the diaphragm that allows abdominal organs to herniate into the thoracic cavity, leading to pulmonary hypoplasia and respiratory distress. It commonly occurs in the posterolateral diaphragm (Bochdalek hernia) but may also present in the anterior diaphragm (Morgagni hernia).

Clinical Features

Newborns with CDH typically present with:

- Severe respiratory distress shortly after birth due to pulmonary hypoplasia and hypertension
- Cyanosis and signs of respiratory failure
- Scaphoid abdomen, as abdominal organs are displaced into the chest
- Asymmetrical breath sounds, with decreased air entry on the affected side
- Shifted cardiac sounds due to mediastinal displacement
- Diminished breath sounds on the ipsilateral side
- Bowel sounds in the chest
- Deviated heart sounds due to mediastinal shift
- Paradoxical movement of the abdomen (retraction with inspiration)

Investigations

- *X-ray* shows bowel loops in the thoracic cavity, mediastinal shift, and absence of a diaphragmatic outline along with paucity of abdominal gas shadow.
- Ultrasound (prenatal and postnatal) is used for diagnosis and assessment of associated anomalies.
- Magnetic resonance imaging (MRI)/fetal MRI helps evaluate lung volume and predict postnatal outcomes.
- Echocardiography assesses pulmonary hypertension and cardiac anomalies.
- Arterial blood gas (ABG) reveals respiratory acidosis and hypoxemia.

Treatment (Figs. 2 and 3)

Initial stabilization:

- Immediate endotracheal intubation and mechanical ventilation to prevent gastric distension and respiratory compromise
- Avoidance of bag-mask ventilation, which may worsen lung compression.
- Gastric decompression with a nasogastric tube
- High-frequency oscillatory ventilation (HFOV) or extracorporeal membrane oxygenation (ECMO) in severe cases.

Surgical repair:

- It is delayed until cardiorespiratory stabilization is achieved.
- It involves repositioning herniated abdominal organs and repairing the diaphragmatic defect either primarily or often with a patch for large defects.

Postoperative Care

- Ventilatory support until adequate lung function is established
- Pulmonary hypertension management with nitric oxide or sildenafil
- Nutritional support and monitoring for complications such as gastroesophageal reflux and recurrent hernia

EMPYEMA THORACIS

Empyema thoracis is a collection of pus within the pleural cavity, usually occurring as a complication of pneumonia, lung abscess, or thoracic surgery. It progresses through three stages: Exudative (early fluid accumulation), fibrinopurulent (thickening and septation), and organizing (fibrosis and lung entrapment). Prompt diagnosis and management are essential to prevent respiratory compromise and systemic complications **(Fig. 4)**.

Clinical Features

- Fever and chills
- Pleuritic chest pain
- Dyspnea
- Decreased breath sounds
- Dullness to percussion
- Decreased chest expansion
- Tachypnea and respiratory distress

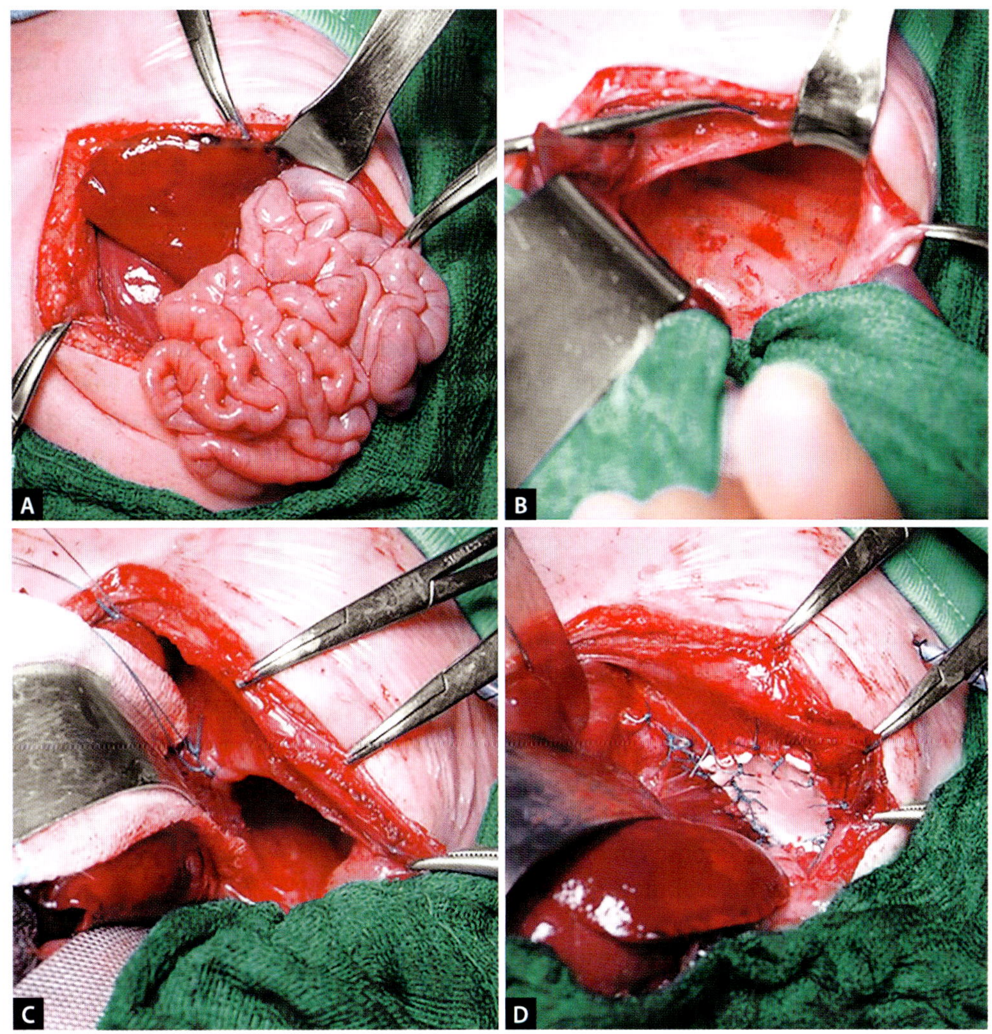

Figs. 2A to D: Open and thoracoscopic repair.

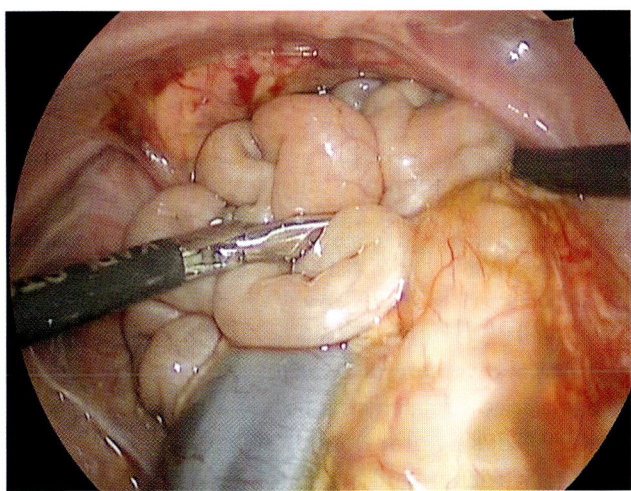

Fig. 3: Thoracoscopic repair.

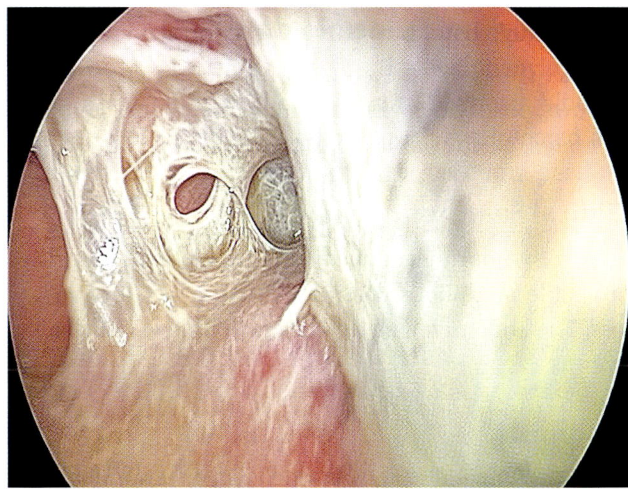

Fig. 4: Thoracoscopic view of empyema.

Investigations

- *Chest X-ray:* Shows pleural effusion with loculation
- *Ultrasound:* Identifies fluid pockets for drainage
- *Computed tomography thorax:* Defines pleural thickening, septations, and underlying lung pathology.

Pleural Fluid Analysis (Thoracentesis)

- *Appearance:* Turbid or purulent.
- *Biochemistry:* Low glucose and high lactate dehydrogenase (LDH).
- *Microbiology:* Gram stain, culture, and sensitivity to identify pathogens.

Treatment

- Broad-spectrum intravenous antibiotics targeting common organisms (e.g., *Streptococcus pneumoniae* and *Staphylococcus aureus*).
- *Tube thoracostomy (chest tube drainage):* To remove pus and re-expand the lung.
- *Intrapleural fibrinolytics:* To break down septations in loculated empyema.

Surgical Management (For Complicated Cases)

- *Video-assisted thoracoscopic surgery (VATS):* For debridement and drainage.
- *Open decortication:* In cases of lung entrapment or chronic empyema.
- Early intervention improves prognosis, prevents fibrothorax, and restores normal pulmonary function.

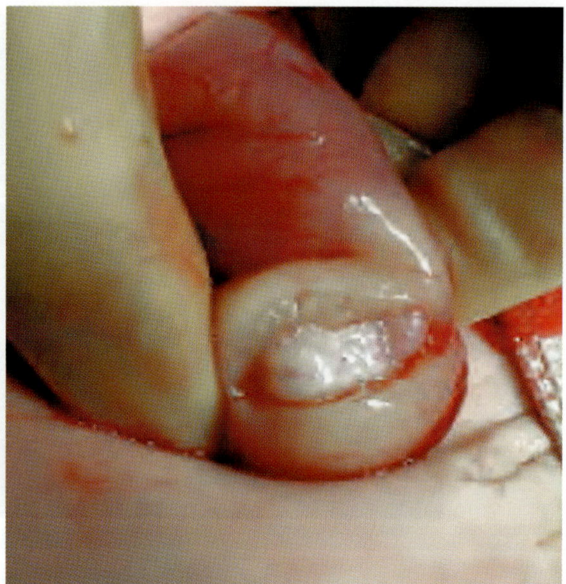

Fig. 5: Open Ramstedt's pyloromyotomy with mucosal bulge.

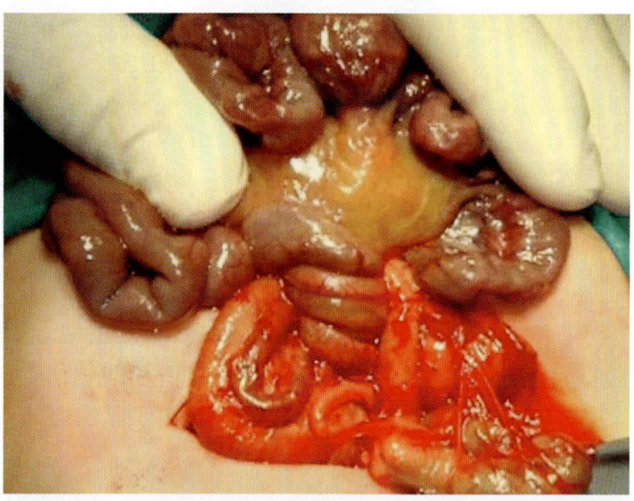

Fig. 6: Malrotation with volvulus.

HYPERTROPHIC PYLORIC STENOSIS

Definition and Epidemiology

Pyloric stenosis is a condition wherein the pylorus narrows, obstructing gastric outflow, and is most common in infants (gastric outflow obstruction).

Clinical Features

Robust first-born term male child typically presents with projectile nonbilious vomiting, dehydration, and weight loss. The abdomen may feel distended due to a thickened pylorus.

Diagnosis

Diagnosis is usually made through clinical examination—an olive shaped mass in the hypochondrium, and confirmed by abdominal ultrasound, demonstrating thickening of the pyloric muscle (4 mm thick) and increase (16 mm) in length of pyloric channel **(Fig. 5)**.

Management

- Preoperative care focuses on correcting electrolyte imbalances and dehydration.
- Ramstedt's pyloromyotomy is performed to relieve the obstruction and allow normal passage of gastric contents.

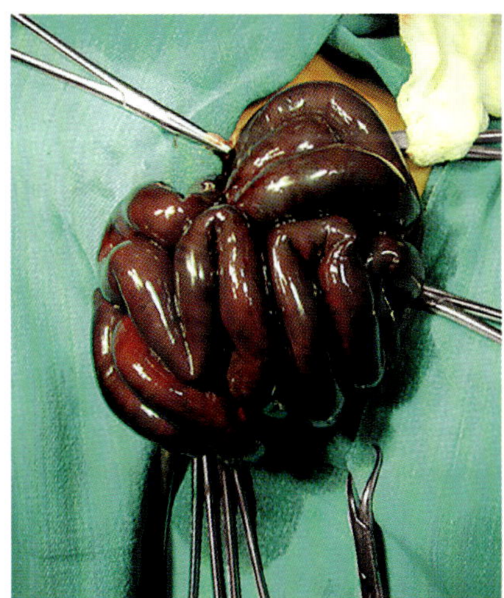

Fig. 7: Malrotation with volvulus and gangrene.

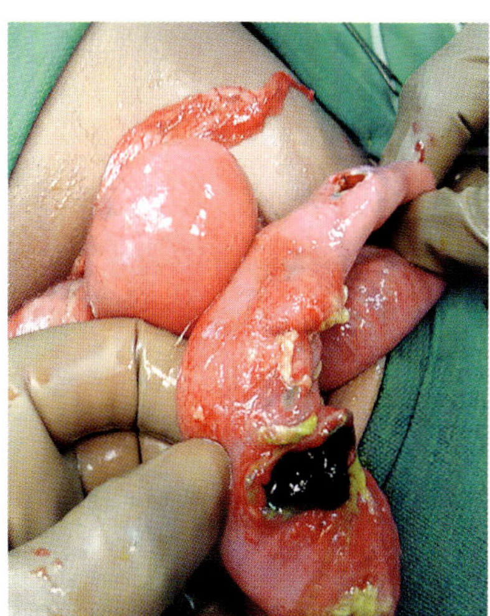

Fig. 8: Necrotizing enterocolitis (NEC) with ileal perforation.

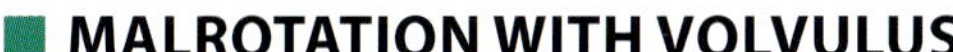

MALROTATION WITH VOLVULUS

Definition and Epidemiology

Malrotation with volvulus is a congenital anomaly of the intestinal rotation and fixation which can lead to life-threatening bowel ischemia and necrosis **(Figs. 6 and 7)**.

Clinical Features

Patients typically present with sudden, severe abdominal pain, and bilious vomiting (hallmark symptom irrespective of age group). Symptoms can vary based on the severity of the obstruction.

Diagnosis

Diagnosis necessitates a clinical suspicion, often confirmed through imaging studies, including an ultrasound that shows altered superior mesenteric artery (SMA) and superior mesenteric vein (SMV) axis and upper gastrointestinal series, which shows abnormal position of duodenojejunal (DJ) flexure.

Management

Urgent surgical intervention is critical to detorse the malrotated bowel and assess for viable bowel segments.

Ladd's procedure includes detorsion, division of Ladd's bands, straightening of duodenum, widening of duodenocolic isthmus, placement of small bowel to the right, and large bowel to the left ± appendectomy.

Associated necrotic segments might need resection to restore intestinal function and blood supply.

NECROTIZING ENTEROCOLITIS

Definition and Epidemiology

Necrotizing enterocolitis (NEC) is a serious gastrointestinal disease that predominantly affects premature infants and is characterized by inflammation and infection of the intestines **(Fig. 8)**.

Clinical Features

- Early signs include feeding intolerance and abdominal distension, white bloody stools occur at later stage.
- Symptoms may progress to lethargy and signs of sepsis as the disease advances.

Diagnosis

Diagnosis is often clinical, supported by imaging studies (abdominal X-rays) showing signs of intestinal perforation or air in the intestinal wall (pneumatosis intestinalis).

Management

- Management includes withholding enteral feedings, providing supportive care, and broad-spectrum antibiotics.
- *Surgical indications:*
  - Pneumoperitonitis
  - Fixed bowel loops (in consequent X-rays)
  - Blood in stools

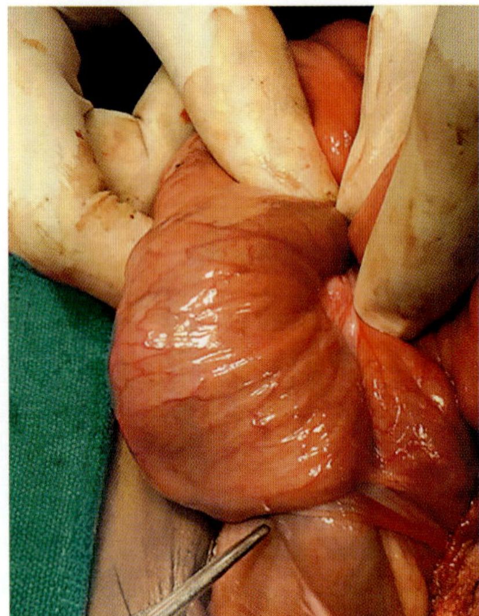

Fig. 9: Open intussusception reduction.

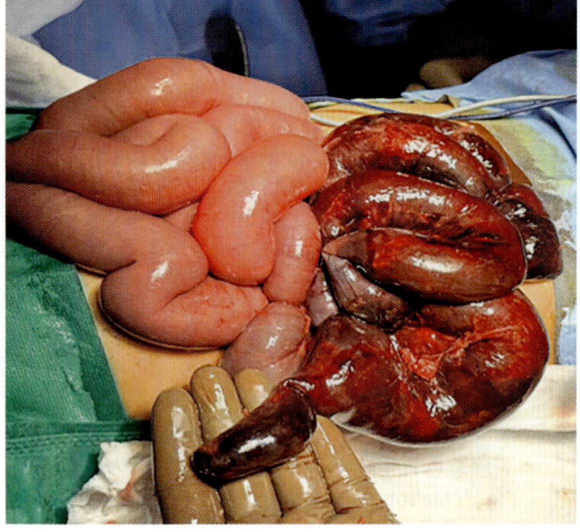

Fig. 10: Meckel's gangrene.

INTUSSUSCEPTION

Definition and Epidemiology

Intussusception is a condition where a portion of the intestine telescopes into an adjacent segment, commonly affecting children aged 3 months to 3 years **(Fig. 9)**.

Clinical Features

- The hallmark symptoms include sudden-onset, colicky abdominal pain, vomiting, and passage of "red currant jelly" (usually in later stages) stools.
- Children may experience intermittent severe pain episodes, leading them to pull their legs toward their chest for relief.

Diagnosis

Diagnosis is primarily achieved through ultrasound, which highlight the intussusception with a classical target sign or bowel within bowel appearance.

Management

- Nonsurgical reduction methods, such as air contrast enema/hydrostatic reduction are often successful if initiated early.
- Surgical intervention is reserved for cases where noninvasive measures fail or if significant complications arise, such as bowel necrosis.

MECKEL'S DIVERTICULUM

Definition

Meckel's diverticulum is a congenital true diverticulum of the small intestine, resulting from the incomplete obliteration of the vitelline duct (omphalomesenteric duct). It is typically located on the antimesenteric border of the ileum, approximately 2 feet (60 cm) proximal to the ileocecal valve **(Fig. 10)**.

Clinical Features

Meckel's diverticulum is often asymptomatic but can present with complications, which include:

- *Painless lower gastrointestinal bleeding (LGIB):*
  - Most common symptom in children
  - Results from peptic ulceration due to ectopic gastric mucosa producing acid
  - Bright red or maroon-colored stool (hematochezia)
- *Intestinal obstruction (second most common complication):*
  - Due to intussusception, volvulus, or adhesions
  - Presents with abdominal pain, distension, vomiting, and constipation.
- *Meckel's diverticulitis:*
  - Mimics acute appendicitis
  - Right lower quadrant (RLQ) pain, fever, nausea, and vomiting
  - Differentiation from appendicitis is clinically difficult.

- *Perforation and peritonitis:* Can result from diverticulitis or ulceration.
- *Neoplasia (Rare):* Carcinoid tumor, adenocarcinoma, or sarcoma can arise within the diverticulum.

Diagnosis

- *Technetium-99m pertechnetate scan (Meckel's scan)*
    - Highly sensitive for detecting ectopic gastric mucosa
    - Best initial test in pediatric patients with painless rectal bleeding.
- *Contrast-enhanced CT (CECT) abdomen:* Useful for diagnosing complications such as diverticulitis, obstruction, or perforation.
- *Diagnostic laparoscopy or laparotomy:* Definitive diagnostic and therapeutic approach, particularly in complicated cases.

Management

- *Asymptomatic Meckel's diverticulum:*
    - *Incidental finding:* Surgical resection (diverticulectomy) is not routinely recommended unless:
        - Ectopic mucosa is present
        - Narrow base of diverticulum (prone to obstruction)
        - Patient is undergoing abdominal surgery for another reason
- *Symptomatic Meckel's diverticulum*
    - *Diverticulectomy* (simple excision of the diverticulum) if the base is narrow
    - *Segmental small bowel resection with primary anastomosis* if:
        - Broad-based diverticulum
        - Complications such as obstruction, perforation, or diverticulitis

ACUTE APPENDICITIS

Definition and Epidemiology

- Acute appendicitis, an inflammation of the vermiform appendix, is considered one of the most common surgical emergencies among pediatric patients **(Figs. 11A and B)**.

Clinical Features

- Symptoms typically begin with vague abdominal pain that later localizes to the right lower quadrant (RLQ).
- Accompanying symptoms can include nausea, vomiting, and a low-grade fever.
- In younger children, the symptoms can be nonspecific, including irritability and refusal to feed.
- Classic signs may include rebound tenderness and guarding, although these are more reliable in older children.
- Need to be addressed early as chances of perforation is early and high in pediatric population.

Diagnosis

- Diagnosis integrates a clinical assessment supported by laboratory tests such as complete blood count (CBC) showing leukocytosis and elevated C-reactive protein (CRP).
- Imaging methods such as ultrasound are frequently used to confirm the diagnosis and assess for complications.

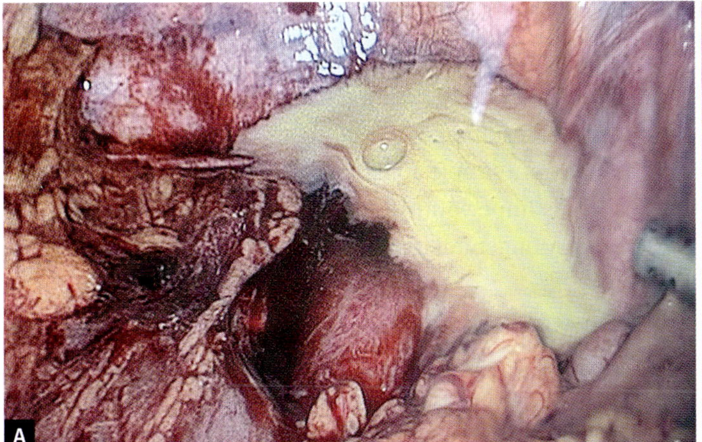

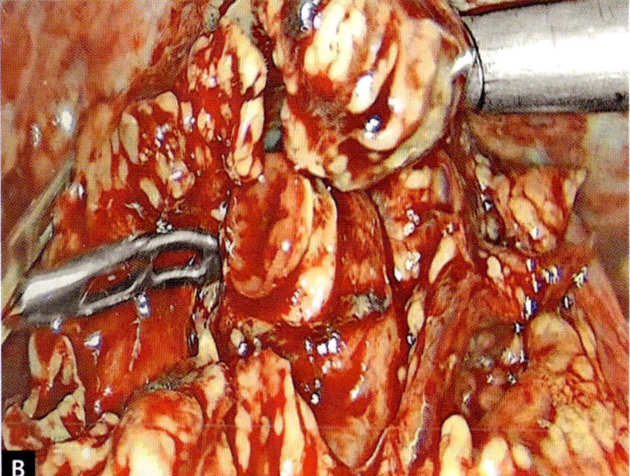

Figs. 11A and B: Appendicular perforation with abscess.

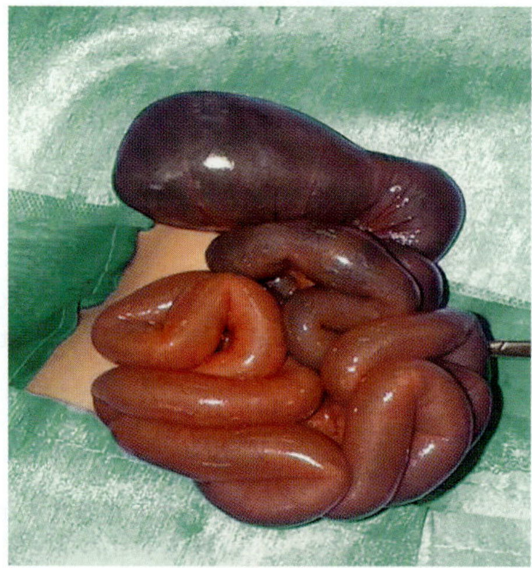

Fig 12: Jejunoileal atresia.

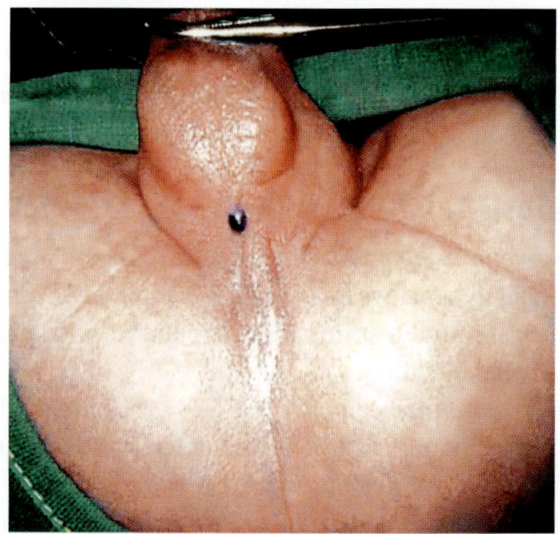

Fig. 13: Meconium speck in perineum.

Management

- Preoperative care should include fluid resuscitation and broad-spectrum antibiotics to address polymicrobial flora.
- Surgical treatment mainly involves appendectomy, usually laparoscopic due to benefits such as reduced recovery time and postoperative pain.
- Postoperative care focuses on pain management, encouraging early mobilization, and monitoring for complications.

INTESTINAL ATRESIA

Intestinal atresia is characterized by a complete obstruction or absence of a segment of the intestine due to developmental failure during fetal life. It commonly affects the small intestine, particularly the duodenum, jejunum, or ileum, though it may also involve the colon **(Fig. 12)**.

Clinical Features

- *Prenatal indicators:* Polyhydramnios (especially in duodenal atresia) detected on ultrasound.
- *Neonatal presentation:* Bilious vomiting, abdominal distension, and failure to pass meconium within the first 24–48 hours of life.
- *Associated conditions:* Duodenal atresia often coexists with Down syndrome, while jejunoileal atresia may be linked to vascular insults in utero.
- Scaphoid abdomen with gastric distension (proximal atresia).
- Generalized distension (distal atresia)

Investigations

- *Duodenal atresia:* "Double bubble" sign.
- *Jejunoileal atresia:* Dilated loops with air-fluid levels.
- *Contrast studies:* Used to define the site of obstruction
- X- ray abdomen.

Treatment

Surgical correction:

- *Duodenal atresia:* Kimura's Duodenoduodenostomy.
- *Jejunoileal atresia:* Resection of the atretic segment with primary anastomosis.
- *Colonic atresia:* Requires resection and possible colostomy/primary anastomosis.

ANORECTAL ANOMALIES

Anorectal anomalies (ARAs) are a group of congenital malformations affecting the development of the anus and rectum, resulting in partial or complete obstruction. They range from simple anal stenosis to complex malformations such as imperforate anus with fistulae connecting to the urinary or genital tract **(Figs. 13 and 14)**.

Clinical Features

- *Absence of normal anus:* The anal opening may be absent, misplaced, or stenotic.
- *Perineal abnormalities:* Presence of a fistula, abnormal skin dimpling, or ectopic anal opening.

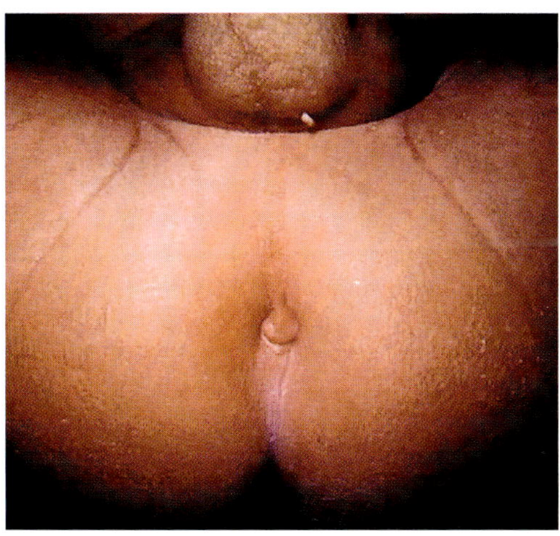

Fig. 14: High anorectal malformation (ARM).

- *Distended abdomen:* Due to bowel obstruction, especially in high-type anomalies.

Diagnosis

- *Radiological imaging:* Abdominal X-ray (invertogram or cross-table lateral X-ray); determines the level of rectal pouch in relation to the levator ani muscle complex.
- *Screening:* Echocardiography (for congenital heart defects).
  - Spinal ultrasound or MRI (to assess spinal dysraphism)
  - Renal ultrasound (to detect urogenital anomalies)

Surgical Treatment

- *Low-type anomalies (e.g., perineal fistula, anal stenosis):* Primary anoplasty.
- *High-type anomalies (e.g., rectourethral or rectovaginal fistula):*
  - *Stage 1:* Colostomy creation
  - *Stage 2:* Definitive corrective surgery [posterior sagittal anorectoplasty (PSARP)]
  - *Stage 3:* Colostomy closure after healing

Postoperative Care

- Bowel management programs for continence.
- Long-term follow-up for functional outcomes.
- Early diagnosis and appropriate surgical intervention lead to good functional and cosmetic outcomes, though some children may require lifelong bowel management support.

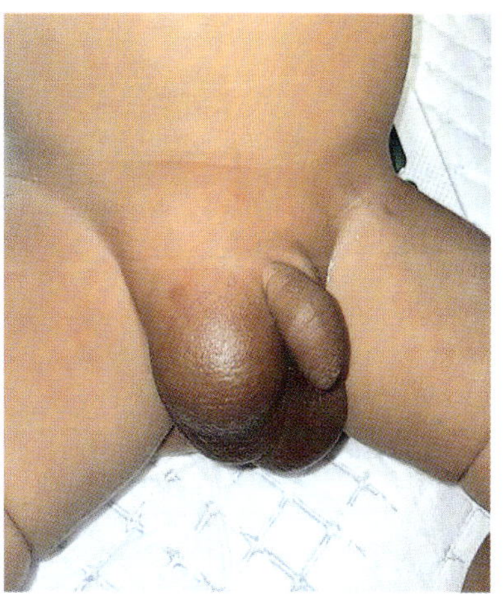

Fig. 15: Irreducible inguinal hernia.

IRREDUCIBLE INGUINAL HERNIA

An irreducible inguinal hernia is herniation of abdominal contents, such as bowel or omentum, that become trapped within the inguinal canal. It may be complicated by strangulation or obstruction, requiring urgent intervention **(Fig. 15)**.

Clinical Features

- *Persistent groin swelling:* A firm, nonreducible mass in the inguinal region in a child with inconsolable cry.
- *Signs of bowel obstruction:* Nausea, vomiting, and abdominal distension.

Investigations

Ultrasound: Identifies hernial contents and signs of strangulation.

Treatment.

Surgical intervention:

- Emergency herniotomy to prevent bowel ischemia
- In neonate with strangulation due to narrow inguinal canal, probability of testicular ischemia to be also explained to parents.

TESTICULAR TORSION

Definition and Epidemiology

Testicular torsion is an acute surgical condition where the spermatic cord twists, compromising blood flow to the testicle and requiring immediate surgical intervention to prevent loss of the testicle **(Figs. 16A and B)**.

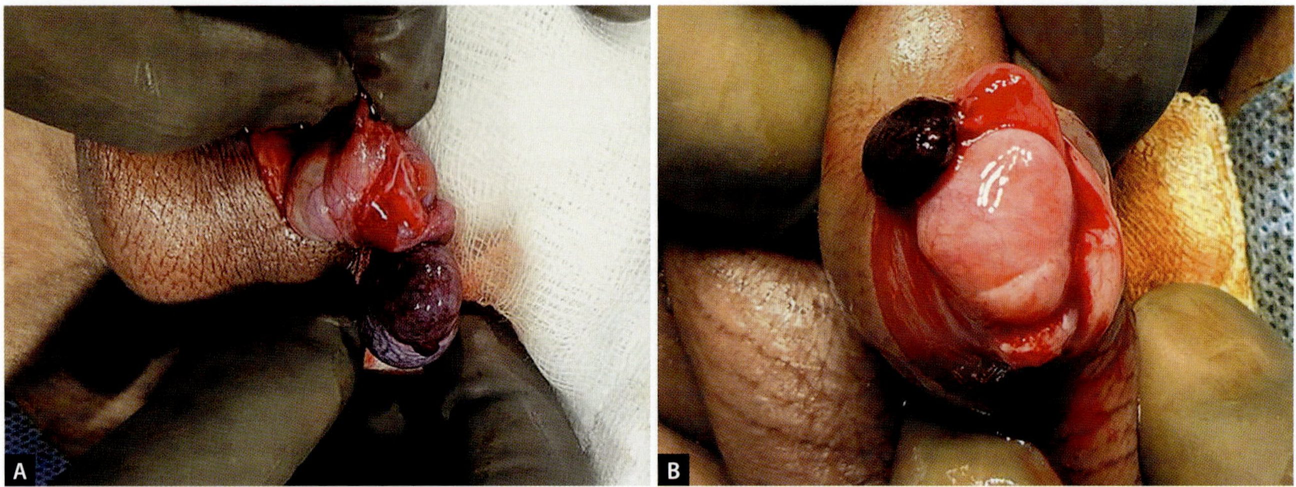

Figs. 16A and B: Torsion appendage testis.

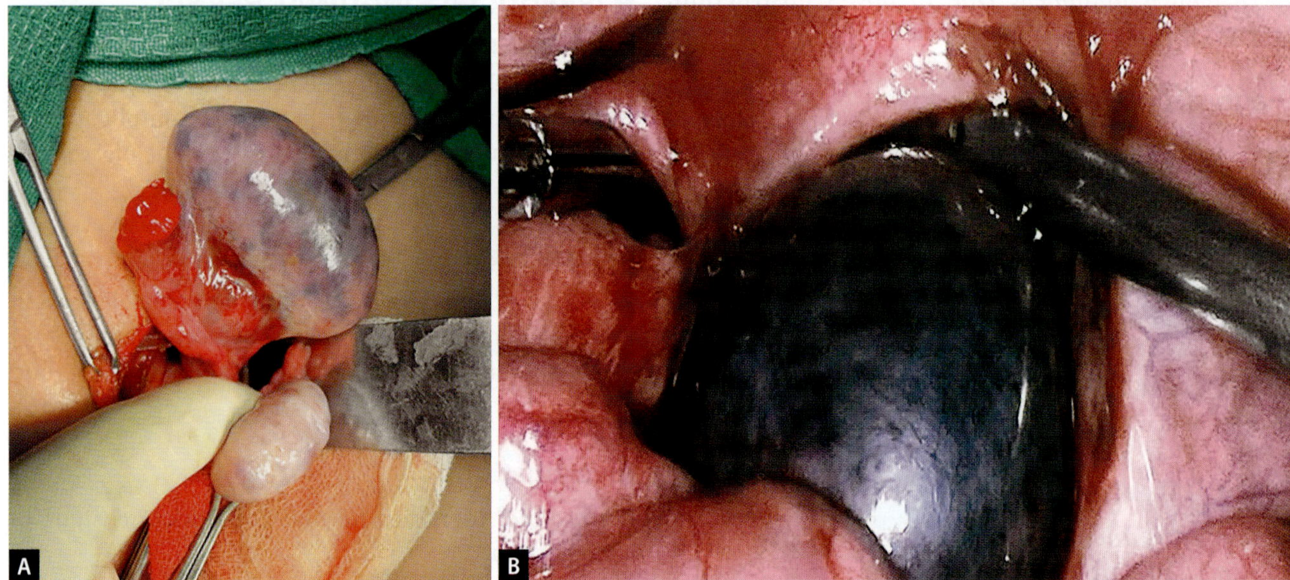

Figs. 17A and B: Ovarian torsion.

Clinical Features

- Symptoms often include sudden onset of unilateral scrotal pain and swelling.
- Nausea and vomiting may accompany the acute pain episode.

Diagnosis

Diagnosis involves physical examination to assess the position of the testicle high riding horizontally placed and may include Doppler ultrasound to evaluate blood flow.

Management

Timely surgical intervention (detorsion and orchidopexy) is the gold standard for treatment to salvage testicular function. Time is critical, as the risk of testicular atrophy increases the longer the torsion persists.

OVARIAN TORSION

Definition and Epidemiology

Ovarian torsion **(Figs. 17A and B)** is a surgical emergency characterized by the twisting of the ovary around the ligaments that support it, compromising its blood supply.

It can be primary or secondary to ovarian lesions (ovarian cyst/malignancy).

Clinical Features

Symptoms typically include sudden onset of unilateral abdominal or pelvic pain and may be accompanied by nausea and vomiting.

Diagnosis

Diagnosis is primarily clinical but can be supported by imaging studies such as ultrasound, which may show an enlarged, edematous ovary and decreased blood flow and augmented by MRI.

Management

Immediate surgical intervention is essential to detorse the twisted ovary. Preservation of the ovary is prioritized post detorsion and oophoropexy is done to prevent recurrence. If secondary to ovarian lesions (ovarian cyst/malignancy), cystectomy/oophorectomy is carried out based on the pathology.

PARAPHIMOSIS

Definition

Paraphimosis is a urological emergency where the retracted foreskin becomes trapped behind the glans penis, leading to edema, venous congestion, and potential ischemia **(Fig. 18)**.

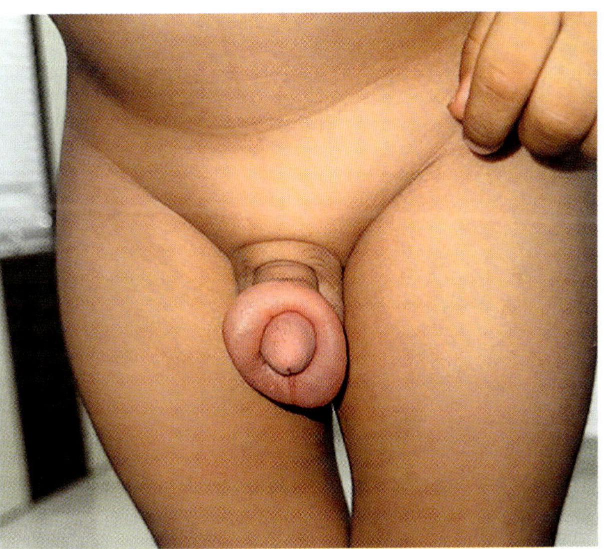

Fig. 18: Paraphimosis.

Clinical Features

- Pain, swelling, and erythema of the glans and foreskin
- Constricting ring of foreskin behind the corona
- Urinary retention in severe cases
- If untreated, can progress to ischemia and necrosis

Diagnosis

- Clinical examination is usually sufficient.
- Doppler ultrasonography if ischemia is suspected.

Management

- *Manual reduction (first-line treatment):*
  - Pain control (local anesthetic or penile nerve block)
  - Edema reduction (ice packs, osmotic agents, or compression)
  - Gradual forward manipulation of the foreskin
- *Surgical management:*
  - Emergency circumcision for recurrent or severe cases
- *Postreduction care:*
  - Antibiotic ointment and foreskin hygiene
  - Consider elective circumcision to prevent recurrence

COMPLICATIONS

- Glans ischemia and necrosis
- Urethral injury
- Recurrent paraphimosis

POSTERIOR URETHRAL VALVE

Definition

Posterior urethral valves (PUV) are congenital obstructing membranous folds in the posterior urethra (at the level of the prostatic urethra) that cause varying degrees of bladder outlet obstruction in male infants. This condition is the most common cause of congenital lower urinary tract obstruction in males and can lead to significant urinary and renal dysfunction if not managed promptly.

Clinical Features

Prenatal Presentation

- Detected via antenatal ultrasound showing:
  - Bilateral hydronephrosis
  - Distended bladder ("keyhole sign")

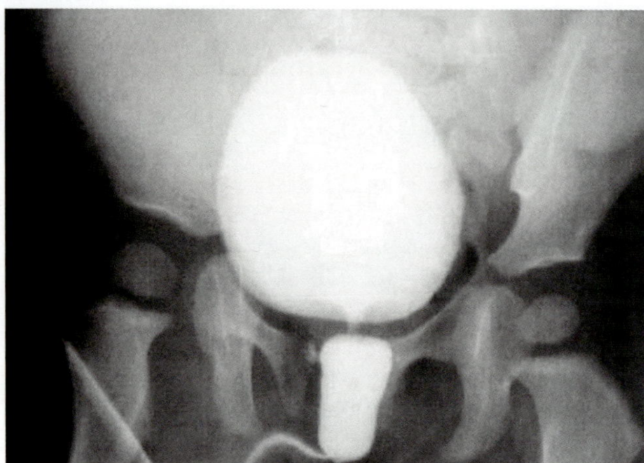

Fig. 19: Voiding cystourethrogram.

- Oligohydramnios and leading to pulmonary hypoplasia (severe cases)

Postnatal Presentation

- *Neonatal period (severe cases):*
  - Poor urinary stream or inability to void
  - Bladder distension
  - Respiratory distress due to pulmonary hypoplasia (Potter sequence)
  - Acute renal failure in severe cases
- *Infants and older children (mild-to-moderate cases):*
- Recurrent urinary tract infections (UTIs)
- Failure to thrive
- Weak urinary stream, straining, or dribbling
- Nocturnal enuresis or incontinence (in milder cases)
- Chronic kidney disease (CKD) in long-standing cases

Diagnosis

Prenatal diagnosis:

- *Fetal ultrasound:* Shows bladder distension, bilateral hydroureteronephrosis, and oligohydramnios
- *Fetal MRI:* Can confirm severity in equivocal cases

Postnatal diagnosis:

- *Voiding cystourethrogram (VCUG)* ***(Fig. 19)*** *is the Gold Standard:*
  - Shows dilated posterior urethra, bladder trabeculation, and vesicoureteral reflux (VUR)
- *Ultrasound Kidneys, Ureters, Bladder (KUB):*
  - Detects hydronephrosis, thick-walled bladder, and possible renal dysplasia
- *Urodynamic Studies* (for long-term bladder dysfunction)
- *Serum creatinine and electrolytes*
  - Assesses renal function, especially in cases with CKD

Management

Initial stabilization (neonates and infants in distress)

- Bladder drainage with a urinary catheter (temporary relief)
- Intravenous (IV) fluids and electrolyte correction (if acute kidney injury present)
- Antibiotic prophylaxis (to prevent UTIs)

Definitive Treatment

- *Endoscopic valve ablation (first-line treatment):*
  - *Transurethral fulguration* or *incision of the valves* using a cystoscope
  - Most effective for relieving obstruction
- *Vesicostomy (temporary diversion in severe cases)*
  - Indicated if endoscopic ablation is not feasible due to small urethral size (preterm babies)
- *Long-term management:*
  - *Urodynamic assessment* for bladder dysfunction
  - *Management of VUR* if present
  - *Monitoring for CKD*
  - *Elective kidney transplantation* in end-stage renal disease (ESRD)

Complications

- Progressive renal failure and CKD
- Bladder dysfunction (detrusor overactivity or hypocontractility)
- Recurrent UTIs and pyelonephritis
- Pulmonary hypoplasia (severe oligohydramnios cases)

URETHRAL CALCULUS IN CHILDREN

Definition

Urethral calculi are rare in children and refers to stones located within the urethra, either originating de novo or migrating from the upper urinary tract. These calculi can cause acute urinary obstruction, dysuria, and significant discomfort. They may be primary or secondary. Risk factors include metabolic disorders (e.g., hypercalciuria and hyperoxaluria), urinary infections, neurogenic bladder, congenital anomalies (e.g., posterior urethral valves and urethral stricture), and previous urological interventions **(Fig. 20)**.

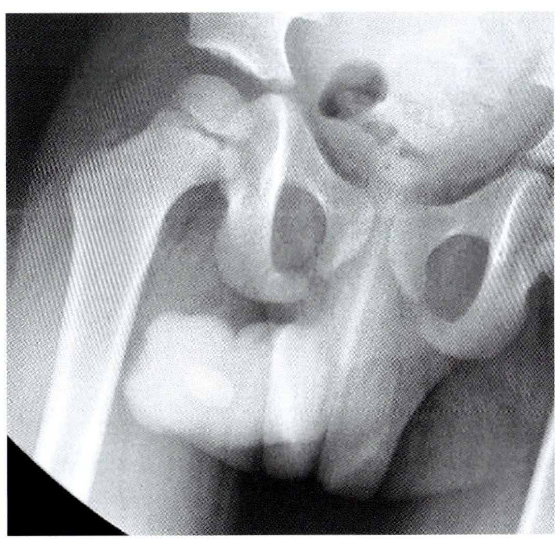

Fig. 20: Urethral calculus in children.

Clinical Features

The presentation of urethral calculus depends on the stone's size, location, and degree of obstruction. Common symptoms include:

- Acute urinary retention
- Dysuria
- Urethral pain
- Hematuria
- Palpable calculus
- Postvoid dribbling
- Penile or perineal swelling

Diagnosis

- *Ultrasonography (USG) of the pelvis and urethra:* First-line imaging to detect urethral stones and bladder involvement.
- *X-ray KUB and retrograde urethrogram (RUG):* Helps visualize radiopaque stones and assess urethral anatomy.
- *Noncontrast CT (NCCT) pelvis:* The gold standard for detecting urethral and urinary tract stones, particularly radiolucent stones.
- *Cystourethroscopy:* Both diagnostic and therapeutic, allowing direct visualization of the calculus and associated pathology.

Surgical Management

The management of urethral calculi depends on stone size, location, degree of obstruction, and underlying conditions.

Endoscopic and Minimally Invasive Techniques

- Endoscopic retrieval:
  - *Cystourethroscopy with stone extraction:* A rigid or flexible cystoscope is used to directly grasp and remove small calculi.
  - *Laser lithotripsy or pneumatic lithotripsy:* Utilized for larger stones that cannot be removed intact.
- Retrograde manipulation into the bladder
- External urethral pressure technique

Open Surgical Approaches

- Ureterolithotomy:
  - Indicated for large or impacted stones that cannot be removed endoscopically
  - Involves a direct incision over the urethra to extract the calculus

Postoperative and Long-term Management

- *Urinary catheterization:* Temporary placement postoperatively to prevent urethral edema and promote healing.
- *Metabolic evaluation:* Identification and management of metabolic risk factors to prevent recurrence.
- *Hydration and dietary modifications:* Increased fluid intake and dietary adjustments based on stone composition.
- *Follow-up imaging:* Routine ultrasound or X-ray to monitor for recurrence, especially in patients with metabolic disorders.

PEDIATRIC TUMOR RUPTURE

Pediatric tumor rupture is a life-threatening event in which a malignant or benign tumor in children undergoes spontaneous or trauma-induced rupture, leading to hemorrhage, peritoneal contamination, or systemic complications. Common tumors associated with rupture include Wilms tumor, neuroblastoma, hepatoblastoma, and germ-cell tumors. Rupture can result in significant morbidity due to hemorrhagic shock, peritonitis, and tumor dissemination **(Fig. 21)**.

Clinical Features

- *Acute abdominal or localized pain:* Sudden onset of severe pain due to capsular breach and bleeding.
- *Rapid abdominal distension:* Caused by intraperitoneal hemorrhage or tumor leakage.

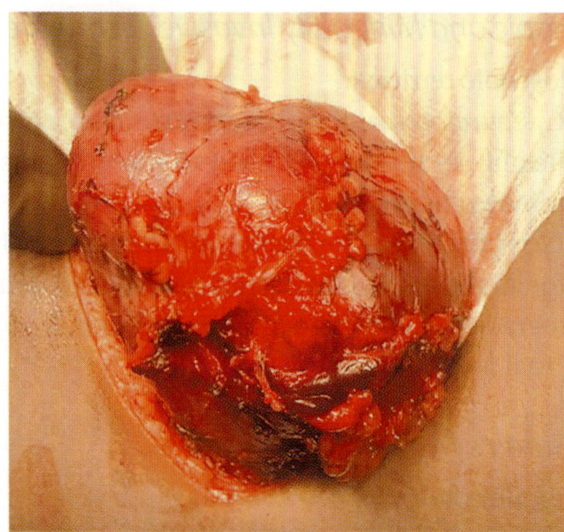

Fig. 21: Wilms tumor rupture.

- Pallor and weakness.
- *Palpable, tender abdominal mass:* Often irregular, firm, and nonreducible.
- Tachycardia, hypotension, cold extremities, and altered mental status.
- *Peritoneal signs:* Guarding, rigidity, and rebound tenderness if rupture leads to peritonitis.
- *Visible bruising or ecchymosis:* Suggesting subcutaneous hemorrhage in some cases.

Investigations

Imaging studies:
- *Ultrasound:* Detects free fluid (hemoperitoneum) and tumor characteristics.
- *Contrast-enhanced CT scan:* Preferred for assessing tumor rupture, extent of hemorrhage, and vascular involvement.
- *MRI:* Provides detailed soft-tissue evaluation, particularly for neuroblastoma.

Treatment

- *Immediate resuscitation:* IV fluid resuscitation and blood transfusion for shock.
- *Emergency laparotomy:* For uncontrolled hemorrhage.
- *Tumor resection or debulking:* If feasible during emergency surgery.
- *Peritoneal lavage:* In cases of peritoneal contamination.

Oncological Management

Chemotherapy or radiotherapy for malignant tumors poststabilization.

Long-term surveillance for recurrence or metastasis is required. Early diagnosis and prompt surgical intervention are critical to reducing mortality and improving long-term outcomes in pediatric tumor rupture.

RUPTURED CHOLEDOCHAL CYST

A ruptured choledochal cyst is a rare but serious complication of congenital bile duct dilatation, leading to bile leakage, peritonitis, and sepsis. Choledochal cysts are classified based on their anatomical location and morphology, with Type I (cystic dilatation of the common bile duct) being the most common. Rupture may occur due to infection, inflammation, trauma, or increased intraductal pressure.

Clinical Features

- Acute abdominal pain
- Fever and chills
- Jaundice
- Nausea and vomiting.

Investigations

- *Ultrasound:* Detects cystic dilatation, free fluid, and thickened bile duct walls.
- *Contrast-enhanced CT Scan:* Identifies cyst rupture, bile leakage, and associated complications.
- *Magnetic resonance cholangiopancreatography (MRCP):* Provides detailed visualization of the biliary anatomy.

Surgical Intervention

- *Definitive surgery (Hepaticojejunostomy):* Excision of the cyst with Roux-en-Y biliary reconstruction.
- *Peritoneal lavage and drainage:* If bile peritonitis is present.
- *Biliary stenting:* Temporary measure in critically ill patients.

SECTION 10 Oncosurgery Emergencies

Emergencies in Oncology

S Dorian Hanniel Terrence

INTRODUCTION

Oncology is a field where there are relatively fewer emergencies than other fields. Yet, it is worthwhile to learn a bit about a few common emergencies, a cancer patient can present with. This will enable you to diagnose and begin the initial management, especially when the patient is admitted under your watch.

SUPERIOR VENA CAVA SYNDROME

Definition

Superior vena cava (SVC) syndrome is the clinical presentation of obstruction of blood flow through the SVC either by compression, invasion, or thrombotic processes in the superior mediastinum.

Anatomy and Pathophysiology

- Superior vena cava drains blood from head, neck, both upper limbs, and upper thorax.
- Extends from the junction of the right and left innominate veins to the right atrium; length: 6–8 cm and width: 1.5–2 cm.
- *Main auxiliary tributary:* Azygos vein.
- Other tributaries that contribute are internal and external jugular veins, subclavian veins, internal mammary veins, intercostal veins, etc.
- The SVC is thin-walled, compliant, and easily compressible. Thus, it is easily involved by any pathologic processes in the mediastinum.
- Superior vena cava obstruction leads to the development of collaterals. Enlarged veins in the neck and chest wall is a typical finding.

Etiology

- Most common cause is malignancy.
- Most common malignancy is lung cancer.
- Most common variants in lung cancer are small cell carcinoma and squamous cell carcinoma.
- Second most common malignancy is lymphoma.
- Most common variants in lymphoma are diffuse large cell lymphoma and lymphoblastic lymphoma.
- *Other malignancies:* Thymic cancer, sarcoma, and mediastinal germ cell tumors.
- Most common metastatic disease to cause SVC syndrome is carcinoma breast.
- *Nonmalignant causes:* Most common causes are intravascular devices such as central line catheters, chemoports, etc. and postcardiac interventions, for example, atrial fibrillation.

Others:

- Inflammatory conditions such as Behçet disease
- Vascular anomalies
- Aneurysms
- Fibrosing mediastinitis
- Castleman disease

Clinical Features

Symptoms:

- Fullness in the face and head
- Facial swelling
- Dyspnea

Signs:

- Dilated veins in the neck and chest
- Facial edema
- Plethora
- Cyanosis
- Upper limb edema
- All symptoms and signs are aggravated by bending forward, stooping, or lying down **(Figs. 1A to C)**.

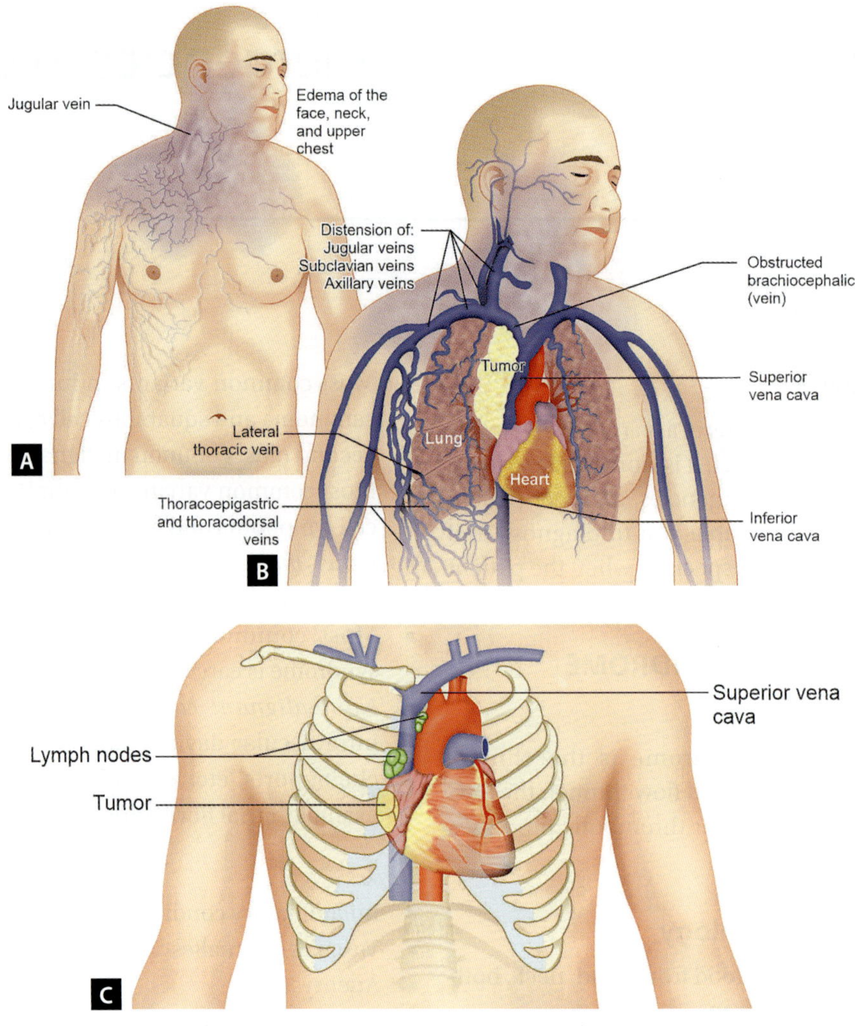

Figs. 1A to C: Superior vena cava (SVC) obstruction.

Investigations

Chest X-ray:

- Superior mediastinal widening
- Pleural effusion

Contrast-enhanced Computed Tomography (CECT) Chest:

- The CECT chest is the diagnostic investigation of choice.
- It gives the status of the SVC and other surrounding structures and the etiology for compression.
- If CECT is contraindicated, magnetic resonance (MR) venography can be used **(Fig. 2)**.

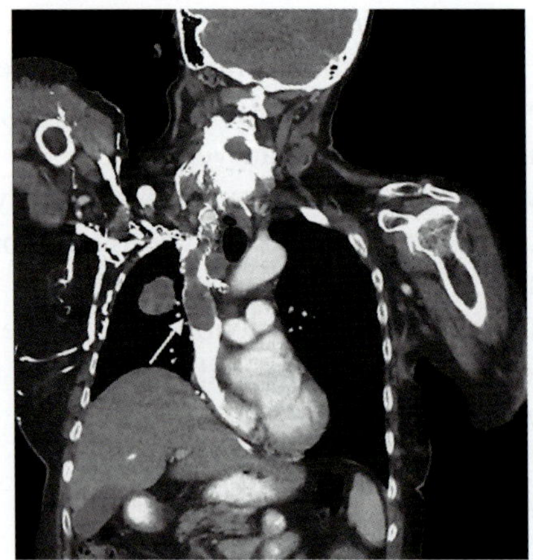

Fig. 2: Superior vena cava (SVC) obstruction in computed tomography (CT).

Role of Positron Emission Tomography–Computed Tomography

If malignancy is confirmed to be the etiologic agent, positron emission tomography-computed tomography (PET-CT) should be done to stage the disease.

Role of Biopsy

If malignancy is confirmed, biopsy proof should be obtained before starting treatment.

Routes of obtaining biopsy:

- CT-guided
- Bronchoscopy—guided biopsy/fine-needle aspiration cytology (FNAC)
- Mediastinoscopy
- Thoracoscopy
- Open thoracotomy

Treatment

Treatment is cause specific.

Basic Measures

- Bed rest
- Head-end elevation
- Supplemental oxygen administration
- Diuretics
- Steroids (after biopsy)

Specific Measures

In case of malignancy: After biopsy proof, staging of the disease should be done using PET-CT. After PET- CT, intent of treatment should be decided (curative vs. palliative) **(Figs. 3A to C)**.

Accordingly, radiation and chemotherapy dose should be given.

Nonmalignant causes:

- Anticoagulation
- Thrombolysis
- Removal of the intravascular device
- Percutaneous transluminal angioplasty
- Stent insertion—covered polytetrafluoroethylene (PTFE) stents

Role of Surgery

Only carried out in fit, young patients with nonmetastatic, nonlymphomatous malignant SVC obstruction.

Approach:

- Sternotomy/thoracotomy
- Resection of the tumor along with then involved portion of SVC is done along with reconstruction.
- Bypass procedures can also be done. Preferred route is from the patient's left internal jugular (or) brachiocephalic vein to the right atrial appendage, bypassing the SVC.

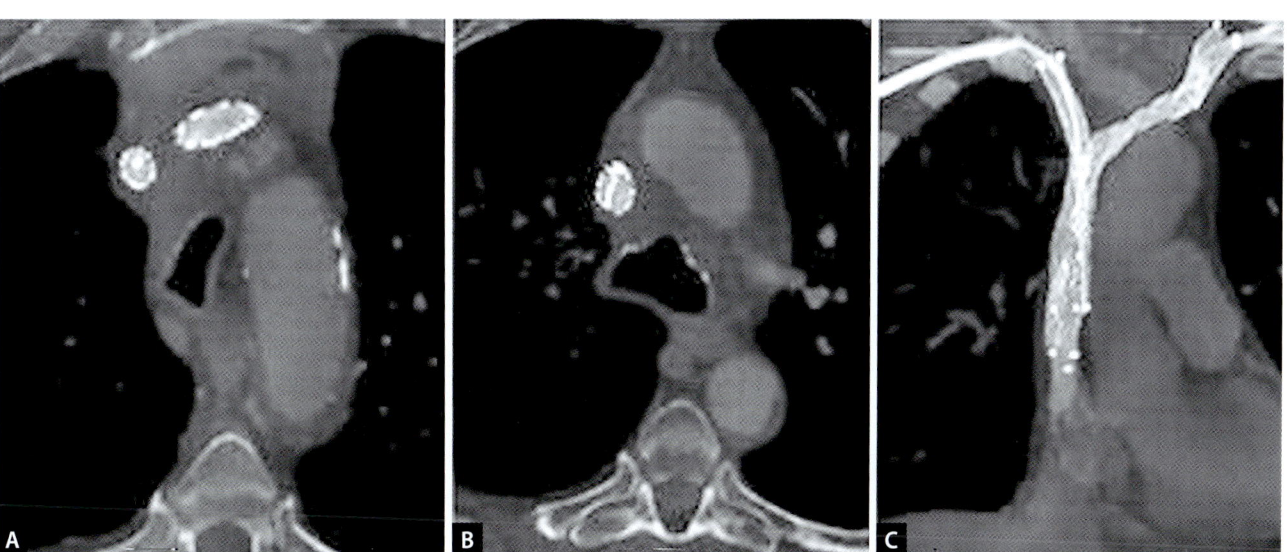

Figs. 3A to C: Superior vena cava (SVC) obstruction treated by stenting.

RAISED INTRACRANIAL PRESSURE DUE TO MALIGNANCY

Intracranial volume is not expandable in adults because of its containment by the skull. The three components inside the skull are brain matter, cerebrospinal fluid (CSF), and blood. An increase in the volume of one component occurs at the expense of the other two (Monro–Kellie Doctrine) **(Figs. 4A to C)**.

Pathogenesis

Increased brain volume may be due to:

- Primary or secondary brain tumors/dural tumors
- Peritumoral edema
- Vasogenic edema due to brain tumor
- Chemotherapy-induced cytotoxic edema
- Intracranial hemorrhage due to coagulopathy in the cancer patient
- Dural venous sinuses thrombosis or compression by primary tumors or metastasis
- Increased CSF volume may be due to imbalance between CSF production, flow, and reabsorption caused by:
  - Mass lesions near the foramen of Monro, aqueduct of Sylvius, etc.
  - Carcinomatosis near the arachnoid granulations resulting in defective reabsorption
  - Increased production of CSF by choroid plexus tumors.

Due to any of the earlier-mentioned reasons, intracranial pressure (ICP) may be raised. When ICP exceeds 40–50 mm Hg, irreversible brain damage occurs.

Etiology

- Brain metastases
- Brain metastases causing intracranial hemorrhage
  - *Most common tumor in adults:* Melanoma and renal cell carcinoma (RCC)
  - *Most common tumor in pediatric age group:* Ewing's sarcoma, rhabdomyosarcoma, and melanoma
- Primary brain tumors with predilection for subependymal or intraventricular locations
- Cancer related coagulopathy and disseminated intravascular coagulation (DIC) leading to intracranial hemorrhage can occur in acute lymphoblastic leukemia (ALL) and acute myeloid leukemia (AML).
- *Post-treatment for cerebral metastases, i.e., after surgery or radiotherapy:* Hemorrhage, infection, inflammation, brain abscess, etc.
- Postbrain radiation-induced fibrosis of arachnoid granulations
- Neoplastic meningitis
- All-trans retinoic acid used for the treatment of leukemia

Clinical Features

- Most common symptom is headache—severe, resistant to common analgesics, and more in the morning (due to reduced venous return from the brain in lying down position)
- Nausea and vomiting
- Somnolence
- Ultimately, patient becomes drowsy and comatose

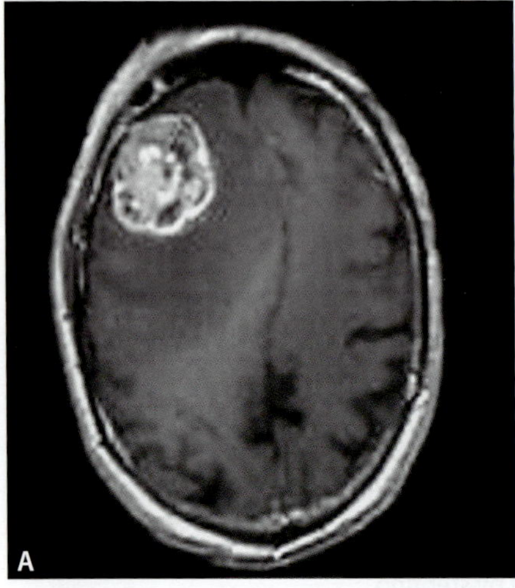

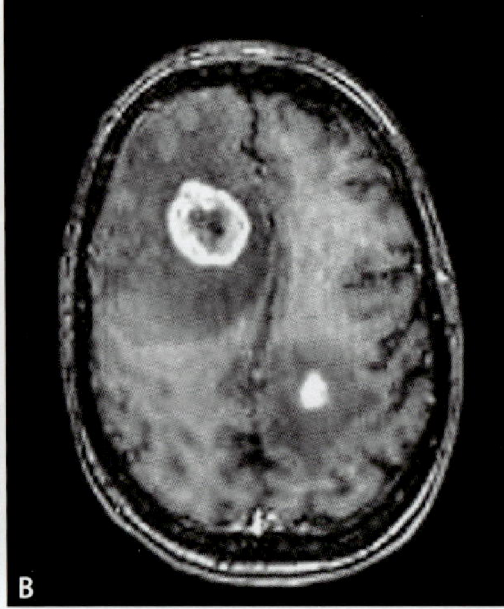

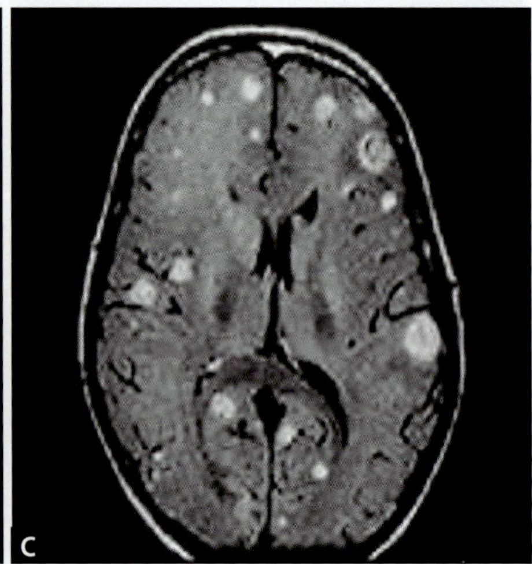

Figs. 4A to C: Brain metastasis.

Signs:
- Papilledema
- *Focal neurologic deficits such as*
  - Cognitive complaints
  - Gaze paresis
  - Hemiparesis
  - Hemianesthesia
  - Intraocular muscle palsies
  - Doll's eye movements
  - Decorticate posturing, etc.
- *Indirect complications:*
  - Hyponatremia due to syndrome of inappropriate antidiuretic hormone (ADH) secretion (SIADH) **(Fig. 5)**
  - Sphincter incontinence
  - Kernig's sign or Brudzinski's sign
- *Cushing's reflex:*
  - Irregular breathing patterns, hypertension, and bradycardia

Investigations

- *Initial investigation:* Plain CT is done to initiate emergency management.
- Magnetic resonance imaging (MRI), either contrast enhanced or diffusion weighted, is the investigation of choice **(Figs. 6A to C)**.

Others:
- Scintigraphic cisternography
- Lumbar puncture
- Transcranial doppler
- EEG (Electroencephalogram)

Treatment

- Head end elevation at 30°
- Antipyretics
- Isotonic fluids to maintain hydration. Hypotonic fluids are avoided to ensure free water does not enter the brain.

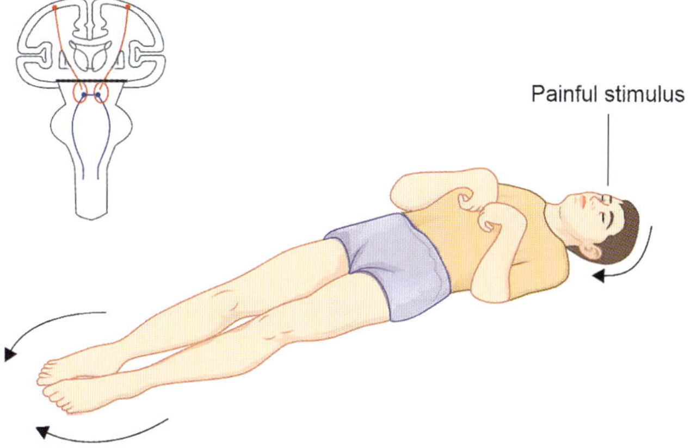

Fig. 5: Decorticate posture.

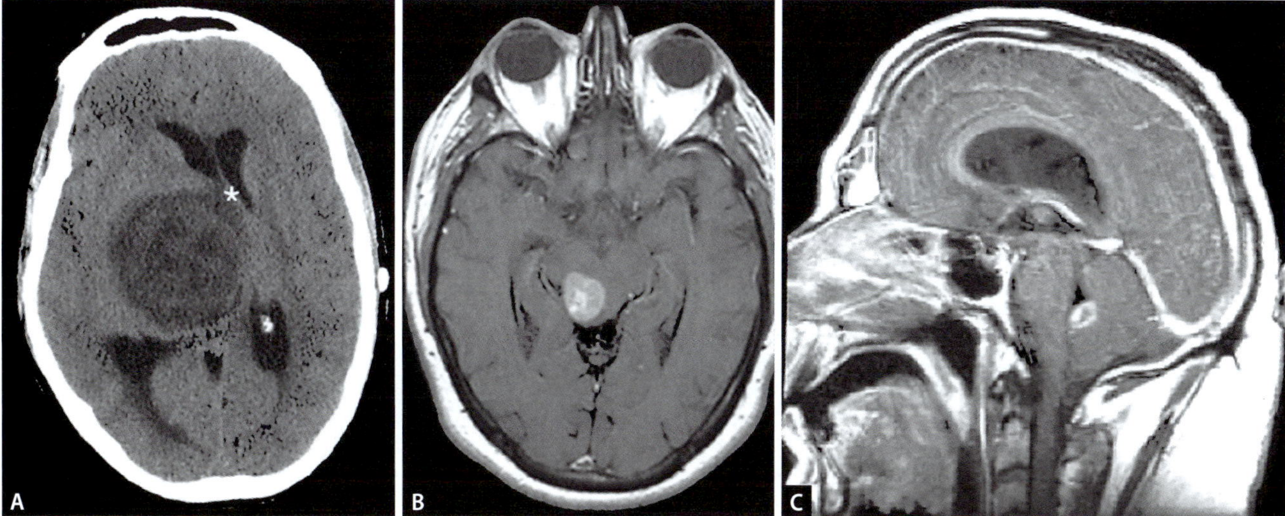

Figs. 6A to C: (A) A 45-year-old patient with an anaplastic astrocytoma of the right thalamus. Computed tomography revealed obstruction at the level of the foramen of Monro (*); (B) A 55-year-old patient with a midbrain metastasis from an adenocarcinoma of the lung. There is partial obstruction at the level of the cerebral aqueduct. The temporal horns of the lateral ventricles are dilated [T1-weighted magnetic resonance image (MRI) with gadolinium]; (C) A 38-year-old patient with seeding of nonsmall cell lung cancer to the floor of the fourth ventricle. He presented with intractable headaches, nausea, vomiting, and severe back pain, indicative of obstructive hydrocephalus and leptomeningeal spread to the spinal canal (T1-weighted MRI with gadolinium, sagittal view).

- *Corticosteroids:* Dexamethasone bolus 10 mg followed by 4–6 mg every 6 hours is used. Steroids are avoided until biopsy is taken in suspected central nervous system (CNS) lymphoma **(Fig. 7)**.
- *Osmotic diuretics:* Mannitol/glycerol
- Intubation with mechanical hyperventilation

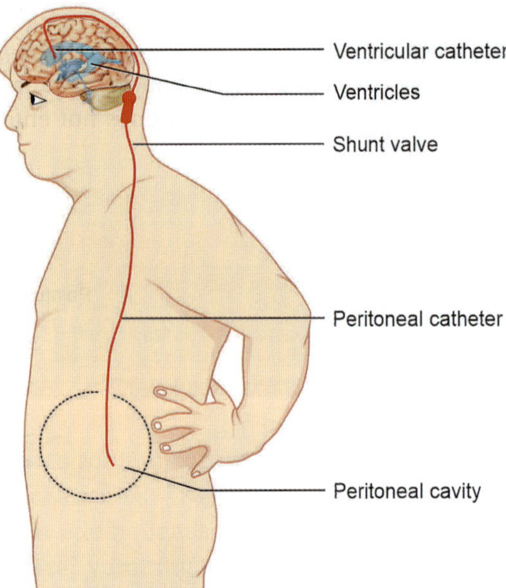

Fig. 7: Placement of a ventriculoperitoneal shunt.

Surgical interventions:

- External ventriculostomy
- Ventriculoperitoneal shunt
- Decompressive craniectomy
- Drainage of abscesses/hematomas

Other measures:

- Correction of coagulopathies
- Hydration
- Antibiotics
- Acetazolamide is used for the treatment of all-trans retinoic acid induced raised ICP.

Cancer specific therapy:

- Resection
- Radiation
- Cytotoxic chemotherapy

MALIGNANT SPINAL CORD COMPRESSION

The spine is the most common site of bone metastases. Approximately 10% of patients with spine metastases will develop malignant spinal cord compression. The thoracic spine is the most common vertebra to be involved. It is because of the greater number of vertebrae in the thoracic spine **(Figs. 8A to C)**.

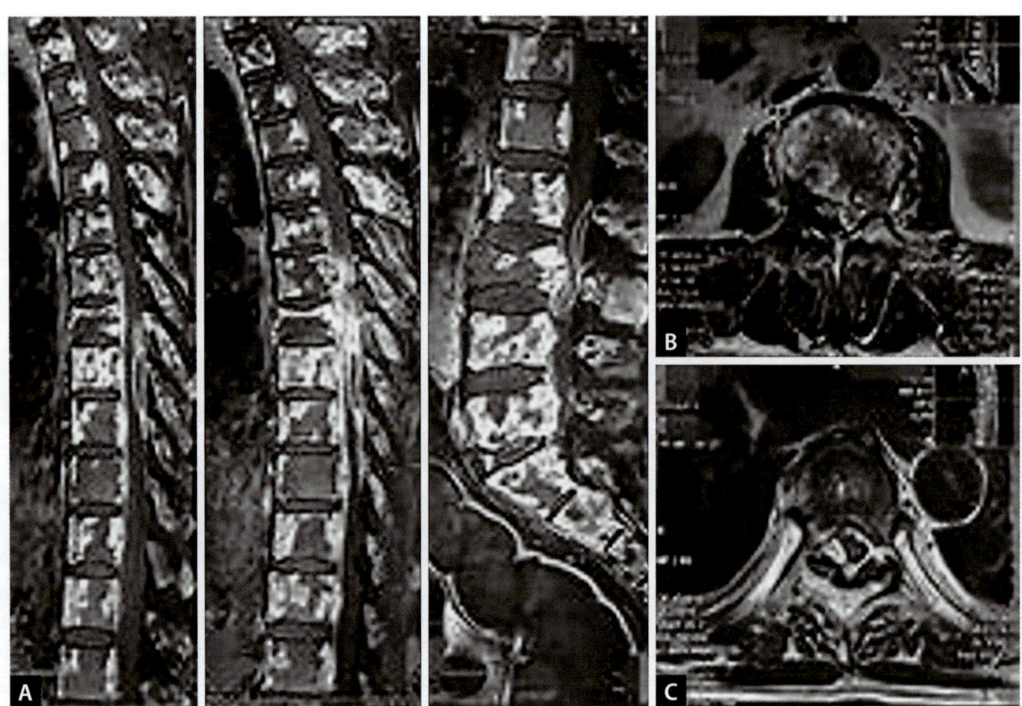

Figs. 8A to C: Malignant spinal cord compression.

Etiology

Adults:
- Lung cancer is the most common cause.
- *Others:*
  - Prostate cancer
  - Multiple myeloma
  - Breast cancer
  - Lymphoma

Pediatric age group:
- Ewing's sarcoma
- Neuroblastoma
- Osteosarcoma
- Germ cell tumors
- Lymphoma

Pathophysiology

Mechanisms of cord compression:
- Direct tumor extension from the vertebral column
- Pathologic fracture of bone, resulting in pushing of structures inside the spinal canal
- Leptomeningeal spread
- Intradural tumors of the spinal cord, e.g., meningioma
- Hematogenous metastasis to the cord

Cord compression results in obstruction of the epidural venous plexus leading to edema of the white and grey matter. This progressively results in spinal cord infarction and neurologic compromise. It results in paralysis distal to the compression **(Figs. 9A to D)**.

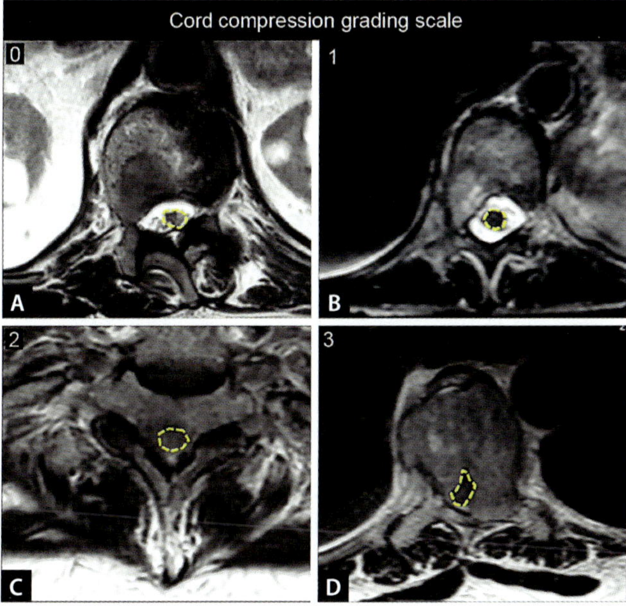

Figs. 9A to D: Cord compression grading scale.

Clinical Features

- Pain is the most common symptom. In patients with cancer, new-onset back pain with (or) without neurologic deficit must be considered as spine metastasis.
- Motor dysfunction is the earliest sign. It usually results in weakness and spasticity. As the most common vertebra affected is the thoracic vertebra, patient presents with paraparesis.
- Sensory weakness
- Bowel/bladder/autonomic disturbances
- Cord compression at cervical spine level will result in quadriparesis and/or respiratory dysfunction.

Investigations

- MRI is the investigation of choice. Preferably, the whole spine is imaged.
- Biopsy of the tumor should be done before initiating treatment (excisional biopsy/CT-guided biopsy/surgical resection).

Grading

The commonly used grading system is Bilsky grading system **(Table 1)**.

Treatment

- Obtaining a tissue diagnosis (biopsy) is the first step in the management.
- Corticosteroid treatment is initiated after biopsy.
- The next step will be directed at the specific management of the cord compression, which may include surgery (or) radiotherapy.
- *MNOP algorithm:* Mechanical, Neurologic, Oncologic, and Preferred treatment.

TABLE 1: Bilsky grading system.

Grade	*Feature*
0	Bone—only disease
1	Epidural extension and impingement on the thecal sac without spinal cord compression
2	Epidural extension with spinal cord compression but without obliteration of cerebrospinal fluid (CSF) space
3	Spinal cord compression with deformation of the spinal cord and obliteration of CSF space

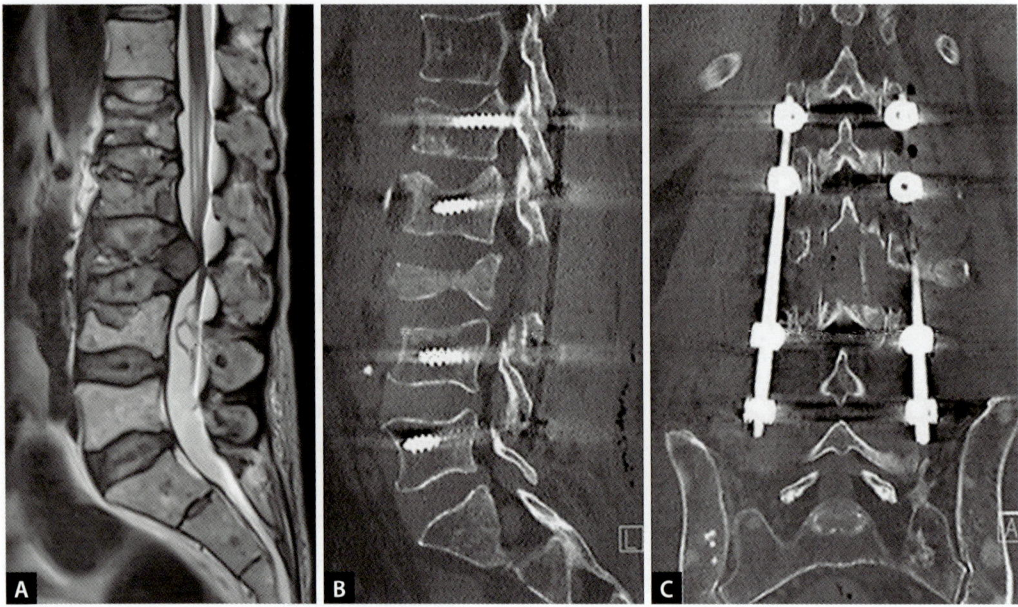

Figs. 10A to C: Fixation of spine.

Mechanical

If the patient has spinal instability, neurosurgical intervention is carried out to fix the spine first. Radiotherapy is usually not started immediately in an unstable spine **(Figs. 10A to C)**.

Neurologic

Grade 0 should be managed similarly to bone-only metastases, whereas other grades should be managed aggressively.

If a patient is presenting with acute decompensation of hours to 3 days, neurosurgery is carried out to resect the tumor. If presentation is >72 hours, recovery of neurologic function is not possible and radiotherapy is usually started to minimize further tumor spread.

Oncologic

After the biopsy report is available, based on the radiosensitivity of the tumor, tumors are classified as:

- *Very radiosensitive tumors;*
  - Lymphoma
  - Multiple myeloma
  - Germ cell tumors
- *Intermediate radiosensitive tumors;*
  - Prostate
  - Breast
  - Gastrointestinal tumors
- *Radioresistant tumors:*
  - Melanoma
  - Sarcoma

Based on the stage of disease, performance status of the patient, life expectancy and various other factors, the intent of treatment may be curative or palliative.

Preferred Treatment

Modalities of treatment used are:

- External beam radiotherapy
- Surgery for fixation or for resection
- Stereotactic Body Radiotherapy (SBRT)
- Radionuclide therapy (e.g., radium, samarium, and strontium)

TUMOR LYSIS SYNDROME

Definition: Tumor lysis syndrome (TLS) is a disorder involving electrolytes, renal function, cardiac, and CNS abnormalities that result from rapid breakdown or lysis of cancer cells **(Fig. 11)**.

It has been classified into two groups: Laboratory and clinical

Laboratory Abnormalities

- Increase in uric acid
- Increase in potassium
- Increase in phosphorous
- Decrease in calcium

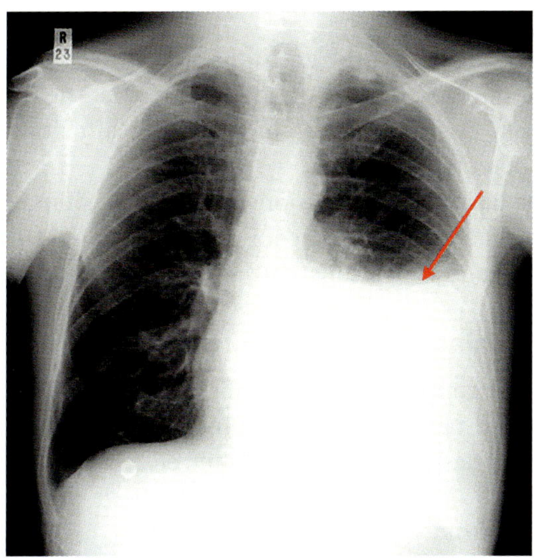

Fig. 11: Chest X-ray—malignant pleural effusion.

Clinical Abnormalities

Laboratory abnormalities with:
- Raised serum creatinine
- Seizures
- Cardiac dysrhythmia
- Death

Cairo-Bishop criteria: Of the 4 laboratory abnormalities, a 25% change from baseline in 2 or more values within 3 days before or up to 7 days after the initiation of therapy.

Cancers Predisposing to Tumor Lysis Syndrome

Usually occurs in rapidly growing chemosensitive hematologic malignancies with a high tumor burden.

Examples are:
- Burkitt lymphoma
- Acute leukemia (AML/ALL)

Pathogenesis

The final end point is kidney damage. It is due to:
- Increased cellular leakage of potassium
- Calcium phosphate crystal deposition in the body leads to hypocalcemia. This leads to increased parathormone secretion, which leads to phosphaturia and renal tubular damage.
- Uric acid release from lysed cells leads to urate crystal deposition in the collecting ducts.

Risk Categories of Tumor Lysis Syndrome

- *High risk:*
  - Medium or high tumor burden (bulky nodes, organomegaly, leukocytosis, and elevated lactate dehydrogenase)
  - Elevated pretreatment uric acid
  - Abnormal organ function (pre-existing nephropathy, hypotension, acidosis, and volume depletion)
- *Established:* Clinical (or) laboratory TLS
- *Others:* Low/intermediate risk

Management

Preventive measures: These should be started 24 hours before chemotherapy administration.
- *Hydration:* 3,000 mL/m^2
- Urine alkalinization

Treatment

- *Hyperkalemia:*
  - Cation exchange resins
  - Dextrose with insulin
  - Calcium gluconate
  - Loop diuretic
  - Hemodialysis
- Hyperphosphatemia:
  - Oral hydration
  - Oral phosphate binders
  - Hemodialysis
- Hyperuricemia:
  - *Allopurinol:* Inhibitor of xanthine oxidase
  - *Febuxostat:* More potent than allopurinol
  - *Rasburicase:* Recombinant urate oxidase can be used if rapid lowering of uric acid is needed. Oxidation of Uric acid by Rasburicase results in the formation of Allantoin, which is 5 times more soluble than uric acid.

HYPERCALCEMIA DUE TO MALIGNANCY

Serum calcium level is >11 mg/dL. The presence of hypercalcemia in a cancer patient signifies a poor prognosis.

High-risk Cancer Patients with Hypercalcemia

- Serum calcium > 12 mg/dL
- Severe nausea and vomiting
- Clinical dehydration
- Altered mentation

- Renal insufficiency
- Cardiac arrhythmia
- Obstipation or ileus
- Frail and elderly patients
- No social support
- Limited access to health care

Types of Hypercalcemia in Cancer

- Local osteolytic hypercalcemia (due to bony metastasis)
- Humoral hypercalcemia of malignancy due to ectopic secretion of parathormone related peptide
- 1,25 dihydroxy cholecalciferol secreting lymphomas
- Ectopic hyperparathyroidism.

Most common type is humoral hypercalcemia of malignancy

Most common cancer to cause is carcinoma lung.

Cancers with high frequency for bony metastasis:

- Carcinoma breast
- Carcinoma prostate
- Carcinoma lung
- Carcinoma thyroid
- Renal cell carcinoma

Management of Hypercalcemia

- Targeting the underlying malignancy
- Correction of dehydration
- *Bisphosphonates:* Drug of choice is zoledronic acid
- *Receptor activator of nuclear factor kappa-β (RANK) ligand inhibitors:* Denosumab (fully human monoclonal antibody).
- Calcitonin
- Hemodialysis
- *Treatment of bony metastasis:*
  - External beam radiotherapy
  - Stereotactic body radiotherapy (SBRT)
  - *Radium 223:* Calcium mimetic that localizes to bone metastasis and emits alpha particles.
  - Systemic radionuclides such as strontium 89, samarium 153, phosphorous 32, rhenium 186, and tin 117; all of the beta emitters.

MALIGNANT PLEURAL EFFUSION

Most common causes:

- Carcinoma lung
- Carcinoma breast
- Lymphoma
- Malignant pleural effusions are always exudative in nature. In India, malignancy is the second most common cause of exudative effusions after tuberculosis.
- Mediastinal compression with tracheal shift and low cardiac output can occur due to malignant pleural effusions, which constitute an emergency.

Diagnosis

Clinical examination that are most important are reduced vocal and tactile fremitus, dullness on percussion and absent breath sounds, tracheal shift, etc.

Chest X-Ray

- *Obliteration of costophrenic sulcus:* 200 mL
- *Obscuration of diaphragm:* 500 mL
- *Effusion up to fourth rib:* 1,000 mL
- *Massive effusion:* Complete opacification

Other features of malignancy such as irregular pleural thickening and nodular lung opacities may be seen **(Fig. 11)**.

Computed Tomography Thorax

Usually, findings are visualized after drainage of effusion **(Fig. 12)**.

Findings:

- Pleural thickening or mass
- Lung mass/nodules
- Mediastinal/hilar lymphadenopathy

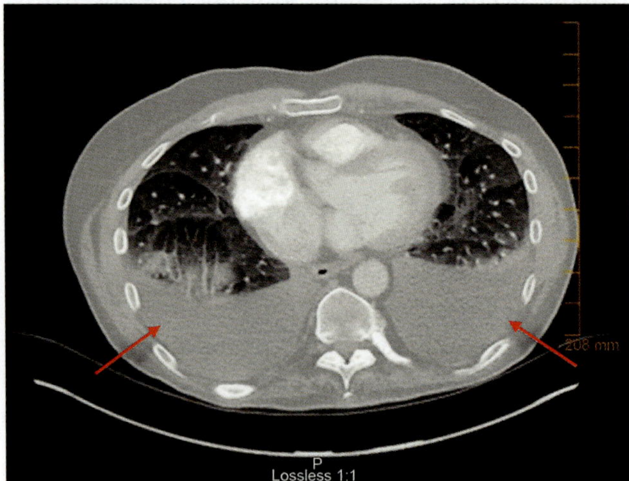

Fig. 12: Computed tomography (CT) thorax.

Treatment

- *Thoracocentesis:*
  - It is both diagnostic and therapeutic
  - Usually, malignant pleural effusion is exudative, hypercellular and blood stained. cytology may be positive for malignancy.
  - Therapeutic aspiration should be done using 8-14 Fr catheters, which drain fluid slowly, in order to avoid re-expansion pulmonary edema (RPE).
  - Maximum drainage level is recommended to be around 1,500 mL at one setting.
  - Thoracocentesis can be used as a bridge to stabilize the patient, until definitive management can be done.
- Tube thoracostomy—intercostal chest drain (ICD) insertion.
- Indwelling pleural catheters—manual removal of pleural fluid by the patient.
- Video-assisted thoracoscopic surgery (VATS) Can help in:
  - Complete drainage of fluid
  - Debridement of loculations
  - Decortication of trapped lung
  - Biopsy
  - Adequate distribution of sclerosants
- *Pleurodesis:* It is the apposition of visceral and parietal pleural surfaces, in order to prevent pleural fluid from accumulating again **(Fig. 13)**.
  - *Chemical agents:*
    - Talc slurry
    - Tetracycline
    - Doxycycline

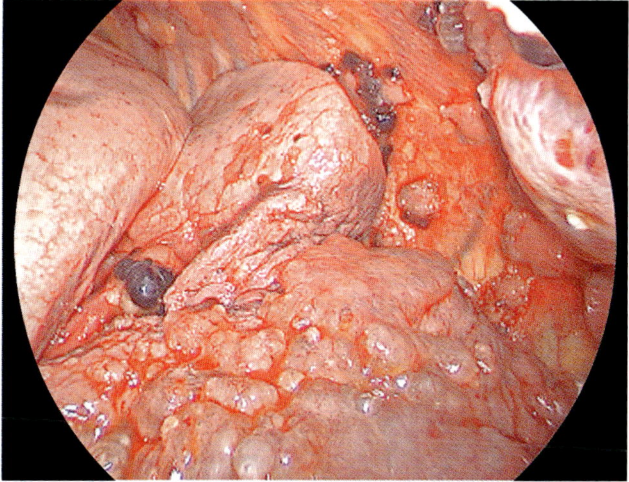

Fig. 13: Both parietal and visceral pleura studded with metastasis—view on video-assisted thoracoscopic surgery (VATS).

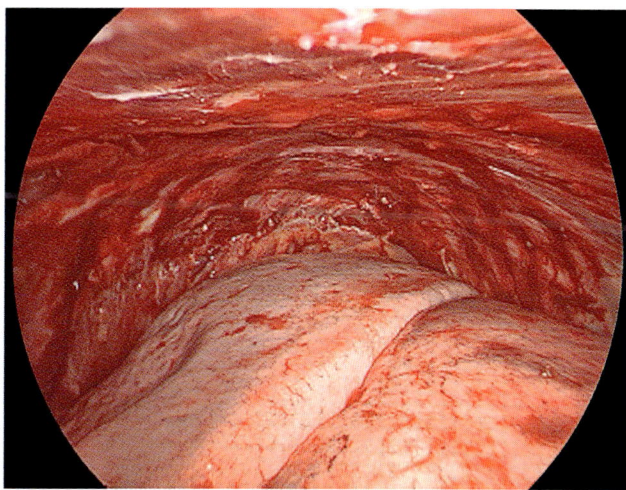

Fig. 14: Partial parietal pleurectomy.

    - Bleomycin
    - Iodine
  - *Mechanical means:*
    - *Pleurectomy:* VATS/Thoracotomy. It is the creation of abrasions on the parietal pleura.
- *Decortication:*
  - It is indicated when the lung is trapped by fibrosis or malignant nodules on the visceral pleura. A trapped lung cannot expand.
  - Decortication is the removal of parietal pleura alone. It allows the affected lung covered by visceral pleura to expand **(Fig. 14)**.

PARANEOPLASTIC SYNDROME OF INAPPROPRIATE SECRETION OF ANTIDIURETIC HORMONE

Syndrome of inappropriate secretion of antidiuretic hormone is a disorder of sodium and water balance characterized by a hypotonic euvolemic hyponatremia.

Basic Physiology

Basic physiology is given in **Flowchart 1.**

Syndrome of inappropriate secretion of antidiuretic hormone results when the ADH levels are not suppressed despite a low plasma osmolality.

Most common malignancy to cause SIADH is small cell carcinoma of lung.

Clinical Features

- Excess water in the body enters the cells, leading to cellular edema. Brain is the most common organ to be affected.

Flowchart 1: Basic physiology.

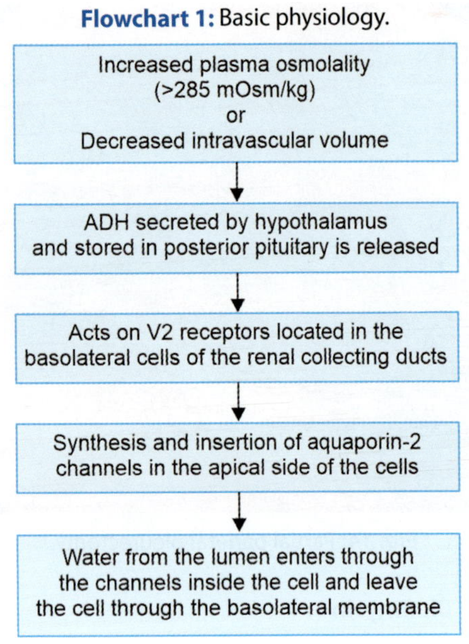

(ADH: antidiuretic hormone)

- Plasma sodium concentration is reduced leading to hyponatremia.
- Brain edema leads to neurologic features such as nausea, vomiting, headache, seizures, respiratory arrest, and death.

Diagnostic Criteria

- Effective plasma osmolality <285 mOsm/kg
- Urine osmolality >100 mg/kg of water—inappropriate urine dilution
- Clinical euvolemia (no volume overload or volume depletion)
- Urine sodium >40 mmol/L with normal dietary salt intake
- Normal thyroid and adrenal function
- No recent use of diuretics.

Treatment

- Cancer specific therapy should be initiated
- Fluid restriction to 800 mL/day
- *Pharmacological management:*
  - Oral salt tablets
  - Oral urea 30 g daily causes osmotic diuresis and increased water excretion.
  - Loop diuretics cause water excretion.
  - Demeclocycline decreases the responsiveness to ADH in the collecting ducts.
  - Vasopressin (ADH) receptor antagonists—Vaptans—block the activation of V2 receptors by ADH.

Drugs:

- Tolvaptan
- Lixivaptan
- Satavaptan
- Conivaptan
- *Hypertonic saline infusion:*
  - It is done in patients with CNS symptoms
  - 3 % NaCl is used.
  - *Maximum sodium correction:* 8–12 mmol/L during the first 24 hours.
  - Hypertonic saline should be discontinued when serum sodium reaches 120 mmol/L or once the total magnitude of correction reaches 18 mmol/L.
  - If hyponatremia is corrected too rapidly, it will lead to the development of osmotic demyelination syndrome.

NEUTROPENIA AND NEUTROPENIC SEPSIS

Neutropenia is the most common side effect of cytotoxic chemotherapy-induced myelosuppression. Neutropenia-induced infections and sepsis during the course of treatment for leukemias, lymphomas, and solid tumors may adversely impact the treatment in the following ways:

- Increased mortality
- More frequent hospitalizations
- Increased treatment cost
- Reduction of dosage of chemotherapy given
- Discontinuation of treatment

Neutropenia

Neutrophil count ≤ 1,500/mm^3

Neutropenic Infection/Febrile Neutropenia

Any fever episode occurring when the neutrophil count is <1,000/mm^3

Fever is defined as a single oral temperature ≥38.3°C or a temperature ≥ 38°C sustained for 1 hour.

Neutropenic Sepsis

Any neutropenic infection in which there is spread of pathogens in the blood stream along with features of the systemic inflammatory response syndrome.

TABLE 2: Risk factors for chemotherapy-induced neutropenia.

1	Type of chemotherapy
2	Age >60–65 y
3	Advanced disease
4	Poor performance status
5	Previous chemotherapy
6	Previous episodes of neutropenic infections
7	Myelophthisis
8	Number of comorbid conditions
9	Abnormal liver enzymes
10	Abnormal creatinine clearance
11	Low neutrophil count at the beginning of the treatment
12	Lymphopenia
13	Hemoglobin
14	Presence of an ongoing infection

TABLE 3: Myelopoietic growth factors.

Granulocyte macrophage colony stimulating factors (GM-CSF)		
1	Sargramostim	*Uses:* • Prevention of neutropenia and neutropenic infections • Stem cell mobilization • Dendritic cell proliferation as adjuvant in immunotherapy
2	Molgramostim	
3	Regramostim	
Granulocyte colony stimulating factor (G-CSF)		
Short acting		
1	Filgrastim	*Uses:* Prevention of chemotherapy-induced neutropenia and neutropenic infections
2	Lenograstim	
3	Tbo-filgrastim	
4	Filgrastim-sndz	
Long acting		
1	Pegfilgrastim	*Uses:* Prevention of chemotherapy-induced neutropenia and neutropenic infections

Risk Factors for Chemotherapy-Induced Neutropenia

Table 2 gives the well-studied risk factors for chemotherapy-induced neutropenia.

Myelophthisis refers to the displacement or destruction of bone marrow cells by infiltrating malignant or nonmalignant cells leading to impaired hematopoiesis. Myelophthisis is particularly common in patients with lymphoma, breast cancer, and prostate cancer.

Management of Neutropenia

Goals of Treatment

- Reduction in the incidence and severity of infectious complications
- Maintenance of dose intensity of chemotherapy at ≥85%

Delaying of treatment: At neutrophil counts <1,500 cells/mm^3

Role of Prophylactic Antibiotics

Current recommendation: Duration of neutropenia is = expected to be >7 days

Antibiotics used:

- Trimethoprim–sulfamethoxazole
- Levofloxacin

They usually reduce the overgrowth of gram-negative organisms, which are the most common cause of bacterial septicemia in neutropenia.

Usage of Myelopoietic Growth Factors

Myelopoietic growth factors are given in **Table 3**.

Management of Febrile Neutropenia

- Guidelines recommend usage of a beta-lactam that has activity against *Pseudomonas aeruginosa*, according to the local resistance patterns.
- Most common drug used is piperacillin tazobactam.
- Vancomycin or linezolid should be added if Gram positive infection is suspected.

Indications for adding vancomycin:

- Hemodynamic instability
- Pneumonia
- Catheter-related infection
- Severe mucositis
- Methicillin-resistant *Staphylococcus aureus* (MRSA) colonization

Duration of treatment: Weeks (or) until resolution of neutropenia

OTHER EMERGENCIES

- Airway obstruction due to laryngeal/pharyngeal growth presenting as stridor. Emergency CT scan with tracheostomy is done.
- Post neck dissection—carotid blow out. Ligation of external carotid artery is done distal to the origin of superior thyroid artery **(Fig. 15)**.

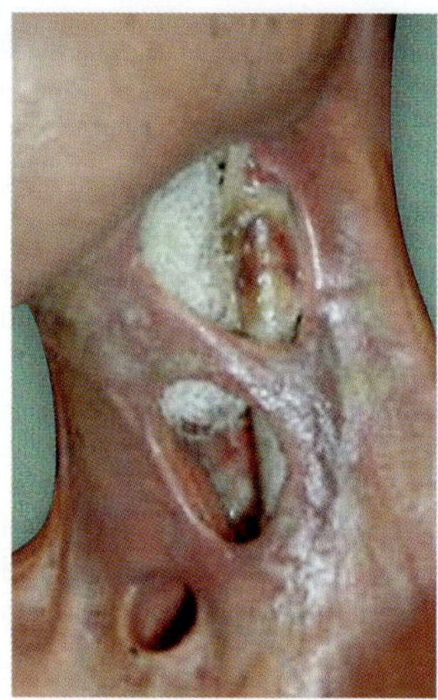

Fig. 15: Partial neck dissection with wound infection and skin loss with exposed carotid artery—high risk for blow out.

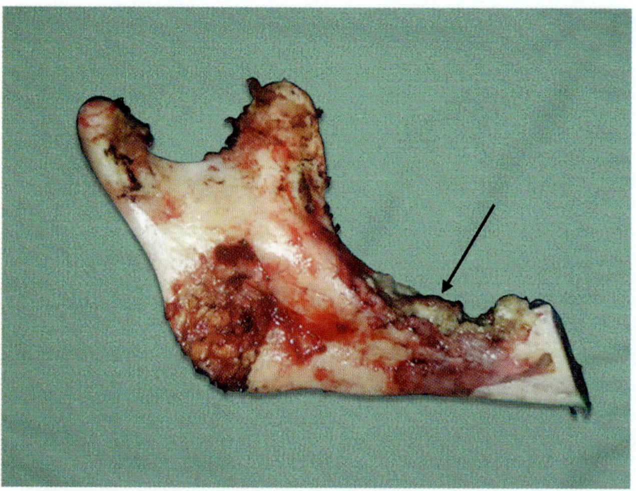

Fig. 16: Hemimandibulectomy specimen in osteoradionecrosis.

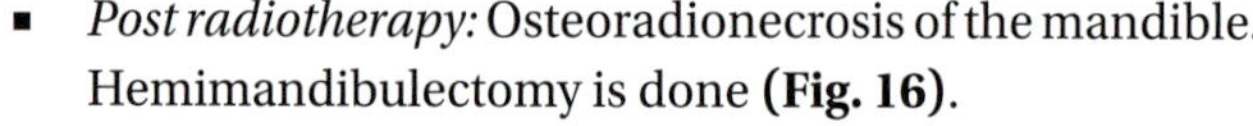

- *Post radiotherapy:* Osteoradionecrosis of the mandible. Hemimandibulectomy is done **(Fig. 16)**.
- Gastrointestinal malignancies presenting as intestinal obstruction/perforation—rarely definitive surgery is done in the primary setting. Usually, diversion ileostomy/colostomy is done.
- Biliary/pancreatic malignancies presenting with cholangitis.
- Fungating inguinal nodal disease presenting with femoral artery erosion.
- Carcinoma cervix presenting with anuria due to encasement of bilateral ureters. Emergency percutaneous nephrostomy (PCN) is done **(Fig. 17)**.

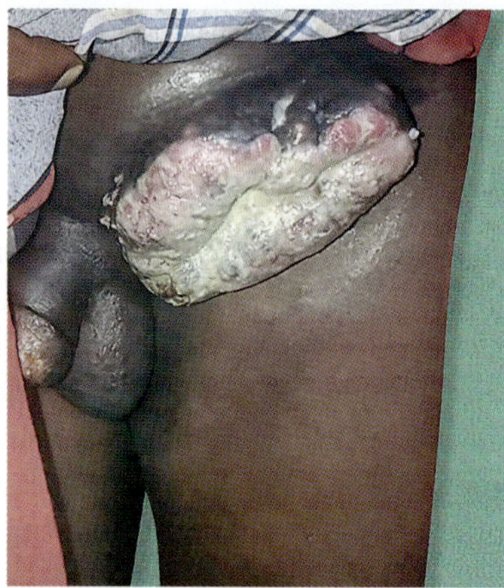

Fig. 17: Carcinoma penis with fungating inguinal nodal metastasis.

Index

Page numbers followed by *b* refer to box, *f* refer to figure, *fc* refer to flowchart, and *t* refer to table.

D

E

I

J

K

L

M

N

T

U

V

W

X

Z